ART OF
ABDOMINAL CONTOURING
Advanced Liposuction

ART OF ABDOMINAL CONTOURING
Advanced Liposuction

Sanjay Parashar MS (Gen. Surgery) DNB (Plast)
MCh (Plast) FICS (Plast)
CEO and Director
Consultant Plastic Surgeon and Laser Specialist
Consultant Plastic and Reconstructive Surgeon
Fellowship, Aesthetic Surgery (Australia)
Fellowship, Plastic and Craniofacial Surgery (Australia)
Cocoona Centre for Aesthetic Transformation
Dubai, UAE

Forewords

Prof. Luiz S Toledo
Prof. Ashok Govila

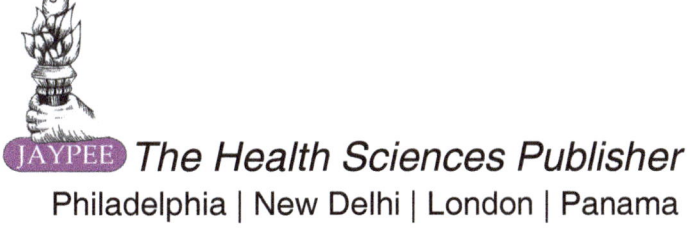

JAYPEE *The Health Sciences Publisher*

Philadelphia | New Delhi | London | Panama

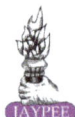 **Jaypee Brothers Medical Publishers (P) Ltd**

Headquarters
Jaypee Brothers Medical Publishers (P) Ltd.
4838/24, Ansari Road, Daryaganj
New Delhi 110 002, India
Phone: +91-11-43574357
Fax: +91-11-43574314
E-mail: jaypee@jaypeebrothers.com

Overseas Offices

J.P. Medical Ltd.
83, Victoria Street, London
SW1H 0HW (UK)
Phone: +44-20 3170 8910
Fax: +44(0)20 3008 6180
E-mail: info@jpmedpub.com

Jaypee Medical Inc.
325 Chestnut Street
Suite 412
Philadelphia, PA 19106, USA
Phone: +1 267-519-9789
E-mail: support@jpmedus.com

Jaypee-Highlights Medical Publishers Inc.
City of Knowledge, Bld. 237, Clayton
Panama City, Panama
Phone: +1 507-301-0496
Fax: +1 507-301-0499
E-mail: cservice@jphmedical.com

Jaypee Brothers Medical Publishers (P) Ltd.
17/1-B, Babar Road, Block-B, Shaymali
Mohammadpur, Dhaka-1207
Bangladesh
Mobile: +08801912003485
E-mail: jaypeedhaka@gmail.com

Jaypee Brothers Medical Publishers (P) Ltd.
Bhotahity, Kathmandu, Nepal
Phone: +977-9741283608
E-mail: kathmandu@jaypeebrothers.com

Website: www.jaypeebrothers.com
Website: www.jaypeedigital.com

Inquiries for bulk sales may be solicited at: jaypee@jaypeebrothers.com

Art of Abdominal Contouring: Advanced Liposuction

First Edition: 2016

ISBN: 978-93-5250-023-9

Dedicated to

*My mom, Late Mrs Malti Parashar, my father, Mr Yadunath Parashar
and my wonderful wife, Sangeeta (who I call iron lady of my house and organization)
and kids, Sanjana and Sidhant.*

Foreword

It is with great pleasure that I write this foreword introducing Dr Sanjay Parashar's work. Dr Parashar has been a colleague and a friend for many years. He has been working in plastic surgery for over 20 years. In 1995, he passed two exams in plastic surgery in Mumbai University and National Board of Examination, New Delhi, working in Mumbai, New Delhi and Nagpur. He then traveled the world working in some of the leading institutes in Australia, USA, Bahrain, and South Korea to refine his skills in craniofacial surgery, aesthetic surgery and laser surgery.

Dr Parashar has now been living in Dubai for many years and has established a solid successful career in plastic surgery, specializing in body contouring, breast surgery and craniofacial surgery and has evolved his skills to other areas of aesthetic medicine, such as the use of Botox, and filler injections for face.

Since moving to Dubai, he understood the benefits of day-surgery procedures in reducing cost and stress to patients. Following this new tendency in the medical world, he opened Cocoona, a center of competence, specializing primarily in cosmetic surgery, and nonsurgical aesthetic procedures. Recently, he added the specialties of orthopedic and bariatric surgeries.

Dubai is becoming known as a center of excellence for medical tourism and Dr Parashar has been contributing to this phenomenon, attracting patients from different countries and producing fine work in his clinic and gathering a number of specialists from other areas to cover many aspects of medicine.

Since 2013, when I as Scientific Director of the Emirates Plastic Surgery Society (EPSS), started organizing monthly meetings in Dubai, he has been very active as a lecturer and has helped to elevate the standards of plastic surgery in the region by sharing his experiences and teaching young plastic surgeons and his colleagues in the UAE. He is one of the most active local members of the International Society of Aesthetic Plastic Surgery (ISAPS), participating in our local ISAPS course in Dubai as an excellent teacher and lecturer.

I recognize in Dr Parashar, the skills of someone with a young spirit, keen to learn and to teach, spreading his knowledge in all medical fields and thinking constantly on how to make things better for the benefit of the patient. He is doing both here in Dubai and with his charity work back in his home country, India. He has covered for my clinic many times in Dubai and I have only heard good things about his skills and bedside manners. It is indeed a pleasure to write this foreword, and I am sure this book will help many young doctors to become as successful and upright as Dr Sanjay Parashar.

Prof. Luiz S Toledo MD
Consultant Plastic Surgeon
Author and Innovator
Dubai, UAE

Foreword

I know Dr Sanjay Parashar, author of the book since his college life in plastic surgery as an artist. His attempt to compile a book of this dimensions that has covered the detailed anatomy of the abdominal wall in the context of liposuction and abdominoplasty procedures deserves all possible compliments.

Art of Abdominal Contouring: Advanced Liposuction is a textbook that covers abdominal contouring in an extensive, detailed and scholarly manner.

Each chapter is not only replete with the latest scientific information, but also accessible and practical for clinicians.

The book covers the history and modern methods of liposuction. The information is state-of-the-art and incorporates the most current information on virtually every aspect of body contouring.

The chapter on aesthetic subunits is unique and informative, and it gives a different perspective to the surgeon operating on the abdominal wall.

There are extensive discussions on essentially all problems and potential complications of body contouring surgery.

I am sure our colleagues will find this new offering to be not only the most extensive and convenient compilation of information in our field, but also the most clinically practical and up-to-date resource in aesthetic surgery.

I wish him a great success with this dream project.

Prof. Ashok Govila MS FAIS MCh FRCS (Glasgow)
Majestica Cirúrgia Plástica
Consultant Plastic and Aesthetic Surgeon
Dubai, UAE

Preface

I learnt as a student "Publish or Perish" while that is true this is not the sole reason to publish this book. During my training as a surgeon and plastic surgeon, I read many books and acquired a lot of knowledge, but there is always something that you learn without books. Your practical experience, teaches you a lot and this is what I wanted to put together in the form of a book.

Liposuction is one of my favorite operations, although it appears simple and I thought, it is the easiest operation to learn. It took me two decades to understand the concept of liposuction and how to effectively apply it on a patient. One of my mentor said "I hate doing liposuction as patient do not see the difference" and that gave me an opportunity, he passed on all the liposuction that he hated to do and I developed that as my forte.

One of the reason, I learnt a lot was that I had the opportunity to see the patient regularly on the follow-up period. The positive result was very motivating and my passion grew stronger. After a journey of more than 15 years and performing nearly 8000 liposuction procedures, I decided to put my thoughts together for my fellow colleagues and trainees.

In this book, I have tried to cover all the aspect that is important for abdominal contouring. Each chapter has clinical relevance and my own thought process as well. The key element is the understanding of aesthetics of abdomen and how to apply it in various body weight people to achieve a dramatic change that persists for long-time.

I have discussed, almost all the modalities of liposuction that I had opportunity to work with. I have also included a chapter on nonsurgical management of fat, so as plastic surgeon, we look at this option without cynicism and include that in our armamentarium.

I have also discussed about the complications, why it occurs and what we can do to prevent it. This is to re-emphasize that complications can be reduced to negligible, if we follow a standard protocol.

This book will help to stimulate your thoughts to advance the concept of liposuction and body contouring. This will help the younger trainees to think with different perspectives and understand this art. It will also be useful to colleagues who are not performing this procedure very frequently. Finally, will be appealing to fellow colleagues with great experience in the field of liposuction and will allow me to have a healthy discussion with them.

It took me over a year to complete this book, and I kept adding content as I felt I have to tell more. In a conference when I present, I always feel that I have insufficient time to express myself. But I have found this a wonderful platform to "express it all" to "share it all".

The challenges I have faced to write this book was collecting photos and videos. This has taught me to record all the procedures meticulously as we perform the surgery and organize it well.

I sincerely hope that all the readers will find the information useful and help them perform the procedure safely with high quality result.

Sanjay Parashar MS (Gen. Surgery) DNB (Plast)
MCh (Plast) FICS (Plast)

Acknowledgments

I have thank my teachers and mentors who have helped me learn and made into the surgeon, that I am today.

Dr Mukund Jagannathan, my lecturer from BYL Nair Charitable Hospital, Mumbai is my greatest inspiration. I am a successful person because of him. Dr Uday Bhat, my senior colleague helped me understand anatomy better. My first exposure to liposuction was with Dr Ashok Gupta (1996), in fact my journey in aesthetic surgery began with him. I have learned a huge lot from him and I sincerely thank him being my mentor.

But, what made me a fine aesthetic surgeon was my experience with Dr Tariq Saeed in Bahrain from 1997. That was the turning point of my life. He made me believe complications are not acceptable in aesthetic surgery. This is where I was introduced to first generation Ultrasonic Liposuction and we performed several ultrasonic assisted liposuction (UAL) and believe me, we did not have a single complication. I cannot thank him enough for this valuable lesson.

When I was working with Prof IT Jackson as a craniofacial fellow in providence hospital, USA, I realized, how important it is to perform aesthetic surgery to keep a balance and run our domestic economy. I assisted him in liposuction and other aesthetic surgery after hours completing the routine operating list of craniofacial surgery.

My subsequent exposure was with Dr Tony Moore (2004) in Australia. He taught me time management and efficient ways of performing surgery. Abdominoplasty appeared very simple in his hands and it did not take the time, I would think. And that was it, after that I was on my own. And then I was sharing operating room with the mighty Dr Luiz Toledo in Dubai, UAE. I think, I absorbed a lot of energy from him by merely being in the same operating premise.

My biggest strength is my team, my staff who has tirelessly worked with me to provide the greatest care a patient can receive before and after the surgery. My nurses, Ellen Baldivino, Mini Johnson, Asha , Lizi, Arya, Caleen, Rahat, Shiny have provided unending support to our patients and to me. I am thankful to them from the bottom of my heart. I wish to express my heartfelt thanks to my patient co-ordinators, Brenda Castino, Dr Dhey, Rhoda and Smita Molla for logistically assisting me and the patient to accomplish the surgeries successfully.

Special thanks to my administrative team, Shahid, Kashif, Shima and rest of the team for being ever enthusiastic and supportive. I would also like to thank my team of aestheticians under Dr Dalia Ibrahim and Smita Sonovane who have helped our patient postoperatively to improve the results. They are also key people to provide nonsurgical weight loss program to the patient. Front desk team including Shayma, Christina, Russel, Mary Jane for facilitating patient consultations and follow-ups. A special thanks to Jay Peralta Repayo, my videographer/graphic designer for helping me with images, videos and illustrations.

We would also like to thank Mr Jitendar P Vij (Group Chairman), Mr Ankit Vij (Group President), Ms Chetna Malhotra Vohra (Associate Director), Ms Angima Shree (Development Editor), and the production team of Jaypee Brothers Medical Publishers (P) Ltd, New Delhi, India.

Sincere thanks to Dr Mazen Arafat, who worked with me as specialist plastic surgeon and as colleague and friend.

Last but not the least my family. Sangeeta Parashar, my wife continuous support to me both at home and in the office. Being a doctor, she understands my pain, tantrums, and challenges and have been tolerating me. I am thankful to her. My daughter, Sanjana and son, Sidhant have always been understanding and supportive. I regret spending time away from them, but feel proud that they understand me. Thank you!

Contents

DVD Contents

1. Infiltration Technique
2. Strokes of Liposuction
   a. Short- and Long-Strokes
   b. Fanning Strokes
   c. Skin Pinching
   d. Deep Liposuction
3. Three-Dimensional Abdominal Liposuction
4. Lipoabdominoplasty
5. Waist Liposculpturing
6. Laser Liposuction
7. Ultrasonic Liposuction
8. RFAL Lipo

CHAPTER 1

History

*"The sooner you make your first five thousand mistakes
the sooner you will be able to correct them"*

—*Kimon Nicolaides*

INTRODUCTION

Kimon Nicolaïdes was a Greek–American artist of 18th century. During World War I, he served in the US Army in France as a camouflage artist. He advocated a three-pronged way of learning to draw: through (1) slow and meticulous contour drawing, (2) free and rapid gesture drawing, and (3) vigorous tonal drawings of weight or mass. The same creative intellectual endeavor is required to mold the bodily morphology of the patients.

But be wiser and learn from others' mistakes! Do whatever it takes to prevent mistakes and that is why history is important.

In 1921, Charles Dujarrier, a French surgeon, curetted a ballerina's knees to create a better shape, but the patient developed gangrene and required an amputation.[1] Think! What would have gone wrong? Anything from improper cannula, technique, direct vascular injury, postoperative compression, lack of follow-up. What do we learn from this?

In 1964, Joseph Schrudde developed curettage and suction.[2] In 1976, Georgio and Fischer, Italian surgeons, developed a fat-removing system with a hollow cannula and an internally rotating planatome and cellusuctiontome.[1,3] They also introduced the concept of cross-tunneling for more uniform results. The concept of cross-tunneling is still applicable and a uniform contour cannot be achieved by two incisions that allows cannula movement in same direction.

Other cannulas were developed by Kesselring and Meyer (1978) and Illouz (1977); the latter also developed the wet technique. Dr Ives Gerard Illouz took a major step ahead in the field of liposuction by introducing negative pressure device with high suction power connected to a cannula. He also developed the wet technique in which he used hypotonic saline solution and hyaluronidase in order to perform dissecting hydrotomy for bloodless fat removal.[1,2,4]

Pierre Fournier (1983)[5-7] favored the syringe technique and instructed physicians to use the cross-tunneling technique. He relied on the dry method without subcutaneous infiltration.

The dry technique uses general anesthesia without any preoperative infiltration of vasoconstrictive solution. The wet technique achieves a moderate reduction in blood loss by using a small amount of epinephrine.

In 1984, Hetter introduced epinephrine into solutions. The superwet infiltration technique, the use of 1.5 mL of solution for each 1 mL of aspirated fat, has been utilized since 1986, popularized by Fodor.[8]

In 1987, Jeffery Klein discussed the tumescent technique that used massive infiltration of the subcutaneous tissue.[9] The proportion of infiltrated liquids to aspirated liquids has developed as follows: dry liposuction, 0:1; wet, 1:1; superwet, 1.5:1; tumescent >2:1.

With these modifications, liposuction has become a safe and effective procedure. Nevertheless, with traditional liposuction, the treatment of fibrous area (as in dorsum, gynecomastia, and secondary liposuction cases) may become difficult.

ENERGY-BASED LIPOSUCTION

In the late 1980s, Zocchi introduced the use of ultrasonic device to release continuous energy to break the fat cells. Scuderi popularized the use of first-generation ultrasonic device which delivered ultrasound energy through blunt solid cannula. This was the beginning of ultrasonic assisted liposuction (UAL).[10,11]

The second-generation UAL introduced a hollow cannula for simultaneous liposuction with an internal diameter of only 2 mm.[12] This was not very efficient.

The ultrasound assisted liposuction had increased the risks of burns and related complications. Hence ultrasonic device became unpopular due to the increased risk of burns and skin damage. There was a need to improvise on the technology. The third generation UAL device was developed that later became popular as VASER (vibration amplification of sound energy at resonance). It uses small-diameter titanium probes (2.9 mm and 3.7 mm) with grooves near the tip to increase fragmentation efficiency by redistributing energy. So there was less energy at the tip reducing the risk of burns. The machine also uses pulsed energy as compared to continuous energy.

SUPERFICIAL LIPOSUCTION

Performance of superficial lipoplasty with standard lipoplasty cannulas, as reported by Souza pinto,[13] Gasperoni, and Gasparotti,[14,15] expanded the boundaries of body contouring by enabling the removal of fat from the superficial layers. However, there is a significant risk of dermal damage, scarring, waviness, and contour irregularities, as well as cutis marmorata when excessive fat removal was performed. It is a long learning curve to understand the technique of superficial liposuction without causing dermal damage. Some suggested to leave 1 cm of fat under the dermis.[15,16]

Scheflan and Tazi[17] reported the superficial application of ultrasound energy to produce "skin stimulation" for purposes of retraction was associated with burns, scarring, waviness, and contour irregularities. Jewell et al.[18] first reported on the clinical application of a third-generation ultrasound lipoplasty device that utilized pulsed low-power ultrasound and high-efficiency, small-diameter solid titanium probes.

HIGH-DEFINITION LIPOSUCTION

Mentz and Ersek[19,20] pointed out that traditional lipoplasty techniques often fail to achieve the aesthetic goal of a "washboard" abdominal contour because "subdermal fat obscures the muscular detail." The Mentz technique called "abdominal etching" used differential lipoplasty to detail abdominal musculature, specifically the rectus abdominis muscle, between the linea alba and the linea semilunaris, while also addressing the tendinous inscriptions (intersectiones tendineae) of the rectus abdominus muscle. However, abdominal etching was designed specifically for male body builders with between 8% and 15% body fat, and was limited to only the anterior abdominal wall.

In 2003, Hoyos[21] presented a new technique at a Colombian National Congress, that he termed "high-definition liposculpture" (HDL). The term "liposculpture" defined the technique as not simply fat removal but as an artistic approach designed to emulate surface anatomy. As Gasparotti mentioned, "I recognized that working superficially I had the ability to go well beyond the simple removal of fatty bulges... Why not use it as a sculpting tool to obtain the imaginary shape, the ideal profile we dream about creating?"[22]

HDL was developed through the study of art and anatomy of the human musculature, as an artistic treatment of the human form to create not only a slim figure, but also the appearance of a highly developed musculature.

High-definition liposculpture elevates the Mentz concept of abdominal etching to a three-dimensional approach. In this approach, one needs to consider the muscular anatomy of the region and hence it can be applied to any body parts including torso, legs, arms, and back. The differing aesthetic goals of male and female body contouring are integrated into this method, as are key areas such as the pectorals in male and the gluteal area in female.

However, it requires a lot of training, experience, and understanding to achieve exceptional results by HDL. Yet another challenge is the long and exhausting surgical hours, postoperative discomfort and healing period, and long term and close follow-up to avoid undesirable results.

Vibration amplification of sound energy at resonance is very useful and complementary to achieve HDL because it emulsifies the fat uniformly just like an artists' "clay." That will make it easy to sculpt and enhance muscular anatomy and minimize discomfort and healing time. This started the era of VASER-assisted high-definition liposculpture that uses combination of VASER and HDL.

VASER-assisted high-definition liposculpture embodies the ultimate understanding of how superficial anatomy influences external appearance. Developed through the study of "surface anatomy" of human musculature much as an artist would view the human form,[23,24] VASER-assisted high-definition liposculpture begins where superficial lipoplasty ends. It highlights the importance of contributions made to the aesthetics of the human form by both the superficial and deep fat layers when these layers are properly proportioned both between and over the muscle groups.

HISTORY OF ABDOMINAL AESTHETICS

The technique has evolved tremendously over decades but the major improvement was to minimize complications, improve scars, and improve shape of umbilicus. But there were more challenges: patients wanted better results, better aesthetic outcome, and certainly longer-lasting results.

In the year1995, Matarasso[25] published extensive work on the aesthetics of abdomen and described methods to improve the results. Such as upper abdomen was not considered in abdominoplasty and hence it would bulge out postoperatively and in long-term. So, Matarraso recommended simultaneous liposuction along with abdominoplasty to improve the contour for long-term.

He suggested that omitting the rejuvenation of one of the abdominal aesthetic units can result in disproportion, disharmony, and patient discord. To avoid this problem, related abdominal aesthetic units should be addressed in both open and closed abdominal contour procedures.

REFERENCES

1. Flynn TC, Coleman WP, III, Field LM, et al. History of liposuction. Dermatol Surg. 2000;26:515-20.
2. Fischer G. First surgical treatment for modeling body's cellulite with three 5 mm incisions. Bull Int Acad Cosm Surg 1976;2:35-37.
3. Fischer G. Liposculpture: the "correct" history of the liposuction. Part I. J Dermatol Surg Oncol. 1990;16:1087-9.
4. Avelar JM, Illouz YG. Histórico da técnica lipólise: lipoaspiração. In: Illouz YG (Ed). Lipoaspiração, 1st edition. São Paulo, Brazil: Hipócrates; 1986. pp. 24-31.
5. Bisaccia E, Scarborough DA, Swensen RD. Syringe-assisted liposuction: a cosmetic surgeon's office technique. J Dermatol Surg Oncol. 1988;14(9):982-9.
6. Fournier PF, Otteni F. Liposuction in body sculpturing: the dry procedure, Presented at the Annual Meeting of the American Society and Reconstructive Surgeons, Honolulu, Hawaii, October, 1982.
7. Edelstein J Craig Fielding liposuction, the syringe technique by Pierre F Fournier. Obesity Surg. 1996;6(1):72.
8. Fodor PB, Watson J. Wetting solutions in ultrasound assisted lipoplasty. Clin Plast Surg. 1999;26:289.
9. Klein JA. Anesthesia for liposuction in dermatologic surgery. J Dermatol Surg Oncol. 1988;14:1124-32.
10. Zocchi ML. Ultrasonic-assisted lipoplasty. Technical refinements and clinical evaluations. Clin Plast Surg. 1996; 23:575.
11. Scuderi N, Devita R, D'Andrea F, et al. Nuove prospettive nella liposuzione la lipoemulsificazone. Giorn Chir Plast Ricoster ed Estética. 1987;2:33-9.
12. Jewell ML, Fodor PB, Souza Pinto EB, et al. Clinical application of VASER-assisted lipoplasty: a pilot clinical study. Aesthet Surg J. 2002;22(2):131-46.
13. De Souza Pinto EB, Abdala PC, Maciel CM, et al. Liposuction and VASER, Clin Plast Surg. 2006;33(1):107-15.
14. Gasparotti M. Superficial liposuction: a new application of the technique for aged and flaccid skin. Aesthetic Plast Surg. 1992;16:141-53.
15. Gasperoni C, Gasperoni P. Subdermal liposuction: long-term experience. Clin Plast Surg. 2006;33:63-73.
16. Lee YH, Hong JJ, Bang CY. Dual plane lipoplasty for superficial and deep layers. Plast Reconstr Surg. 1999;104:1877-84.
17. Scheflan M, Tazi H. Ultrasonically assisted body contouring. Aesthet Surg J. 1996;16:117-22.
18. Jewell ML, Fodor PB, de Souza Pinto EB, et al. Clinical application of VASER-assisted lipoplasty: a pilot clinical study. Aesthet Surg J. 2002;22:131-46.
19. Mentz H, Gilliland M, Patronella C. Abdominal etching: differential liposuction to detail abdominal musculature. Aesthetic Plast Surg. 1993;17(4):287-90.
20. Ersek RA, Salisbury AV. Abdominal etching. Aesthetic Plast Surg. 1997;21:328-31.
21. Hoyos AE, Millard IA. Vaser assisted high definition lipoplasty. Aeste Surg. 2007;27:594-604
22. Gasperotti M. Superficial liposuction: A New application of the technique for aged and flaccid skin. Aeste Plastic Surg.
23. Simblet S, Davis J. Anatomy for the Artist. New York, NY: DK Publishing; 2001.
24. Rubins DK. The Human Figure: An Anatomy for Artists. New York, NY: Penguin Books; 1976.
25. Matarasso A. Liposuction as an adjunct to a full abdominoplasty. Plast Reconstr Surg. 1995;95:829-36.

CHAPTER 2

Abdominal Wall Anatomy

▌ INTRODUCTION

This chapter will review the anatomy of abdominal region with regards to its significance in aesthetics, importance in surgical restoration and cautions to prevent complications. Do not skip this as you may find interesting facts in between the lines.

▌ RELEVANT ANATOMY

The abdominal wall is embryonically derived in a segmental manner, and this is reflected in blood supply and innervation. This is important to understand when you plan abdominal contouring procedures, redo surgeries, or surgeries in patient with old scars of cholecystectomy, etc. This knowledge is also useful for local infiltrative anesthesia.

The transition of an embryo from a trilaminar disk to a three-dimensional structure on the 22nd day of gestation initiates the formation of abdominal wall. The abdominal wall becomes a definitive structure after the umbilical cord is separated.[1]

Abdominal Planes

The anatomic planes of the abdominal wall are made of multiple muscular and fascial layers that interdigitate and unite to form a sturdy, protective musculofascial layer. The musculofascial layer of abdomen protects the visceral organs and provides strength and stability to the body's trunk. This anatomy varies with respect to the different topographic regions of the abdomen; thus, a firm understanding of these layers, their blood supply, and their innervation is essential to surgical management of the abdomen.

The abdominal cavity is the largest hollow space in the body. It is bound cranially by the xiphoid process of the sternum and the costal cartilages of ribs 7–10; caudally, by the anterior ilium and the pubic bone of the pelvis; anteriorly, by the abdominal wall musculature; and posteriorly, by the L1–L5 vertebrae.

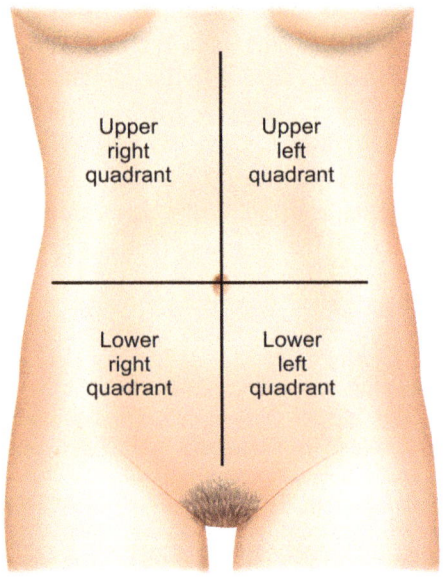

Fig. 2.1: Abdominal wall is divided by vertical and horizontal lines that pass through the umbilicus forming right upper and lower, and left upper and lower quadrant.

The abdominal planes change with age and many changes occur during a lifetime. Excess fat deposition occurs in different planes of the abdominal wall as well as in the intra-abdominal region. The abdomen bulges anteriorly, laterally, and in the lumbar area as well.

Pregnancy causes stretching of the abdominal wall and it weakens musculoaponeurotic system.

Abdominal Regions

The flat abdominal plane is broken up only by the costal margins, anterior superior iliac spines, and the umbilicus.

The most common and widely accepted system for identification of various regions of the abdomen pertaining to the abdominal viscera is a simple division of the abdomen into four quadrants by a vertical and horizontal line bisecting the umbilicus and forming the right and left upper and lower quadrants (Fig. 2.1).[1] This division is more important for diagnosis of intra-abdominal pathologies and abdominal wall tumors and hernias.

It may help an aesthetic surgeon to assess the symmetry and contour deformities.

ABDOMINAL SKIN

Langer Lines

Elsewhere on the human body, the abdominal skin is transgressed by Langer lines, also called cleavage lines. This is a term used to define the direction within the skin along which the skin has the least flexibility and corresponds to the alignment of the collagen fibers within the dermis. Across the superior half of the anterior abdominal skin, these lines are oriented in a transverse direction. In the inferior half of the abdominal skin, the Langer's lines begin to assume a slightly more oblique course in an inferior medial direction toward the groin, paralleling the inguinal crease.

Stretch marks also called as striae gravidarum, are caused by excessive stretching of the abdominal skin during pregnancy. The striae gravidarum are usually found running perpendicular to the Langer lines. The skin with expansion stretches more in the vertical direction and dermal tear occurs when expanding horizontally.

Umbilicus

The umbilicus is a midline fibrous cicatrix formed by folds of skin. In young adults, it is located at level of third and fourth vertebra. The level of umbilicus is lowered in people with large amount of extra abdominal fat and is often associated with hanging panniculus.

Umbilical stalk consists of umbilical ligaments (median, medial, and lateral). The median is remnant of urachus; medial is obliterated umbilical arteries; and lateral is inferior epigastric vessels. Since it is a weak spot umbilical hernia can occur if intra-abdominal volume or pressure is high.

Rarely, umbilicus may receive Meckels diverticulum or round ligament of liver. It is important to be aware of these anomalies that may pose challenges. A shallow and flush umbilicus is sign of increased intra-abdominal volume.

SUPERFICIAL FASCIA

The superficial fascia of the abdominal wall is the next layer encountered just deep to the skin. It consists of connective

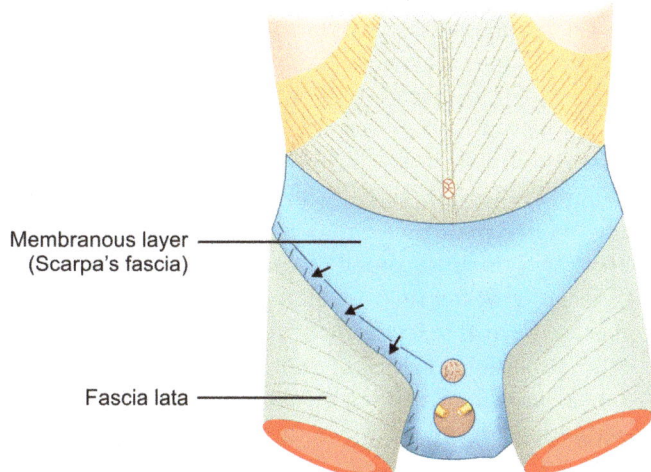

Fig. 2.2: Scarpa's fascia overlying the lower part of the abdomen.

Membranous layer
(Scarpa's fascia)

Fascia lata

tissue that contains a variable amount of fat. This layer can vary in thickness from < 1 cm to > 15 cm, depending on a person's body habitus.

Camper and Scarpa Fasciae

Superior to the umbilicus, the superficial fascia consists of a single layer. Inferior to the umbilicus, it splits into two layers. The more superficial and fatty layer is the Camper fascia and the deeper, more fibrous layer is the Scarpa fascia.

Campers fascia contains fatty tissue and its thickness depends upon the extent of fat deposition. In males, it continues inferiorly as dartos fascia and is devoid of fat. In females, it continues into the labia majora and also has variable amount of fat.

The Scarpa fascia is a membranous layer and contains very little fat. It is continuous in both the superficial fascia of the thigh known as the fascia lata and the superficial fascia of the perineum known as the Colles fascia. The space between Scarpa's fascia and deep fascia of the muscles contains a deep layer of fat. This fat is looser with large globules and less vasculature as compared to more compact and vascular fat in Campers fascia. This is most likely akin to orbital fat or buccal fat with gliding function between the planes of abdomen.

This layer of fat can commonly undergo fat necrosis in extensive abdominal flap elevation during abdominoplasty. Scarpa's fascia is tough structure and has surgical significance. Scarpa's fascia allows secured suturing during abdominoplasty surgery (Fig. 2.2).

Extent of Scarpa's Fascia

It is a single, well-defined continuous membrane. Laterally, it blends with the deep fascia of the external oblique muscle at the level of the anterior axillary line; inferiorly, it crosses the outer part of the inguinal ligament and attaches to the fasciae latae and the fundi form ligament (suspensory ligament); medially and cranially, the margins were not that clearly defined because Scarpa's fascia becomes divergent, creating two or more septal layers approximately at the lateral border of the rectus sheet and at the umbilicus. It appears to be oval in form and oblique in direction.

The superficial fascial system (SFS), the connective tissue network that resides below the dermis, has been implicated as a pivotal structure in body contouring procedures. Surgical repair of the SFS has been claimed to increase wound strength and decrease seroma formation. In a porcine model, Song et al.[2] showed that repair of the SFS layer in addition to dermis repair significantly increased the initial biomechanical strength of wound repair. This could lead to a decrease in early and late wound dehiscence, less widening of the scars, and lasting aesthetic results.

This in vivo model confirms Lockwood's idea that repair of the SFS results in a stable scar that heals without migration. This has the potential of changing or enhancing post-bariatric body contouring outcomes, as the surgeon is dealing with large surface areas of tissue that need to be approximated under significant tension.

The SFS also produces many topographic landmarks of body—surface anatomy. The creases, plateaus, valleys, and bulges of our body are explained by anatomy and relation of SFS to skin and underlying muscles.

Anatomy of Superficial Fascial System

The SFS is a connective tissue network that extends from subdermal plane to underlying muscle fascia and it consists of several thin horizontal membrane sheets separated by varying amount of fat with interconnecting vertical and oblique fibrous septa.

There are zones of adherence where they are tightly adhered to the underlying muscle, linea alba, tendinous intersections, and iliac crest region.[3]

Superiorly, SFS splits into anterior and posterior lamella/capsule of female breasts.

▋ ABDOMINAL MUSCLES

The abdominal wall is composed of five paired muscles: two vertical muscles (the rectus abdominis and the pyramidalis) and three layered, flat muscles (the external abdominal oblique, the internal abdominal oblique, and the transversus abdominis muscles).

These muscles and their fascial attachments interdigitate and unite to form a sturdy, protective musculofascial layer that gives strength and support to the anterolateral abdominal wall.

External Abdominal Oblique Muscle

The external abdominal oblique muscle is the largest and most superficial of the three paired, flat abdominal muscles. It arises from the lower eight ribs and interdigitations of the serratus anterior muscle.

As the external abdominal oblique courses in an inferior medial direction, its muscle fibers change from thick muscle to a fibrous aponeurosis that inserts medially in the linea alba. Inferiorly, the external abdominal oblique aponeurosis folds back on itself to form the inguinal ligament between the anterior superior iliac spine and the pubic tubercle before inserting into the pubic tubercle and the anterior half of the iliac crest. Just medial to its insertion in the pubic tubercle, the aponeurosis divides and forms the superficial (or external) inguinal ring.

The external abdominal oblique is innervated in a segmental pattern by the anterior rami of the inferior six thoracoabdominal nerves.

Internal Abdominal Oblique Muscle

The internal abdominal oblique muscle is the intermediate layer of the three paired, flat abdominal muscles. It originates broadly from the anterior portion of the iliac crest, lateral half of the inguinal ligament, and thoracolumbar fascia. The internal abdominal oblique inserts in the inferior border of the 10–12th ribs, the linea alba, and the pubic crest via the conjoint tendon. The muscle fibers of the internal abdominal oblique course upward in a superomedial orientation, perpendicular to the muscle fibers of the external abdominal oblique.

Like the external abdominal oblique, the internal abdominal oblique forms a broad aponeurosis that fuses into the midline and contributes to the rectus sheath. Superior to the arcuate line (Fig. 2.3A), the internal abdominal oblique aponeurosis splits anteriorly and posteriorly to enclose the rectus muscle and helps form the rectus sheath. However, inferior to the arcuate line, the internal abdominal oblique aponeurosis does not split and only passes anterior to the rectus muscle as part of the anterior rectus sheath (Fig. 2.3 B).

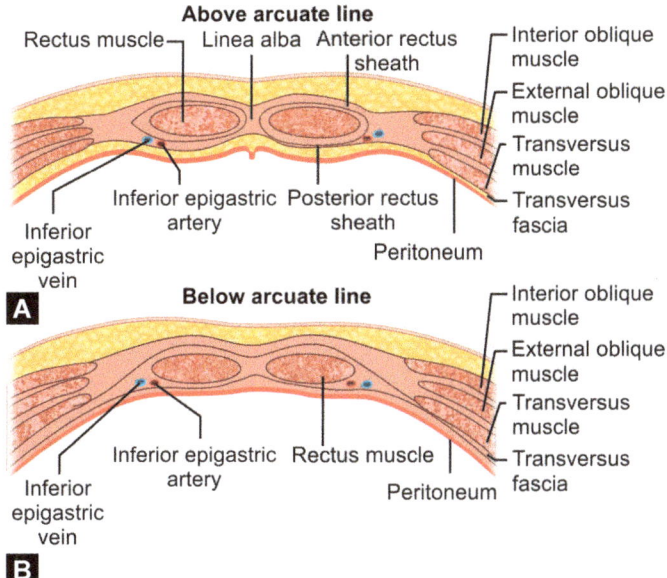

Figs. 2.3A and B: Superior to arcuate line the aponeurosis is present above and below the rectus muscles. Inferiorly the aponeurosis covers only the anterior wall of the rectus muscles and is missing posteriorly.

The inferior aponeurotic fibers of the internal abdominal oblique muscle course over the spermatic cord, through the inguinal canal, and the medial fibers fuse with the aponeurosis of the transversus abdominis muscle to form the conjoint tendon.

The internal oblique is innervated in a segmental pattern by the anterior rami of the inferior six thoracoabdominal nerves (T7–T12) and first lumbar nerves (iliohypogastric and ilioinguinal nerves).

Of note, all the neurovascular structures supplying the abdominal muscles run in the plane between the internal abdominal oblique muscle and the transversus abdominis muscle, except for the iliohypogastric and ilioinguinal nerves. Initially, they lie on the anterior surface of the quadratus lumborum, and then pass laterally into the plane between the transversus abdominis and the internal abdominal oblique. Above the anterior superior iliac spine, they penetrate the internal abdominal oblique to run between this muscle and the aponeurosis of the external abdominal oblique muscle.

Transversus Abdominis Muscle

The transversus abdominis muscle is the deepest of the three paired, flat abdominal muscles. It originates on the internal surfaces of the 7–12th costal cartilages, thoracolumbar fascia, anterior three fourths of the iliac crest, and lateral third of the inguinal ligament.

As with the other flat muscles, the transversus abdominis forms a broad aponeurosis that helps make up the rectus sheath before it fuses into the midline to the linea alba. Above the arcuate line, the transversus abdominis aponeurosis contributes to the posterior rectus sheath. Below the arcuate line, it is fused with the other flat muscles as the anterior rectus sheath (Figs. 2.3A and B).

As its name implies, the muscle and aponeurotic fibers run in a transverse direction, except for the most inferior aponeurotic fibers. These fibers curve in an inferomedial direction to unite with the aponeurosis of internal abdominal oblique to form the conjoint tendon, which attaches to the pubic crest and the pectineal (Cooper) ligament. The inferior aponeurotic fibers are fused to the underlying transversalis fascia, thus forming the posterior wall of the inguinal canal. A small triangular opening in this posterior wall is known as the deep or internal inguinal ring. The spermatic cord is formed at the internal inguinal ring by ductus deferens, testicular vessels and genital branch of Genitofemoral nerve and through which all indirect inguinal hernias develop.

The transversus abdominis is innervated in a segmental pattern by the anterior rami of the inferior six thoracoabdominal nerves (T7–T12) and first lumbar nerves (iliohypogastric and ilioinguinal nerves).

Rectus Abdominis Muscles

The rectus abdominis muscles are paired, long muscles that run just lateral to the linea alba in a vertical direction from the xiphoid process of the sternum and costal cartilage of the 5–7th ribs to the pubic symphysis. These muscles function to tense the abdominal wall, flex the trunk, stabilize the pelvis, and aid in childbirth, defecation, micturition, and forced expiration.

Each muscle is divided along its course by three or four transverse fibrous bands known as tendinous intersections, which essentially divide the muscle into a series of interconnected muscles (Fig. 2.4B). This results in "abs" or "six-pack." The rectus muscles are contained within the rectus sheath, which is formed by the aponeuroses of the external abdominal oblique, internal abdominal oblique, and transversus abdominis muscles.

The rectus muscles have a dual blood supply (Fig. 2.4A). The superior epigastric artery and vein, which are direct continuations of the internal thoracic vessels, supply the superior half of the rectus muscles. The inferior epigastric

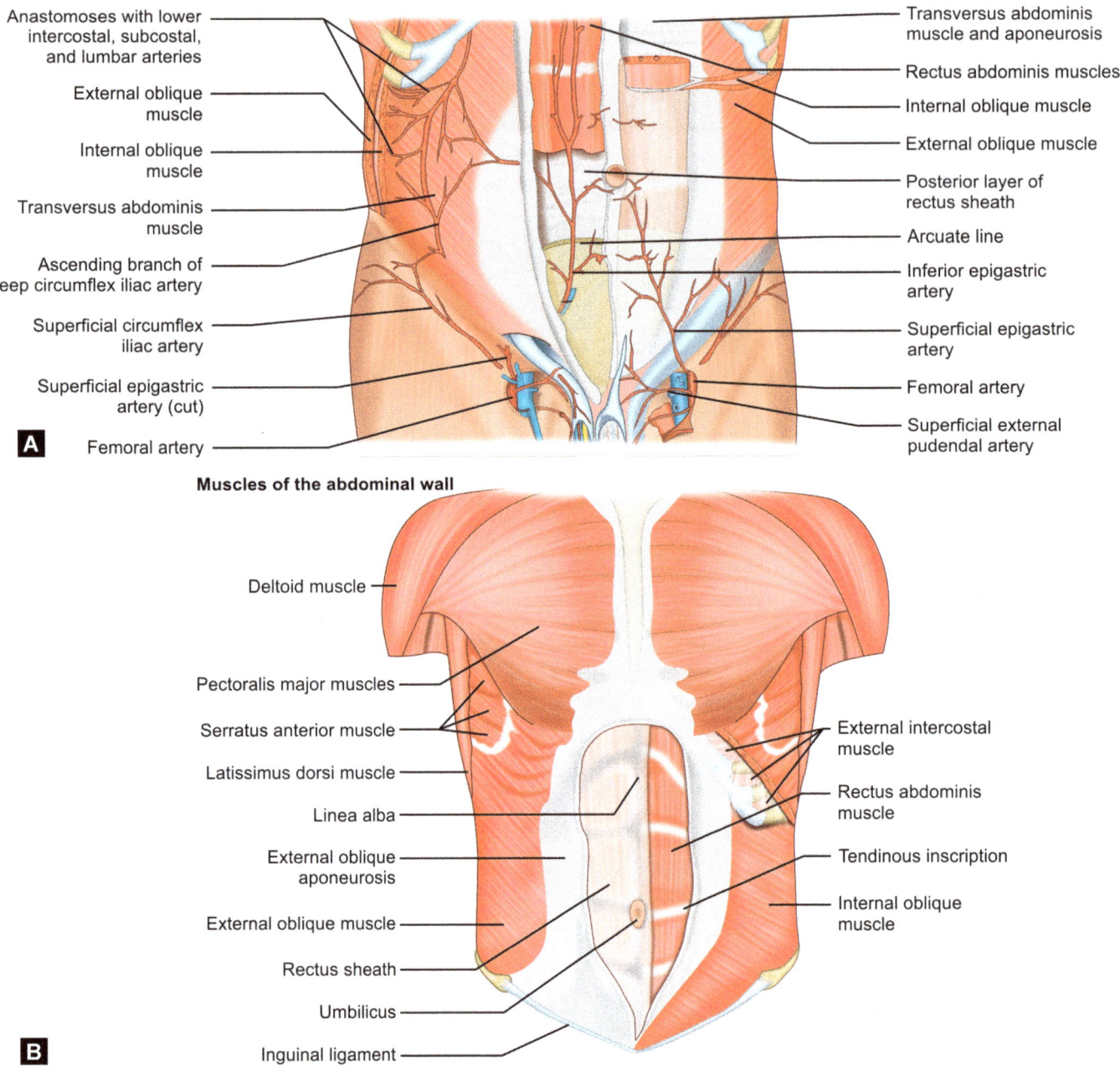

Muscles of the abdominal wall

Figs. 2.4A and B: (A) A blood circulation of abdominal muscles, (B) Anterior abdominal wall muscles, anterior rectus sheath, posterior rectus sheath and arcuate line.
Source: Encyclopædia Britannica, 2008 by Encyclopædia Britannica, Inc.

artery and vein, which arise from the external iliac vessels just proximal to their passage under the inguinal ligament, supply the inferior portion of the rectus muscles and run superiorly until they anastomose with the superior epigastric vessels. In addition, there are numerous small, segmental contributions from the lower six intercostal vessels (Fig. 2.4 A).

The rectus muscle is innervated in a segmental pattern by the anterior rami of the T7–T12 thoracoabdominal nerves.

Pyramidalis Muscle

The pyramidalis muscle is a small, triangular muscle that lies anterior to the inferior aspect of the rectus abdominis muscles. It originates at the pubic symphysis and attaches superiorly at the linea alba. This muscle functions to tense the linea alba and aid in midline stabilization. The pyramidalis muscle is generally considered insignificant in humans and is, in fact, absent in about 20% of the population.[4]

Arcuate Line

Approximately midway between the umbilicus and the pubic symphysis is an arching, transverse anatomic line known as the arcuate line or the semicircular line of Douglas. Superior to this line, the anterior rectus sheath is composed of the fusion of the aponeuroses of the external abdominal oblique and the anterior leaf of the internal abdominal oblique aponeuroses. (The internal abdominal oblique aponeurosis splits to envelop the rectus muscle at this level.)

The posterior rectus sheath above the arcuate line is composed of the fusion of the posterior leaf of the internal abdominal oblique aponeuroses and the transversus abdominis aponeuroses. Inferior to the arcuate line, the anterior rectus sheath is composed of the fusion of all three muscle aponeuroses, and little or no posterior sheath exists, because only the thin transversalis fascia runs posterior to the rectus muscle (*see* Figs. 2.3A and B).

Linea Alba and Linea Semilunaris

The linea alba is a dense, tendinous line created by the decussating aponeuroses of the external abdominal oblique, internal abdominal oblique, and transversus abdominis muscles at the abdominal midline. Between the rectus muscles, it extends superiorly from the xiphoid, continuing inferiorly, where it passes superficially in front of the rectus muscles to attach to the symphysis pubis. Deeper fibers pass behind the rectus abdominis, attaching to the posterior pubic crest to create a triangular lamella known as the "adminiculum lineae albae."[3]

Above the umbilicus, the well-formed linea alba is wider, progressively narrowing and becoming more vague below the umbilicus to its inferior attachments. Widening of the superior linea alba can cause a noticeable midline bulge known as a diastasis recti, or separation of the rectus muscles. Diastasis recti is a common and normal condition in newborns and is very common in women who have had multiple pregnancies.

The linea alba is visible superficially in thin and muscular people and is an important aesthetic landmark that gives an attractive characteristic to the abdomen.

Linea semilunaris (Spigelian line) marks the lateral border of rectus abdominis muscle. There occurs a ledge because the surface level of rectus muscle is slightly elevated above the external oblique muscle. This is also an aesthetic feature in young and fit individual.

▌ TRANSVERSALIS FASCIA

The transversalis fascia is a thin layer of connective tissue lining most of the abdominal cavity between the posterior surface of the transversus abdominis and superficial to the extraperitoneal fat and peritoneum. Superiorly, this fascia continues with the inferior diaphragmatic fascia; inferiorly with the iliac and pelvic fascia; posteriorly with the thoracolumbar fascia; and laterally to the iliac crest.

Above the arcuate line, the transversalis fascia contributes to the posterior sheath along with the posterior leaf of the internal abdominal oblique and the transversus abdominis muscles. Below the arcuate line, the transversalis fascia forms the posterior sheath alone. With attachments to the posterior margin of the inguinal ligament, it contributes to the formation of femoral sheath, contributes the internal spermatic fascia, and becomes the only layer contributing to the inguinal floor. At the deep inguinal ring, the structures of the spermatic cord in males and, in females, the structures of the round ligament of the uterus pass through the transversalis fascia.[4,5]

Abdominal Wall Vasculature

The blood supply of the abdominal wall has been exhaustively described by Taylor and Palmer.[6] The angiosomes and vascular territories as we have learnt in flap surgery are also applicable in abdominal wall surgery.

There are two types of cutaneous blood supply:
1. Direct vessels that directly supply the skin;
2. Indirect vessels that "emerge from the deep fascia as terminal spent branches of arteries whose main purpose is to supply the muscles and other deep tissues." – perforators

In a subsequent study in 1988, Moon and Taylor were able to demonstrate connections between the deep superior and deep inferior epigastric systems and their relationship to the cutaneous circulation.[7] The contributions of the superficial inferior epigastric vessels and the intercostal vessels were also delineated.

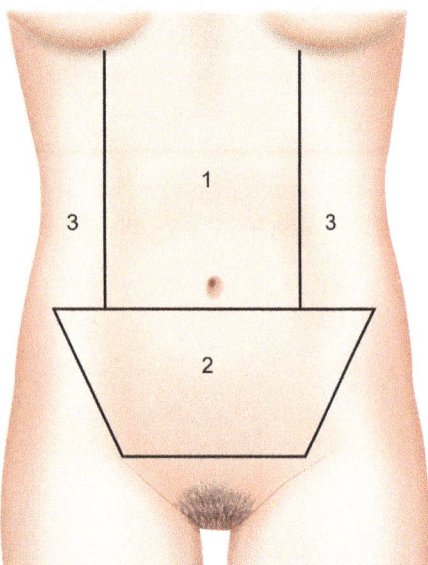

Fig. 2.5: Huger's zones, zone 1 area overlying the upper rectus muscles and vascularised only by deep epigastric arcade, zone 2 overlying the lower abdominal wall and vascularized by superficial epigastric, superficial external pudendal and superficial circumflex iliac system and zone 3 overlies the lateral abdominal wall and vascularised by six lateral intercostals and four lumbar arteries.

A clear understanding of the arterial supply of the abdominal wall is crucial to operative planning, especially when the patient's history includes prior abdominal or chest wall surgeries. Huger's[8] description of the different zones of the blood supply guides the surgeon in planning and performing a safe operation.

▌ HUGER'S ZONES

Zone I: It defined as the area that is fed anteriorly by the vertically oriented deep epigastric arcade (Fig. 2.5).

Zone II: The lower abdominal circulation is provided by the superficial epigastric, superficial external pudendal, and superficial circumflex iliac systems (zone II). A rich plexus between these systems allows collateral flow.

Zone III: It defines as the lateral aspect of the abdominal wall (flanks) that are fed by the six lateral intercostal and four lumbar arteries.

During abdominoplasty, the cutaneous blood supply to zone I and much of zone II is divided, with the abdominal flap circulation fully dependent on zone III. If a scar, such as a subcostal cholecystectomy incision, crosses the elevated flap, the circulation to the tissue distal to the scar is in jeopardy. A vertical midline incision can further jeopardize flap circulation.

The supporting structures of the abdominal wall have been elegantly described by Hartrampf.[9] He describes two static vertical supporting structures (linea alba, two linea semilunaris ligaments) and two static transverse ligaments (anterior rectus sheath, transverse tendinous inscription).

In order to gain a greater understanding of vascular complications during abdominal wall surgery, liposuction or abdominoplasty, we need to understand the microvasculature system. In the upper third the abdominal wall is composed of perforators from superior epigastric systems, while in the central region it is from deep inferior epigastric system.

These two systems anastomosed at midpoint between umbilicus and xiphisternum in most cases. Whereas, in the lower abdomen vascular network is contributed by superficial inferior epigastric artery, superficial circumflex iliac artery, superficial externalpudendal artery and perforators of deep inferior epigastric, intercostal and subcostal arteries.

Inferior Epigastric Artery

The origin of deep inferior epigastric artery is a single branch from external iliac artery and after it enters the rectus muscle it divides into medial and lateral divisions. In 20% cases there is a third branch going straight to the umbilicus. The lateral division of deep inferior epigastric artery is major with maximum perforators as compared to medial division.

On an average there are 4–7 perforators within 4 cm of umbilicus. About 40% are situated in the upper lateral part of umbilicus and 20% in the upper medial part. As these perforators penetrate Scarpa's fascia, they divide and run in vertical direction and form subdermal plexuses (Figs. 2.6 and 2.7). Whereas small musculocutaneous perforators < 0.5 mm have short course and they terminate immediately above rectus sheath in deep subcutaneous fat layer and they contribute to the blood supply of deep fat layer.

Superior Epigastric System

Superior epigastric artery is a branch of internal mammary artery and it enters the abdominal region by passing between costal and xiphisternum origins of the diaphragm.

It divides into multiple branches before penetrating the rectus muscle. In each side of the upper abdomen, there are average four large > 0.5 mm perforators. They are located in a triangle formed by costal margins and the base is at midway between xiphisternum and umbilicus.

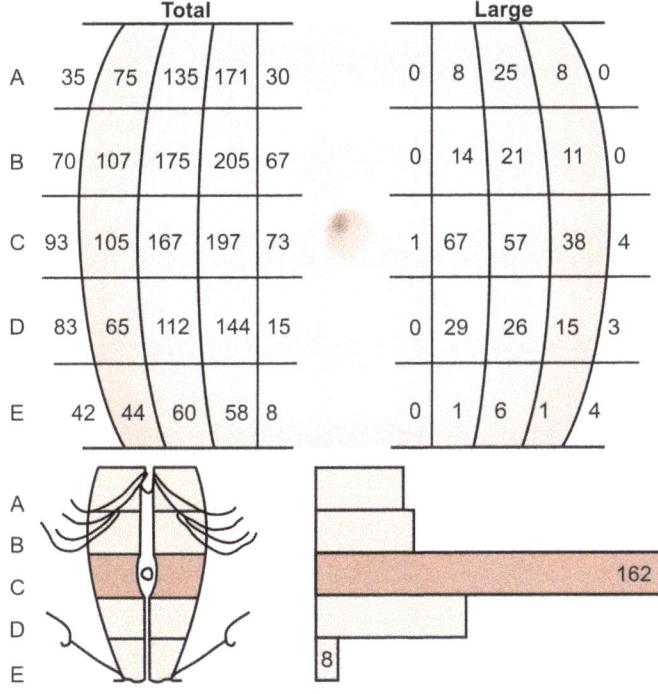

		Total						Large			
A	35	75	135	171	30	0	8	25	8	0
B	70	107	175	205	67	0	14	21	11	0
C	93	105	167	197	73	1	67	57	38	4
D	83	65	112	144	15	0	29	26	15	3
E	42	44	60	58	8	0	1	6	1	4

Fig. 2.6: (*Above*) Division of the rectus abdominis into horizontal fifths and vertical thirds producing 15 zones per muscle (*shaded*). In 50 muscles, the total number of large and small perforators in each zone is shown on the left, and the numbers of large perforators alone are given on the right. The figures in the *unshaded areas* represent the equivalent numbers of perforators passing through the linea alba medially and the external oblique aponeurosis laterally. There are generally fewer perforators in the lateral third of the muscle, and very few large perforators pass through the linea alba or external oblique. (*Below*) Note the paraumbilical concentration of large perforators and their scarcity in the lower one-fifth of the muscle. This histogram plots the total number of large performators located over the rectus muscle in each of the five horizontal zones in 50 fresh cadaver dissections (compare with *above, right*). The average number per side is obtained by dividing these figures in each zone by 50, being 3.2 in the paraumbilical region.
Source: Boyd JB, Taylor GI, Corlette RJ. The vascular territory of the superior epigastric and deep inferior epigastric arteries, published in PRS 1984;73:1. Reprinted with permission.

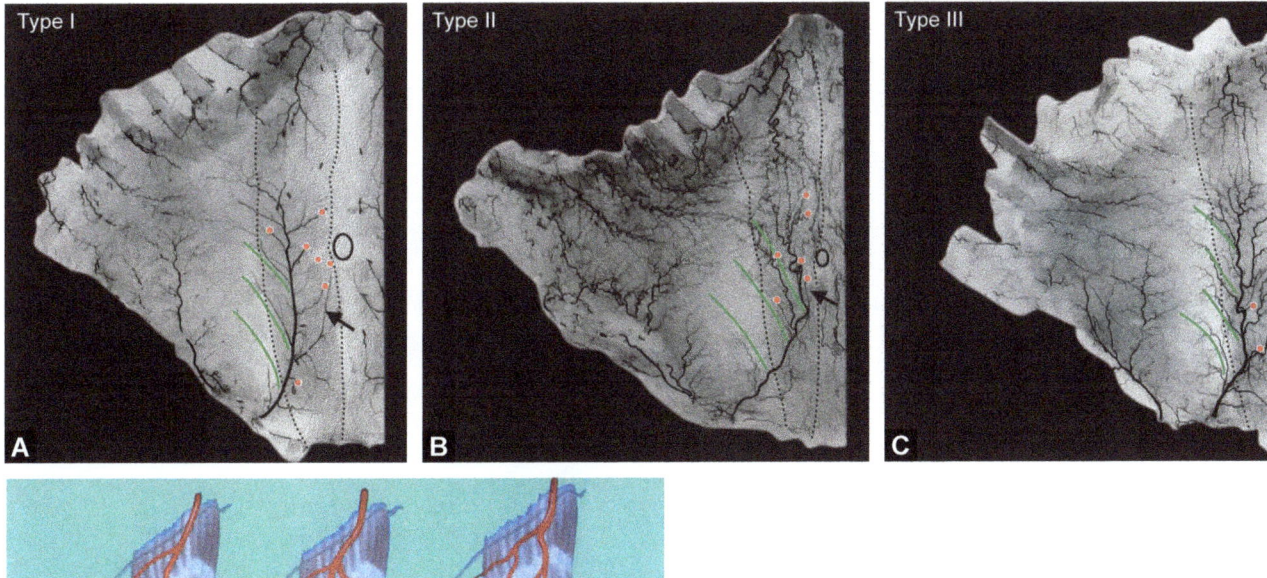

Figs. 2.7A to D: Illustrations from cadaveric studies showing perforators located around the umbilicus. Red dots highlight the origin of the dominant (>0.5 mm) cutaneous perforators. The outline of rectus muscle is highlighted with broken lines in each radiographic cadaver study.
Source: Boyd JB, Taylor GI, Corlette RJ. The vascular territory of the superior epigastric and deep inferior epigastric arteries, published in PRS 1984;73:1. Reprinted with permission.

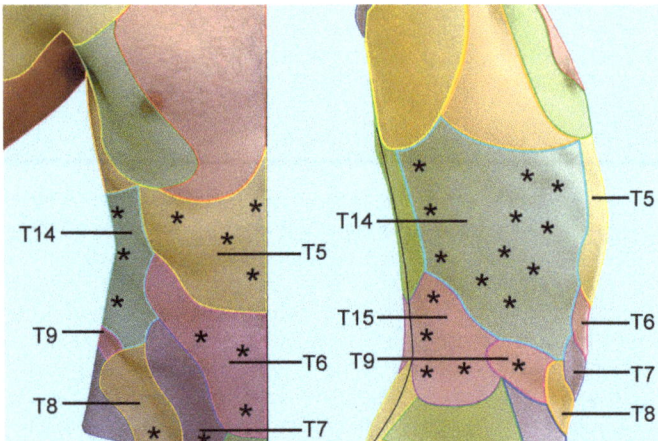

Fig. 2.8: Schematic representation of the vascular territories of the source arteries of the lateral lumbar region. The locations of their typical reliable perforators are marked with asterisks. (Left) Anterior view. (Right) Lateral view. (T5: Superior epigastric artery; T6: Deep inferior epigastric artery; T7: Superficial inferior epigastric artery; T8: Superficial circumflex iliac artery; T9: Deep circumflex iliac artery; T14: Lateral branches of posterior intercostal arteries; T15: Lumbar arteries.
Source: Offman SL, Geddes CR, Tang M, et al. The vascular basis of perforator flaps based on the source arteries of the lateral lumbar region plastic and reconstructive surgery. 2005 May;115(6):1651-59. Reprinted with permission.

One critic of lipoabdominoplasty is the risk of loss of vasculature of central abdominal skin. Dillerud and Heden demonstrated loss of vasculature in pig buttock skin after suction lipectomy.[10] Inceoglu et al. and Blondeel et al. had similar observation with infiltration, conventional, and even ultrasonic assisted liposuction.[11,12]

There are many investigators who demonstrated that the concentration of perforators around the umbilicus and the rich subdermal pleaxus that it forms preserves the vasculature of the lower flap.[13-15] So, the recent understanding is a successful lipoabdominoplasty that can be performed without the risk of devascularization if there is limited tunneling in the upper part of the abdomen to repair the rectus muscle preserving the perforators.[16]

Posterior Intercostal Arteries and Lumbar Arteries

There are nine pairs of posterior intercostals arteries arising from descending aorta and arranged segmentally around the posterior and lateral parts of the trunk. They terminate anteriorly in rectus abdominis muscle. Each posterior intercostal artery has four parts: vertebral, costal groove, intermuscular, and rectus segments.

The important anatomy in relation to abdominoplasty surgery is the lateral and anterior segment. The musculocutaneous perforators arise through interdigitations of serratus anterior and external oblique muscle along the lateral aspect of abdomen and it is important source of cutaneous supply.

The intermuscular segment travels in between transversus abdominis and internal oblique muscles. There are 13 ± 4 perforators along the lateral abdominal wall (Fig. 2.8).[17]

The nerve supply to the abdominal wall is via intercostal nerves VIII–XXII. These nerves pass between the internal oblique and transversus abdominis muscles. The motor branches pass behind the rectus muscles and enter the muscles at the junction of the lateral one third and medial two thirds.

The abdominal skin is innervated in a segmental pattern by the anterior rami of the T7–L1 thoracoabdominal nerves. T7–T9 thoracoabdominal nerves innervate the skin above the umbilicus; T10 thoracoabdominal nerves innervates the skin around the umbilicus; and T11 thoracoabdominal nerves plus cutaneous branches of the subcostal (T12), iliohypogastric, and ilioinguinal (L1) nerves supply the skin inferior to the umbilicus.[1,18]

■ REFERENCES

1. Moore KL, Agur AM, Dalley AF. Essential Clinical Anatomy. Keith Moore (Ed.) 4th edition, Chapter 2, The abdomen. Philadelphia, PA: Lippincott Williams & Wilkins; 2011. pp. 116-35.
2. Song AY, Askari M. Biomechanical Properties of the Superficial Fascial System. A Esthe Urgery J. 2006;26(4): 395-403.
3. Lockwood TE. Superficial fascial system (SFS) of the trunk and extremities: a new concept. Plast Reconstr Surg. 1991; 87(6):1009-18.
4. Gray H. Anterior abdominal wall. In: Standring S (Ed). Gray's Anatomy: The Anatomical Basis of Clinical Practice. 39th edition. Philadelphia, PA: Elsevier Churchill Livingstone; 2005. pp. 1104-11.
5. Rosse C, Gaddum-Rosse P Abdomen. Hollinshead,s Textbook of Anatomy. 5th edition. Philadelphia, PA: Lippincott-Raven; 1997. pp. 518-25, 622-8.
6. Taylor GI, Palmer JH. The vascular territories (angiosomes) of the body: experimental study and clinical applications. Br J Plast Surg. 1987;40:113.
7. Moon HK, Taylor GI. The vascular anatomy of rectus abdominis musculocutaneous flaps based on the deep superior epigastric system. Plast Reconstr Surg. 1988;82(5):815-29.
8. Huger WE, Jr. The anatomic rationale for abdominal lipectomy. Am Surg. 1979;45:612.

9. Hartrampf CR. Hartrampf's Breast Reconstruction with Living Tissue. Norfolk, VA: Hampton; 1991.

10. Dillerud E, Hede´n P. Circulation of blood and viability after blunt suction lipectomy in pig buttock flaps. Scand J Plast Reconstr Surg Hand Surg. 1993;27:9-14.

11. Inceoglu S, Ozdemir H, Inceoglu F, et al. Investigation of the effect of liposuction on the perforator vessels using color Doppler ultrasonography. Eur J Plast Surg.1998;21:38.

12. Blondeel PN, Derks D, Roche N, et al. The effect of ultra-sound-assisted liposuction and conventional liposuction on the perforator vessels in the lower ab dominal wall. Br J Plast Surg. 2003;56:266-71.

13. Emeri JF, Krupp S, Doerti J. Is a free or pedicled TRAM flap safe after liposuction? Plast Reconstr Surg. 1993;92:1198.

14. Teimourian B, Kroll S. Subcutaneous endoscopy in suction lipectomy. Plast Reconstr Surg. 1984;74:708-11.

15. Ozcan G, Shenaq S, Baldwin B, et al. The trauma of suction-assisted lipectomy cannula on flap circulation in rats. Plast Reconstr Surg. 1991;88:250-8.

16. Graf R, de Araujo LR, Rippel R, et al. Lipoabdominoplasty: liposuction with reduced undermining and traditional abdominal skin flap resection. Aesthetic Plast Surg. 2006; 30:1-8.

17. Offman SL, Geddes CR, Tang M. More the vascular basis of perforator flaps based on the source arteries of the lateral lumbar region Plast Reconstr Surg. 2005;115(6):1651-9.

18. John T Hansen, Netter's Clinical Anatomy, Chapter 4, Abdomen, Elsevier Health Sciences 14 Feb, 2014; P.147-8.

CHAPTER 3

Aesthetic Subunits of Abdomen

▍ INTRODUCTION

Aesthetic subunits are important to understand because skin elasticity, fat distribution, and musculoskeletal anatomy vary in the abdominal region. This chapter will describe the subunits, its aesthetic implications, and the related anatomy.

Abdominal contour surgery is one of the commonest aesthetic procedures. Either it is performed as liposculpturing alone or in combination with abdominoplasty.[1]

In order to achieve best results and provide a good contouring to the whole abdominal region, it is important to understand the underlying anatomy, the skin variation in different regions of the abdomen, and the fat distribution pattern. Literature is deplete of detailed anatomical characteristics of skin, subcutaneous tissue and the muscle in different aesthetic subunits of the abdomen. This anatomy is important for an aesthetic surgeon who wants to do abdominal contouring surgery.

Matarasso proposed in his publication to segmentalize the "abdomen" area into several aesthetic units on the basis of underlying anatomy.[2]

Matarasso described seven subunits of the abdominal region in women and six subunits in men.

In women:
1. Upper abdomen
2. Lower abdomen
3. Umbilicus
4. Flanks
5. Mons
6. Sacral area
7. Bra roles
   In men:
1. Upper abdomen
2. Lower abdomen
3. Umbilicus
4. Flanks
5. Mons
6. Sacral area

We have learnt the importance of facial aesthetic units. The concept of facial aesthetic units followed by subunits spurred improvements in aesthetic refinement in nasal reconstruction.[3,4]

Scott Spear and Steven Davison[5] described aesthetic subunits of breasts for a better aesthetic breast reconstruction. Constantino Mendieta described gluteal aesthetic units, in which he described that there are 10 aesthetic units to posterior region with 6 important zones that truly define the buttock shape.[6]

Sanjay Parashar, the author of this textbook would like to emphasize on ten different areas of "the abdomen", both in women and men on the basis of underlying musculoskeletal structures and overlying aesthetic contours.

All the ten subunits of the abdomen needs to be considered while performing abdominal contouring surgery.

The reasons for contouring in all the anatomic areas are as follows:
1. Better aesthetic contouring three dimensionally.
2. Better skin retraction because of extensive undermining thus preventing skin sagging.
3. Some patients come back with areas of disproportion after liposuction of limited areas and it is difficult to go back into the same areas due to excessive fibrosis and the final outcome is not satisfactory.
4. The fat left behind in any of the abdominal subunits after liposuction can expand and get stored if patients gain any additional weight that can sometimes cause disfigurement.

This is the basis of high-definition liposuction, waste sculpting, and liposculpturing of the abdominal region.

▍ ANATOMICAL VARIATION OF ABDOMINAL REGION

Anterior Abdominal Wall (Figs. 3.1A and B)

Skin

There are anatomical variations of the skin, underlying musculoskeletal framework and their adhesions in different regions of the abdominal area.

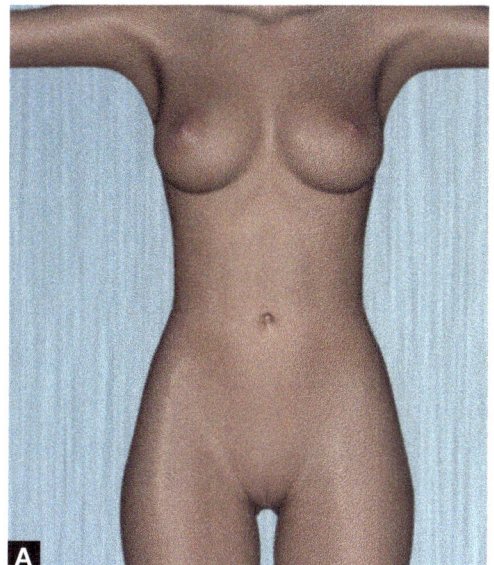
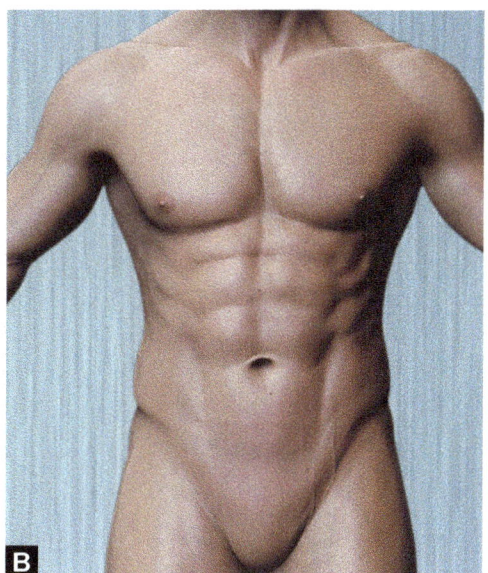

Figs. 3.1A and B: Anterior abdominal wall in woman and man.

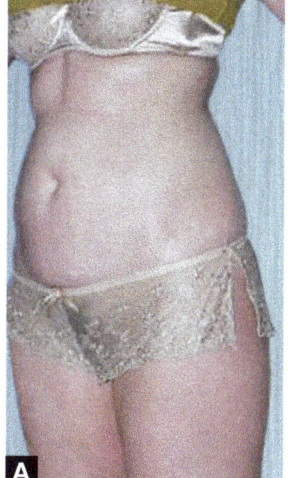
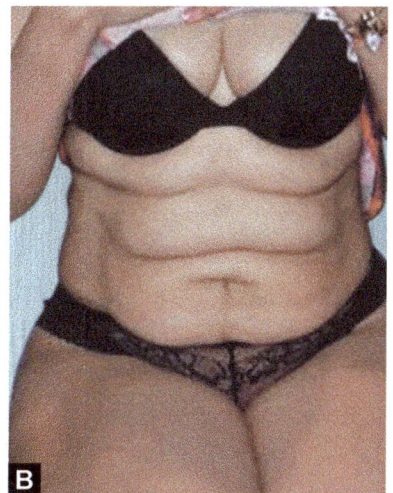
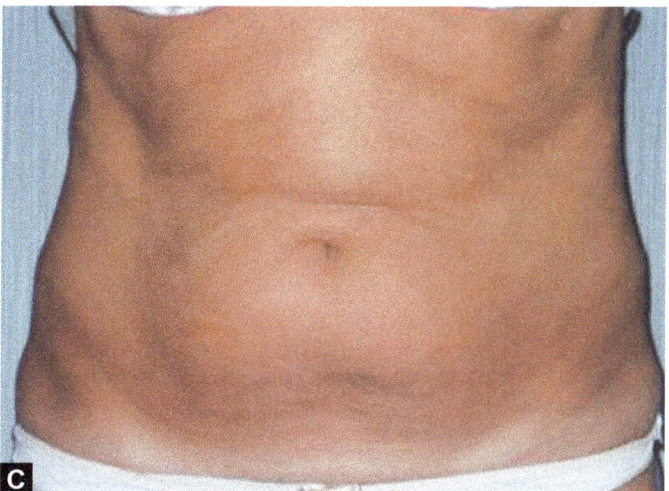

Figs. 3.2A to C: (A) Flexion crease in the upper abdomen, (B) Multiple flexion creases and rolls, (C) Supraumbilical flexion crease.

Skin has normal adhesions overlying the bony areas such as xiphoid bone, costal margin superiorly, and pubic bone and iliac crest region inferiorly that are relatively fixed points of skin. The skin is fairly mobile in between these fixed points. Centrally it is anchored by umbilicus.

Skin has soft tissue adhesions such as linea alba region, intersections of rectus muscle, and inguinal region, particularly noted in thin-built male patient. These adhesions get obliterated with fat accumulation masking the aesthetics of the abdomen.

There are abnormal adhesions, which can be termed as "flexion creases", that are formed due to sitting in flexed position and vary from individual to individual depending upon the fat rolls (Figs. 3.2A to C).

There is expansion of skin due to fat accumulation and post pregnancy changes. The skin elasticity or physical force is largely determined by biomechanical properties of the skin itself. It significantly varies in different regions of the abdomen.[7,8]

The supraumbilical skin is more rigid and expands less than the lower abdominal region. This is evident by the fact that majority of women have lax skin, panniculus, and stretch marks in the lower part of their abdomen as compared to their upper part.

Abdominal rolls are formed by fat deposits and skin excess that is limited by deep adhesions "flexion creases". The abdominal rolls can form above or below the umbilicus.

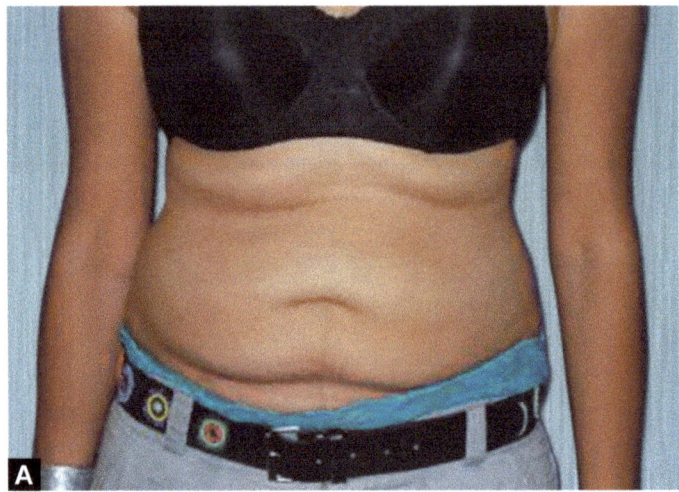 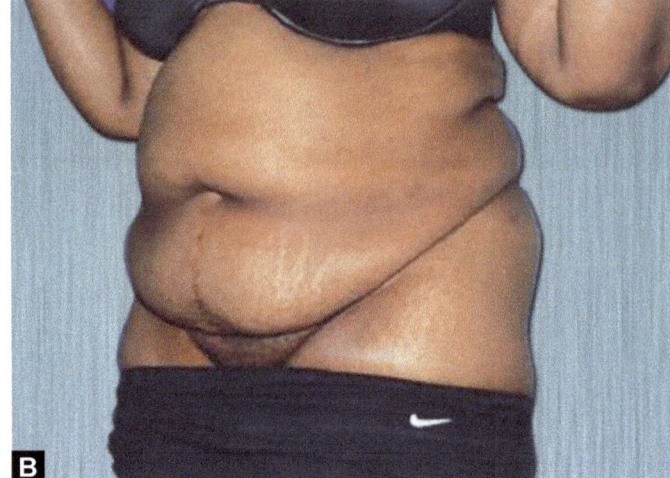

Figs. 3.3A and B: Lower abdominal rolls and skin adhesion.

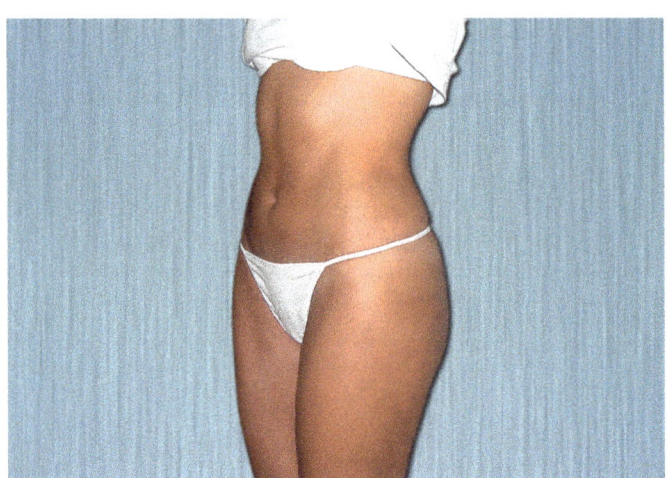

Fig. 3.4: Concave upper abdomen and convex lower abdomen in women.

The lower abdominal skin forms a fold that stops at the lower abdominal area and inguinal region due to the skin adhesions or, in some cases, is continuous with the pubic region (Figs. 3.3A and B). Poor-quality skin with extensive stretch marks has poor capability of retracting.[9]

Musculoskeletal Anatomy

The bulge of the bony areas and rectus muscle anatomy cause a curve silhouette in women particularly. The upper abdomen is concave above the umbilicus and is convex in the lower abdomen because of absence of posterior rectus sheath below the accurate line. (Fig. 3.4). The skin adhesions at the linea alba and tendinous intersections give an aesthetic and toned look to the tummy.

Some patients have flaring and prominent costal framework. The rib prominences may be masked by overlying fat. This poses a challenge during liposuction procedure potentially risking inadvertent cannula penetration in thoracic cage.

Fat Distribution

Fat distribution and consistency vary in the anterior abdomen. In the lower abdomen, the fat consistency is different than the upper abdomen. In the lower abdomen, fat layer above the Scarpa's fascia is more compact, the multiple fibrous septae. The fat below the scarpa's fascia is more loosely arranged with sparse fibrous septae. While performing liposuction under local anaesthesia and sedation the infiltration procedure is more painful in the upper abdomen. In the lower abdomen the infiltration process is relatively less painful in subscarpal plane. The technique of liposuction varies in the upper and lower abdomen, which is described later in this book.

Lateral Abdominal Wall (Fig. 3.5)

Skin

Skin is relatively thicker in this region and unless there is a very large amount of fat accumulation or intra-abdominal increase in volume the dermis remains intact. There are adhesions in bony areas—costal margin superiorly and iliac crest inferiorly.

Soft tissue adhesions in men are on the iliac crest region and during contouring it needs to be preserved

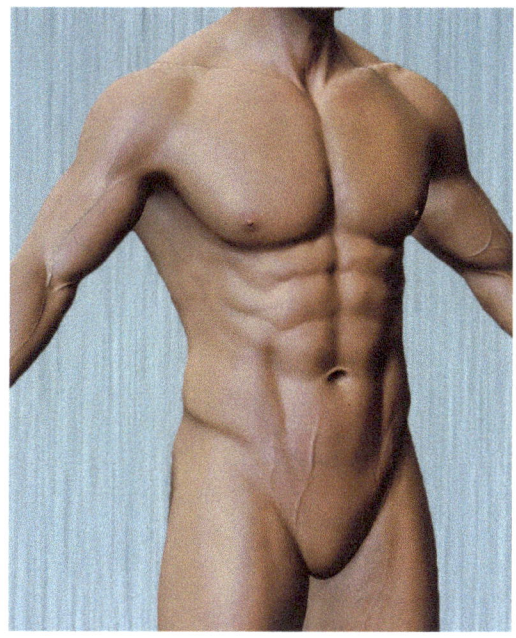

Fig. 3.5: Lateral abdominal wall.

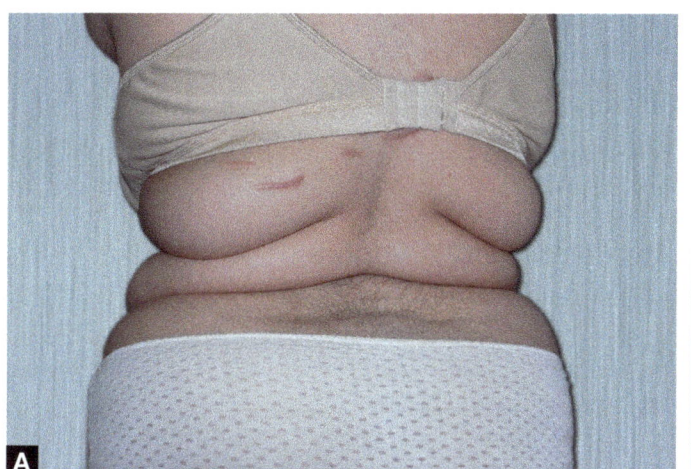

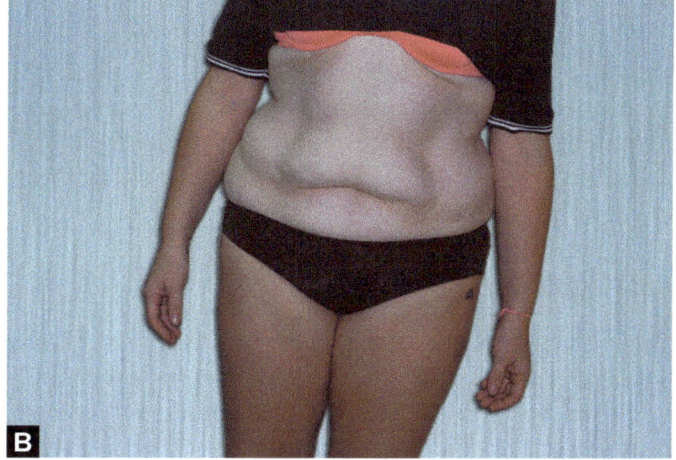

Figs. 3.6A and B: (A) Lateral abdominal rolls extending in the back region as "bra rolls" and "waist rolls", (B) Lateral abdominal rolls in flank region

to prevent feminization. Where as in women it is in the mid-buttock area and often is responsible for "guitar" shaped deformity and requires special attention during contouring.

Flexion creases are often developed with fat accumulation forming rolls (Figs. 3.6A and B). Waist is defined as the narrowest part of the body between the thorax and hips. The body gradually widens above and below the waist line giving an hour-glass appearance, particularly, in healthy people. Waist-hip ratio is the ratio of the circumference of the waist to that of the hips. Waist-hip ratios of 0.7 for women and 0.9 for men have been shown to correlate strongly with general health and fertility.

With the weight gain there is fat deposition in this region that changes the waist-hip ratio of the person. The waist area has three-dimensional aesthetic curves that are visible in aneroposterior view, oblique view, and lateral view (Figs. 3.7A and B).This is an important area to consider in liposuction to reduce the size of the waist and improve aesthetics in three-dimensional fashion. The skin is firmly adhered to the waist region and the underlying fat layer is more fibrous and compact.

Musculoskeletal Anatomy

Underlying musculoskeletal anatomy casues typical concavoconvex silhouette anterolaterally and laterally. There

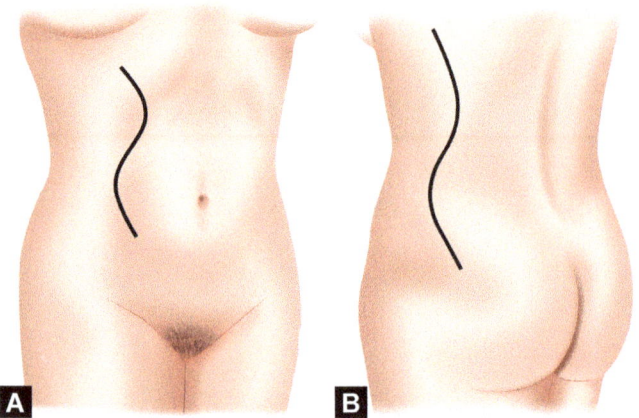

Figs. 3.7A and B: (A) Aesthetic curve in the anterolateral part of abdomen (B) Aesthetic curve in the posterior part of trunk.

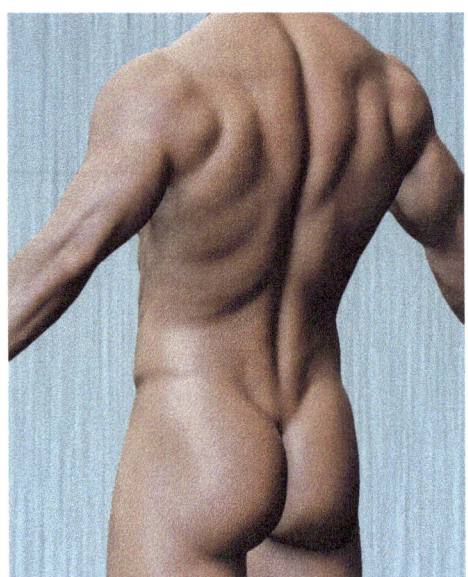

Fig. 3.8: Posterolateral abdomen unit.

is a gentle curve starting at the costal area with a "dip" in subcostal area. This area is obliterated due to fat accumulation. It is convex in the region of waist and gradually becomes curvaceous just above the iliac crest.

Fat accumulation in this area causes the typical "love handle" deformity that extends posteriorly.

The lateral linea semilunaris region is marked by the lateral border of rectus abdominis where there is a depression as lateral abdominal wall muscles are at lower level and often thinner than rectus bulge muscle.

Fat Distribution

There is often tough fibrofatty tissue in the costal region with deep pockets of fat in subcostal region. "Love handles" or flanks bulge often start in this region and extend posteriorly.

In women, the fat accumulation is continuous inferiorly up to mid buttocks where there are deep adhesions. Below this, it continues as trochanteric-region fat, also known as "saddle bags".

In men, this fat ends at the level of iliac crest due to the adhesion in this region.

Posterolateral Region (Fig. 3.8)

Skin

Skin is thicker in this region and very rarely has stretch marks. It has better chances of contraction after liposuction.

Skin is adhered in the costal areas above and posterior iliac crest area inferiorly.

In women the adhesion is located in the mid-buttock area causing bulge above and below that area. In men the adhesion is over the iliac crest region.

There are abnormal adhesions causing side rolls in case of fat deposition. Superiorly it extends along the lower part of breasts to posterior part, often called "bra roll" (Fig. 3.9).

Musculoskeletal Anatomy

Musculoskeletal structure overlying the posterior costal region, lumbar region, and gluteal region is responsible for an aesthetic curve (Fig. 3.10) that is often obliterated with fat deposition.

The muscles in the lumbar region include latissimus dorsi and external oblique and along with iliac crest they form "lumbar triangle" (Fig. 3.11). The aesthetic curve starts from the posterior costal margins with deepest point in the lumbar triangle region and curves down on the iliac crest and gluteus maximus muscle.

Fat Deposition

Fat deposition in this region obliterates the lumbar triangle and is typically in an oblique fashion with deep extensions overlying the lumbar muscles.

Posterior Midline Region (Figs. 3.12A and B)

Skin is adhered over the spinous processes and posterior iliac spine causing a midline groove and dimples inferolaterally.

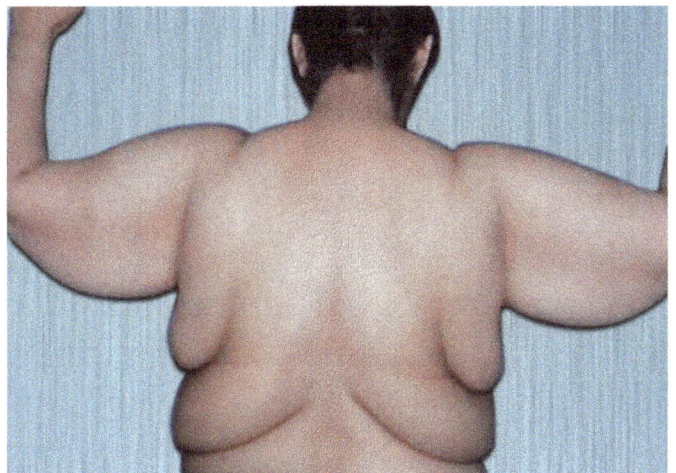

Fig. 3.9: Bra rolls.

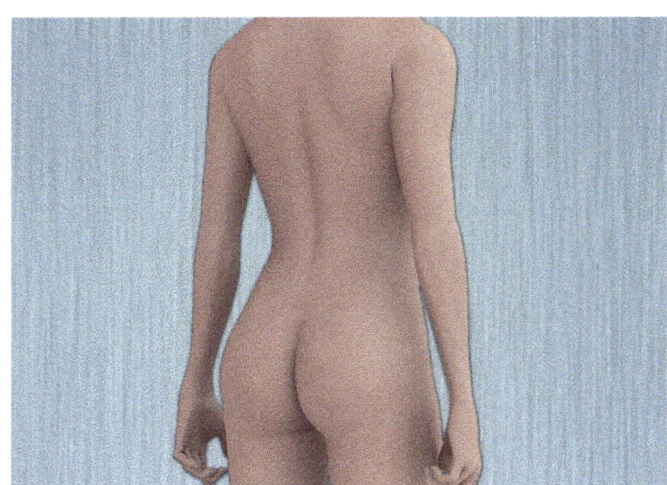

Fig. 3.10: Posterolateral curve in women.

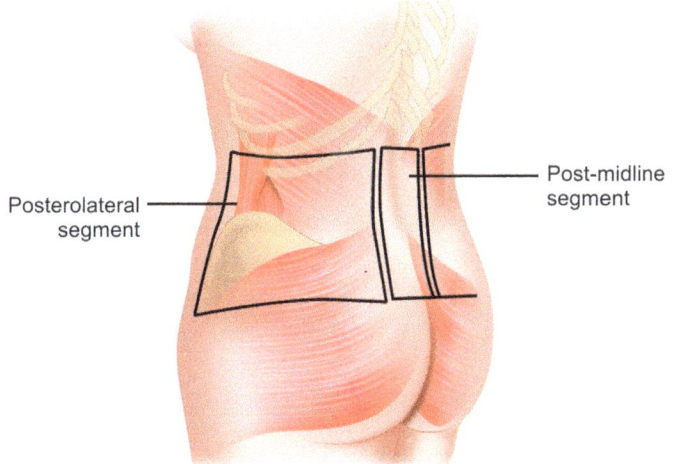

Posterolateral segment

Post-midline segment

Fig. 3.11: Lumbar triangle.

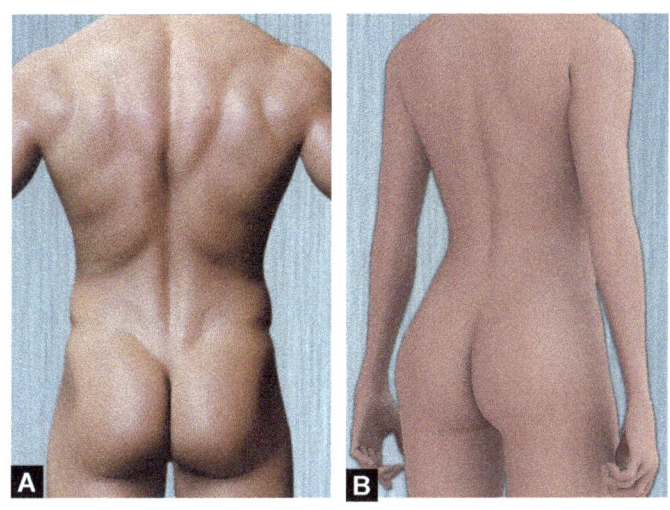

Figs. 3.12A and B: Posterior midline region in male and female.

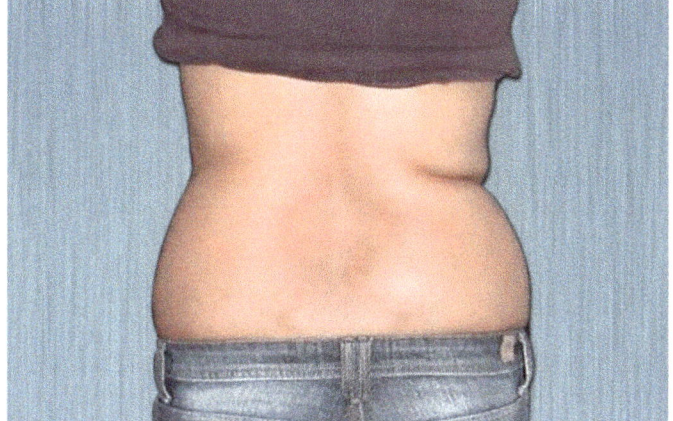

Fig. 3.13: Accumulation of fat in the lower part of posterior midline, called as "lumbar pad".

There is a typical fat deposit inferiorly on the sacral region called "lumbar pad" that obliterates the aesthetic curve posteriorly (Fig. 3.13).

AESTHETIC UNITS OF ABDOMEN (FIGS. 3.14A TO C)

Based on these anatomical characteristics and the typical fat deposition pattern, the abdominal area can be considered to have ten aesthetic subunits including the abdominal region and adjacent areas that significantly affect the aesthetic appearance of the midsection.

1. *Upper midline aesthetic unit*: This unit overlies the midline of the abdomen (linea alba) extending from xiphoid sternum to the umbilicus.

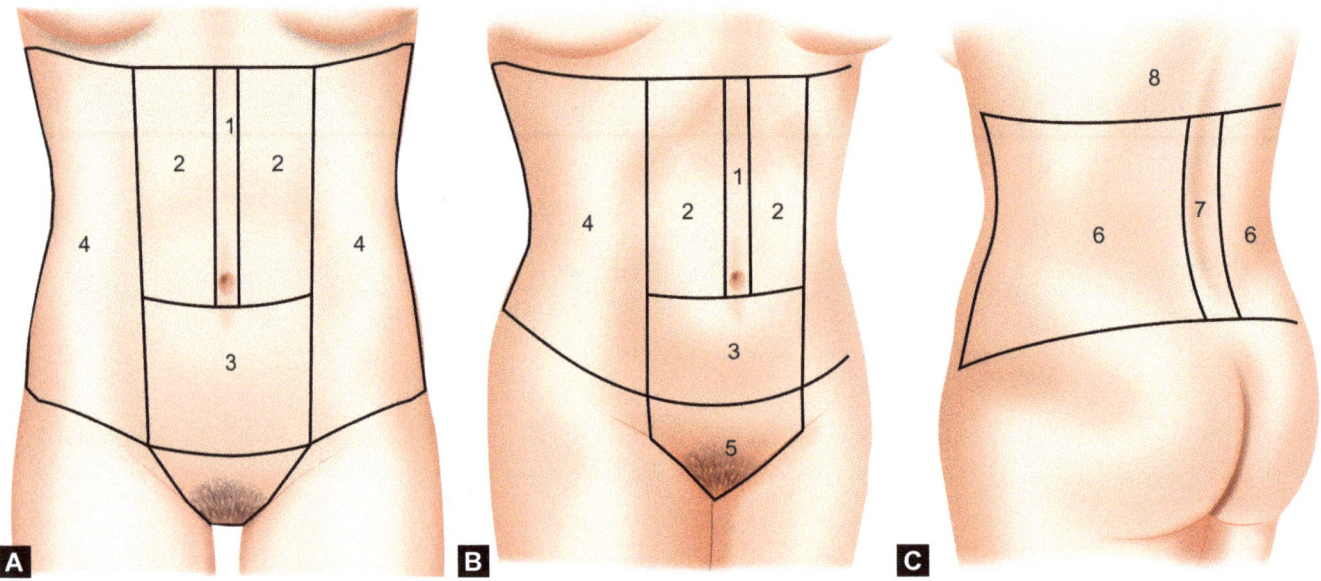

Figs. 3.14A to C: Aesthetic units of abdomen.

2. *Two upper rectus aesthetic units*: There are two upper rectus units overlying the rectus muscles extending from the lower costal margin to the level of umbilicus.

3. *Lower recti aesthetic unit*: Single lower rectus unit overlies both the recti muscles below the umbilicus and extends down to the upper pubic hair line.

4. *Two lateral abdominal aesthetic units*: These units on either side of the rectus units extend from the lower four costal areas superiorly, extend inferiorly over the oblique muscles to the iliac crest and inguinal regions.

5. *Pubic area*: Pubic area unit overlies the pubic region.

6. *Two lumbar aesthetic units*: These units lie overlying the lumbar muscles extending superiorly from the posterior costal region and inferiorly to the gluteal region.

7. *Posterior midline aesthetic unit*: Posterior midline unit is overlying the spinous processes of the lower thoracic and lumbar vertebras and sacral area.

8. *Bra roll area*: Bra roll area unit is above the lumbar aesthetic unit. It involves the upper back region and extends into the infra-axillary region.

These aesthetic subunits have varied anatomy that gives an aesthetic silhouette to a healthy body. Weight gain can alter these subunits in a varying proportion. Consideration of these aesthetic units and understanding the anatomy, skin behavior, and fat deposition pattern can help achieve a great aesthetic result after body contouring procedures with long-term outcome.

Judicious liposuction of these aesthetic units and understanding the perforators can help achieve a better aesthetic outcome in combined lipoabdominoplasty.

REFERENCES

1. American Society for Aesthetic Plastic Surgery, Inc. 1998 Statistics on Cosmetic Surgery. New York, NY: ASAPS; 1999.

2. Matarasso A. Abdominoplasty. In: Guyuron B, Achauer BM, Eriksson E, et al. (Eds). Plastic Surgery: Indications, Operations, Outcomes, vol. 4, 1st edition. Philadelphia, PA: Mosby-Yearbook; 2000.

3. Gonzalez-Ulloa M. Regional aesthetic units of the face. Plast Reconstr Surg. 1987;79:489.

4. Burget GC, Menick FJ. The subunit principle in nasal reconstruction. Plast Reconstr Surg. 1985;76:239.

5. Spear SL, Davison SP. Aesthetic subunits of the breast. Plast Reconstr Surg. 2003;112(2):440-7.

6. Mendieta CG. Gluteoplasty. Aesthet Surg J. 2003;23:441-55.

7. Agache PG, Monneur C, Leveque JL, et al. Mechanical properties and Young's modulus of human skin in vivo. Arch Dermatol Res. 1980;269:221-32.

8. Cua AB, Wilhelm KP, Maibach HI. Elastic properties of human skin. Relation to age, sex, and anatomical region. Arch Dermatol Res. 1990;282:283-8.

9. Dabb RW, Hall WW, Baroody M, et al. Circumferential suction lipectomy of the trunk with anterior rectus fascia plication through a periumbilical incision: an alternative to conventional abdominoplasty. Plast Reconstr Surg. 2004; 113(2):733-4.

CHAPTER 4

Abdominal Fat Pathophysiology

"There is a most intimate interdependence of physiology, pathology and surgery. Without progress in physiology and pathology, surgery could advance but little, and surgery has paid its debt by contributing much to the knowledge of the pathologist and physiologist, never more than at the present". —*William Stewart Halsted (1852–1922).*

■ INTRODUCTION

This chapter is important to understand the fat deposition pattern, predict long-term outcome of body contouring procedure, and to educate patient to understand the concept of fat distribution. Please do not miss this chapter!

Generally speaking, abdominal fat is either visceral (surrounding the abdominal organs) or subcutaneous (lying between the skin and the abdominal wall). Fat located behind the abdominal cavity, called retroperitoneal fat, is generally considered as visceral fat. Several studies indicate that visceral fat is most strongly correlated with risk factors such as insulin resistance, which sets the stage for type 2 diabetes. Some research suggests that the deeper layers of subcutaneous fat may also be involved in insulin resistance (in men but not in women). From clinical and basic investigations, aging, sex hormones, excess intake of sucrose, and lack of physical exercise have been suggested to be determinants for visceral fat accumulation. Since intra-abdominal fat (mesenteric and omentum fat) has been shown to have high activities of both lipogenesis and lipolysis, its accumulation can induce high levels of free fatty acids, a product of lipolysis, in portal circulation that go into the liver.[1]

■ LOCATION OF ABDOMINAL FAT

Visceral Fat (Fig. 4.1)

Fat accumulated in the lower body or upper body is subcutaneous, while fat in the abdominal area can be intra-abdominal (visceral) and subcutaneous in varying proportions.

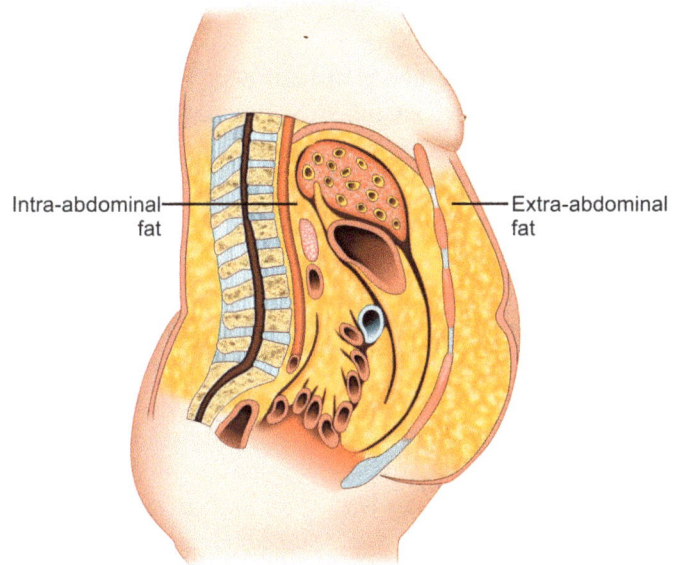

Intra-abdominal fat

Extra-abdominal fat

Fig. 4.1: Distribution of fat: Intra-abdominal or visceral fat and extra-abdominal or subcutaneous fat.

This distribution of abdominal fat is influenced by several factors. Heredity is one: scientists have identified a number of genes that help determine how many fat cells an individual develops and where these cells are stored.[2] There is evidence of genetically programmed developmental differences in adipocytes and their precursors in different regions of the body. This plays an important role in obesity, body fat distribution, and potential differences between internal and subcutaneous adipose tissue.

Recent advances have demonstrated that white adipose tissue plays a central role in the regulation of energy balance and acts as a secretory organ that mediates numerous physiological and pathological processes such as immunological responses, vascular diseases, and appetite regulation. Leptin, the obese gene product, is a hormone that is primarily secreted by mature adipocytes. Leptin plays a crucial role in the regulation of energy balance. Resistin is another adipocyte-secreted product that potentially links obesity to diabetes.[3]

During recent years, it has become evident that adipocytes express and secrete a number of hormones involved in the regulation of energy and substrate metabolism including leptin, adiponectin, resistin, and acylation stimulating protein. Acylation stimulating protein is a hormone produced by adipocytes and is of importance for the storage of energy as fat.[4]

Although there have been considerable recent insights into the control of appetite and energy expenditure as contributing factors to obesity, little is known about the genetic basis for determination of adipocyte number and differences in body fat distribution.

Studies have revealed that both body mass index and waist–hip ratio are inheritable traits, and have some variability. In addition, individual humans observe differences in their own body fat distribution as they gain or lose weight such as in some ethnic groups (Africans) who have been noted for excessive accumulation of fat in the buttocks, a condition known as steatopygia. Some lipodystrophies appear to have segmental or dermatomal distribution.[3]

The rate of lipolysis in adipose tissue taken from subcutaneous sites is lower than that of adipose tissue from visceral sites. Furthermore, the lipolytic effect of catecholamines is weaker and antilipolytic effect of insulin is more pronounced in subcutaneous than in visceral adipose.[5,6] This is evident by the fact that intra-abdominal fat can be reduced by exercise and diet management more easily as compared to subcutaneous fat. Visceral fat is more easily stored and faster to be burned. This is because it has a greater blood supply and is more sensitive to the fat metabolizing hormones (catecholamines) compared to subcutaneous fat.

Brown adipose tissue, previously known to be found only in small mammals and neonates, has only recently been shown to contribute significantly to the metabolic signature in adults. The detection of brown adipose tissue in adults has led to a renewed interest and is now considered to be a potential therapeutic target to prevent excess white fat accumulation in obesity.[7]

Role of Hormones in Fat Distribution and Correlation with Dieting and Exercise

Insulin plays a major role in fat metabolism, and the single biggest influence over the levels of insulin is from starchy and sweet foods. Cortisol (stress hormone) is another important hormone that influences fat storage.[8] Cortisol influences both lipoprotein lipase and hormone-sensitive lipase (HSL). Lipoprotein lipase is responsible for storage of fat and HSL is activated when the body needs to mobilize energy stores, and so responds positively to catecholamines, an adrenocorticotropic hormone. Insulin activity inhibits fat-releasing activity of cortisol.[9,10]

Starch and sugar combined with fat may represent the worst combination for fat gain. Starches and sugar raise insulin levels while fat supplies calories by itself.

Protein and vegetables does not stimulate insulin production. This means less calorie deposition. Adequate sleep aids in fat metabolism by lowering cortisol and increasing human growth hormone (HGH)—a fat-burning and muscle-building hormone. Intense exercise is known to stimulate cortisol and HGH (and testosterone in men).

What Happens in Women?

Sex hormones strongly influence body fat distribution and adipocyte differentiation. Estrogens and testosterone differentially affect adipocyte physiology. Estrogens and estrogen receptors regulate various aspects of glucose and lipid metabolism. Disturbances of this metabolic signal lead to the development of metabolic syndrome and a higher cardiovascular risk in women. Estrogen hormone is insulin sensitizing and helps in metabolizing the fat causing fat loss.

At menopause, estrogen production decreases and the ratio of androgen (male hormones present in small amounts in women) to estrogen increases and that has been linked to increased abdominal fat after menopause. Some researchers suspect that the drop in estrogen levels at menopause is also linked to increased levels of cortisol, a stress hormone that promotes the accumulation of abdominal fat.

What is Wrong with Abdominal Fat?

Adipose tissue is no more just energy-saving structure but research suggests that fat cells—particularly, abdominal fat cells—are biologically active. It is more accurate to think of fat as an endocrine organ or gland, producing hormones and other substances that can profoundly affect our health. As we have seen, leptin is normally released after a meal and dampens appetite. Fat cells also produce the hormone adiponectin, which is thought to influence the response of cells to insulin.

Visceral fat secretes immunogenic chemicals called cytokines—e.g. tumor necrosis factor and interleukin-6—that can increase the risk of cardiovascular disease by promoting insulin resistance and low-level chronic inflammation. Considered to be excess visceral fat is so harmful

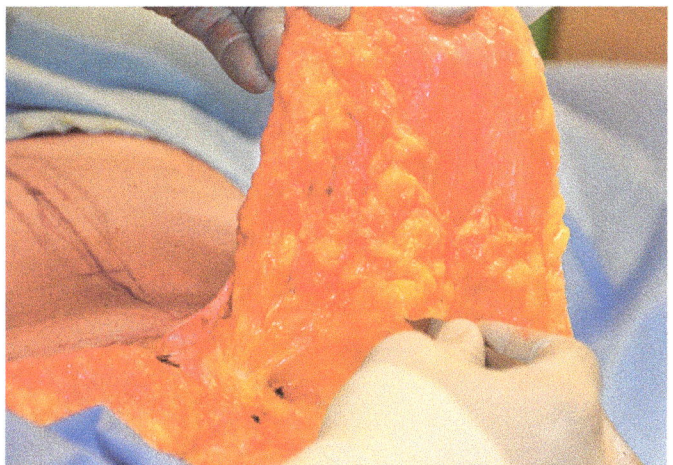

Fig. 4.2: Subcutaneous fat.

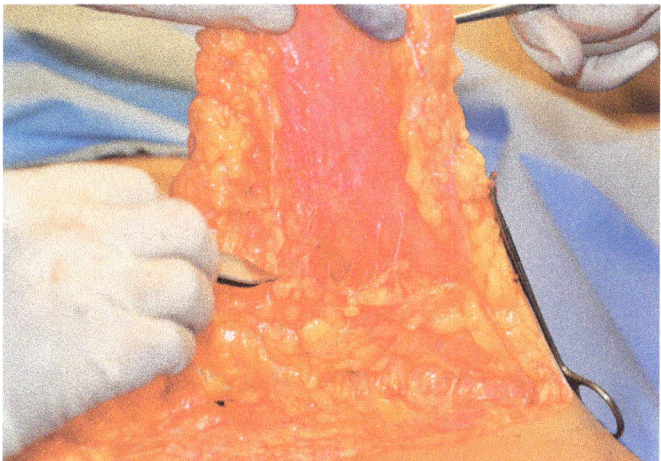

Fig. 4.3: Fat layers below and above Scarpa's fascia.

possibly due to its location near the portal vein, which carries blood from the intestinal area to the liver. Substances released by visceral fat, including free fatty acids, enter the portal vein and travel to the liver, where they can influence the production of blood lipids. Visceral fat is directly linked with higher total cholesterol and low-density lipoprotein (bad) cholesterol, lower high-density lipoprotein (good) cholesterol, and insulin resistance—major risk factors for heart disease and stroke.[11,12] An excess of visceral fat is known as central obesity, or "belly fat," in which the abdomen protrudes excessively. Excess visceral fat is also linked to type 2 diabetes, insulin resistance, inflammatory diseases, and other obesity-related diseases.[13]

The good news is that visceral fat yields fairly easily to exercise and diet, with benefits ranging from lower blood pressure to more favorable cholesterol levels. Subcutaneous fat located at the waist can be frustratingly difficult to reduce. High-intensity exercise is one way to effectively reduce total abdominal fat.[14,15]

Bariatric surgery has been proved not only to reduce the weight of the body but also to correct the metabolic problems associated with obesity.[16]

There are a few studies by Berntorp et al.,[17] Giese et al.,[18] and Gonzalez-Oritz et al.[19] that show liposuction can help in facilitating glucose utilization, increasing insulin sensitivity, thus reducing blood pressure and other metabolic derangement, at least in short-term.

Subcutaneous Fat (Nonvisceral Fat) (Fig. 4.2)

The subcutaneous tissue is also called as hypodermis. The hypodermis consists primarily of loose connective tissue and lobules of fat. It contains larger blood vessels and nerves than those found in the dermis.

The fat globules are grouped together and held firmly by stromal fibrous network. They are arranged in layers forming superficial fat and deep fat. In the lower abdomen, the two layers are separated by Scarpa's fascia (Fig. 4.3), whereas in the upper abdomen there is no distinct fascial layer. In the upper abdomen, the fat is firmly arranged with compact fibrous network with more dense vascular and neural network.

In the upper abdomen, it is more painful to infiltrate fluid if liposuction is performed under local anesthesia. The areas of underlying adhesions have compact tough fibrofatty tissue.

On the other hand, in the lower abdomen the fat layers are less compact and less neurotized. The fat above the Scarpa's fascia is more compact and vascular than below.

Enlargement of these fat cells causes various abdominal protuberances, cellulites, folds, rolls, and panniculus.

Abdominal Roles/Panniculus

There is not much literature about the description of panniculus except that it is layer of fatty tissue occurring in lower abdomen and can hang at various levels from pubic area to knees.

Classical description for panniculus is apron of skin and fat formed at the lower abdomen. Small panniculus is fold of skin that covers the upper part of the pubis. Moderate panniculus extends beyond the pubic area and covers the external genitalia where as large panniculus extends into the thigh region.

It is not uncommon to see upper abdomen folds particularly in patients who have undergone massive weight loss.

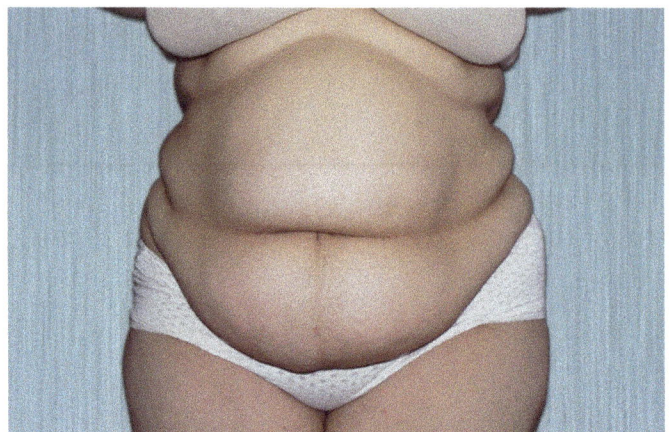

Fig. 4.4: Obese patient with lower abdominal panniculus, side rolls, bra rolls and upper abdominal protuberance.

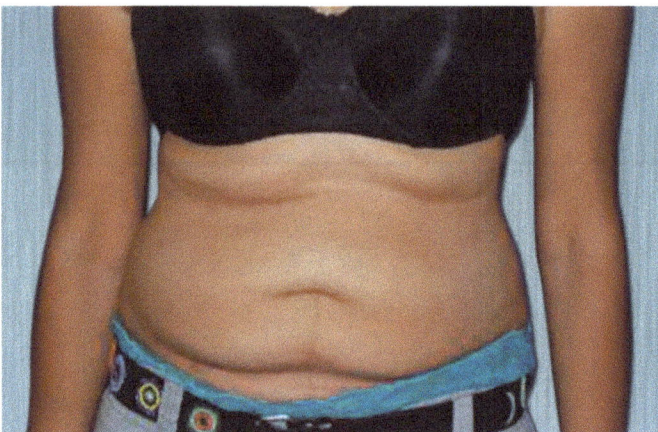

Fig. 4.5: Abdominal rolls formed by flexion creases and underlying tough fibrofatty attachments inferior to the rolls.

Abdominal rolls are formed by disproportionate fat deposits that are surrounded by compact fibrous network causing either circular or oblong bulges, such as upper abdomen protuberances, bra rolls and waist rolls (Fig. 4.4). Abdominal rolls/panniculus are formed by excess adipose tissue deposition and expansion of skin. However, there are deep adhesions that form a firm constriction ring at the lower part of the fold. If the fat continues to deposit the skin fold hangs over the constriction ring. In some patients, their are tight fibrous rings superiorly and inferiorly to the fold. The tight fibrofatty tissue ring needs to be addressed in abdominal contouring procedures (Fig. 4.5). Skin-retaining ligaments, major, and minor anchors the skin to the hypodermis and some fibers run deep to musculoaponeurotic fascia (as described earlier). Disrupting these retaining ligament will help to mobilize the overlying skin and unroll the folds.

▌REFERENCES

1. Matsuzawa Y, Shimomura I, Nakamura T, et al. Pathophysiology and pathogenesis of visceral fat obesity. Obes Res. 1995;3:187S-94S.
2. Gesta S, Blüher M, Yamamoto Y, et al. Evidence for a role of developmental genes in the origin of obesity and body fat distribution. Proc Natl Acad Sci USA. 2006;103(17):6676-81.
3. Gregoire FM. Adipocyte differentiation: from fibroblast to endocrine cell. Exp Biol Med. (Maywood). 2001;226:997-1002.
4. Ahrén B1, Havel PJ, Pacini G, et al. Acylation stimulating protein stimulates insulin secretion. Int J Obes Relat Metab Disord. 2003;27(9):1037-43.
5. Mauriege P, Galitzky J, Berlan M, et al. Heterogeneous distribution of beta and alpha-2 adrenoceptor binding sites in human fat cells from various fat deposits: functional consequences. Eur J Clin Invest. 1987;17:156-65.
6. Bolinder J, Kager L, Ostman J, et al. Differences at the receptor and postreceptor levels between human omental and subcutaneous adipose tissue in the action of insulin on lipolysis. Diabetes. 1983;32(2):117-23.
7. Enerbäck S. The origins of brown adipose tissue. N Engl J Med. 2009;360(19):2021-3.
8. Law J, Bloor I, Budge H, et al. The influence of sex steroids on adipose tissue growth and function. Horm Mol Biol Clin Investig. 2014;19(1):13-24.
9. Kersten S. Physiological regulation of lipoprotein lipase. Biochim Biophys Acta. 2014;1841(7):919-33.
10. Kraemer FB, Shen WJ. Hormone-sensitive lipase: control of intracellular tri-(di-) acylglycerol and cholesteryl ester hydrolysis. J Lipid Res. 2002;43(10):1585-94.
11. Lew EA, Garfinkel L. Variations in mortality by weight among 750,000 men and women. J Chronic Dis. 1979;32:563-76.
12. Reaven GM. Banting lecture: role of insulin resistance in human disease. Diabetes. 1988;37:1595-1607.
13. Mokdad AH, Ford ES, Bowman BA, et al. Prevalence of obesity, diabetes, and obesity-related health risk factors, 2001. JAMA. 2003;289(1):76-9.
14. Coker WR, Kortebein P, Sullivan D, et al. Influence of exercise intensity on abdominal fat and adiponectin in elderly adults. Metab Syndr Relat Disord. 2009;7(4):363-8.
15. Ohkawara K, Tanaka S, Miyachi M, et al. A dose-response relation between aerobic exercise and visceral fat reduction: systematic review of clinical trials. Int J Obes (Lond). 2007;31(12):1786-97.
16. Rubino F, Gagner M. Potential of surgery for curing type 2 diabetes mellitus. Ann Surg. 2002;236(5):554-9.
17. Berntorp E, Berntorp K, Brorson H, et al. Liposuction in Dercum's disease: impact on haemostatic factors associated with cardiovascular disease and insulin sensitivity. J Intern Med. 1998;243(3):197-201.
18. Giese SY, Bulan EJ, Commons GW, et al. Improvements in cardiovascular risk profile with large-volume liposuction: a pilot study. Plast Reconstr Surg. 2001;108(2):510-9.
19. Gonzalez-Oritz M, Robles-Cervant tes JA, Cardenas Camarena L, et al. The effects of surgically removing subcutaneous fat on the metabolic profile and insulin sensitivity in obese women after large-volume liposuction treatment. Horm Metab Res. 2002;34(8):446-9.

CHAPTER 5

Clinical Conditions

▌ INTRODUCTION

In aesthetic practice, one may come across a wide range of patients requesting abdominal contouring. As aesthetic plastic surgeon, we see a large number of patients with protruding abdomen due to obesity, postpregnancy deformities, abdominal wall hernias, etc. At the same time, we also see really petite women, fit men with minor bulges, and localized lipoadiposities requesting abdominal contouring. It is ironic, but we have to be prepared to deal with all situations. To increase your body contouring work, be prepared to deal with the whole gamut of abdominal contouring requests.

Once your expertise in body contouring increases, you will come across people of all weight groups coming to your office.

▌ HOW TO EVALUATE THE PATIENT FOR ABDOMINAL CONTOURING?

Patient Request

When a patient approaches an expert for a consultation, ask him/her about his or her concerns. Let the patient elaborate their concerns, expectations, likes and dislikes about such a procedure. In many situations, the patient is able to spell out exactly what procedure they want; this is relatively easy to deal with as they would have done their own research to understand the procedure and the related risks and benefits. It is challenging when the patient is not sure about liposuction, abdominoplasty, or bariatric surgery.

Medical History

This is the most important part of the consultation. The questionnaire includes the following details:

1. *Past history* of any procedures such as injection lipolysis, cavitation, and liposuction. It is very common to find patients who have visited weight-loss centers and would have undergone some or the other procedures. Patients forget to mention such things as they consider it trivial. Nonsurgical and minimal invasive procedures, including injection lipolysis and cryotherapy can cause scarring and fibrous tissue formation, which is a major hindrance during liposuction affecting the outcome. Similarly, a secondary liposuction is also a very challenging procedure.

2. *Weight fluctuation*: Irregular dietary habit and pregnancy causes significant skin laxity. A leading history of maximum and minimum weight of the patient will give an indication about the skin tone and elasticity. Weight fluctuation causes skin laxity and also helps us to understand the skin elasticity of the patient. Weight fluctuation also gives us an idea about the patient's lifestyle.

3. *Comorbid conditions*: Patients with comorbid condition such as tobacco use, hypertension, diabetes mellitus, coronary artery disease, and pulmonary diseases. should be screened carefully. Patients with multiple diseases are often on blood thinners and they forget to mention that in the list of medications.

4. *Deep vein thrombosis (DVT) and thromboembolic phenomenon* should be specifically inquired as these patients require chemoprophylaxis and sequential compressive devices during the surgery.

5. Even in the absence of history of DVT do enquire about the risk factors for DVT such as chronic venous insufficiency, thrombotic syndromes in family, obesity, trauma, polycythemia, CNS disease, malignancy, pelvic irradiation, birth control pills, and hormone replacement therapy (HRT).

6. *Medications and supplements (list)*: Ask the detail history of medications, allergies to medications and supplements. Several medications and supplements can cause blood thinning increasing the risks of bleeding and hematoma. You may need an expert opinion to check if these medications can be discontinued before and after the surgery without affecting their primary pathology.

COUNSELING

This is the process of discussion where the doctor is carefully evaluating the medical history, understanding the expectations of the patient, assessing the psychosocial reasons for the procedure, and explaining the details about the risks and benefits of the said procedure.

The patient is also explained about the steps required prior to the surgery that include medical tests, documentation, and photographs. It is important to describe the procedure in details and the necessary after care. It is beneficial to realistically describe the expected outcome, limitations, and possible complications of the procedure.

This stage elaborates on the lifestyle changes that should be considered for a better long-term outcome. The patient should also be aware of possible corrections or additional nonsurgical and surgical procedures that may be required to improve the result such as lymphatic massage, radio-frequency skin tightening, and touch-up procedures.

Detail discussion on the financial commitment will minimize disgruntled patients in future. The cost of the procedure, medications prescribed, pressure garments, and any potential additional consumables should be described, so they do not have unexpected expenses. Unexpected expenses are one of the causes of dissatisfaction and medicolegal conflicts.

PHYSICAL EXAMINATION

Detailed physical examination is mandatory to ensure nothing is missed. A systematic way of examination and documentation will not only help to analyze the anatomy, fat distribution, and skin elasticity but will ensure that any abnormalities are not missed.

Measurements are important to document the extent of fat bulges and will help postoperatively to assess the outcome objectively. During the examination ensure that the patient is standing straight so that his/her body posture and symmetry can be assessed.

A systematic examination is than carried out assessing the aesthetic subunits of the abdomen and back. Look for fat bulges, folds, panniculus, and flexion creases that are commonly seen in upper abdomen, at the umbilicus, or in lower abdomen. Sometimes they are asymmetrical depending upon the posture, they commonly acquire while at rest and work, or simply due to asymmetrical fat deposition.

Bra rolls or back rolls are due to fat accumulation and excess skin. Patient is realistically explained on the expected skin tightening after the procedure.

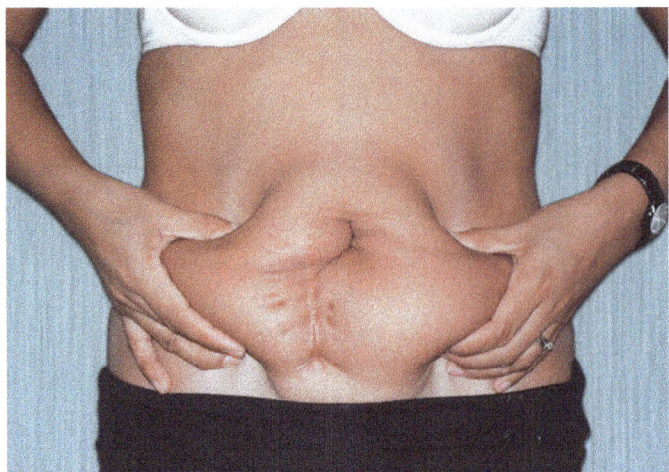

Fig. 5.1: Horizontal pinch test.

Skin examination may also reveal surgical scars, pigmentation changes to the skin, stretch marks, wrinkles, etc. Ensure that the patient is aware of all these changes and document it for future reference.

Pinch the skin and assess the amount of fat deposit; at the same time also note the elasticity of the skin and its turgor (Fig. 5.1). It is possible to distinguish turgid fat bulge from excess skin by feeling the texture of the tissue. The patient are explained about the findings.

This is followed by the examination of the underlying musculofascial structure. Ask the patient to pull the abdomen in by contracting the muscles. Patient will be unable to pull the abdomen in if there is a large volume of intra-abdominal fat. Another method to identify volume of intra-abdominal fat is to ask the patient to lie down. People with less Intra-abdominal fat will appear flat.

Abdominal muscle tone is demonstrated by voluntary contraction. Poor muscle tone of the abdominal wall will bulge out on relaxation and is retracted on contraction. On the other hand in athletic and physically fit individuals there is not much change in muscle position.

MEASUREMENTS

Body Mass Index

Body mass index (BMI) is a fairly reliable indicator of body fat for most people. It does not measure body fat directly, but research has shown that it correlates to the direct measure of body fat, such as underwater weighing and dual energy X-ray absorptiometry.[1,2]

Body mass index is easy to use in our practice and helps us to classify patients and form relevant protocols to manage them.

Formula: Weight (kg)/Height (m²)

With the metric system, the formula for BMI is weight in kilograms divided by height in meter squared. Since the height is commonly measured in centimeters, divide the height in centimeters by 100 to obtain the height in meters.

Formula: Weight (lb)/Height (in²) × 703

Calculate BMI by dividing weight in pounds (lb) by height in inches (in) squared and multiplying by a conversion factor of 703.

For adults of 20 years old and older, BMI is interpreted using standard weight status categories that are the same for all ages and for both men and women (Table 5.1).

The correlation between the BMI number and body fat is fairly strong; however, the correlation varies with sex, race, and age. These variations include the following examples:[3,4]

- At the same BMI, women tend to have more body fat than men
- At the same BMI, older people, on average, tend to have more body fat than younger adults
- Highly trained athletes may have a high BMI because of increased muscularity rather than increased body fatness.

Circumferences

The evaluation of waist circumference is supported by research and literature to assess the risk factors in normal and overweight people. Abdominal, measurement of circumference is important to evaluate the outcome after body contouring surgery.

The following measurements will help planning for body abdominal contouring with either liposuction or combined abdominoplasty surgery. This is also useful measurement to plan postoperative garments for the patient.

1. At inframammary level
2. The narrowest waist
3. At the level of umbilicus
4. At level of pubis
5. Widest hips

Pinch Measurement

Horizontal pinch measurement using a caliper in all aesthetic units except anterior and posterior midlines will

Table 5.1: Interpretation of body mass index with weight status

BMI	Weight status
Below 18.5	Underweight
18.5–24.9	Normal
25.0–29.9	Overweight
30.0 and above	Obese

allow us to evaluate the symmetry and amount of fat. This can be compared postoperatively to evaluate the outcome.

Measurement of Skin Excess

There is a scarcity of data in the literature about objectively assessing the skin excess. Abdominal skin in young people is more elastic and reshapes better after weight loss as compared to older people. The predictability factor is reduced in patients with history of excessive weight loss, pregnancy, and obesity. By and large history of excessive weight loss (>30% of body weight) and multiple pregnancies indicate poor skin tone. Signs of stretched skin such as extensive striae and thinning of the skin are also indicators of poor skin elasticity. I think we need to have more data and studies on skin measurement for accurate assessment of excess skin.

A measurement of excess skin is performed in all patients for abdominal contouring surgery according to standardized clinical practices at our center. Measurement of vertical and horizontal skin excess will allow us to understand the amount of skin excess and predict the outcome. The measurement is also important to make the patient aware of the skin excess and then to realistically explain the potential of skin contraction. Evidence of extensive stretch mark is a forewarning that the dermis is already breached and skin may not contract significantly. Extensive superficial liposuction may be contraindicated in such patients.

Following measurements are recorded:
1. *Xiphoid process to umbilicus* with and without maximum stretching.
2. *Umbilicus to upper border of pubic hair line* with and without stretching.
   If there is a panniculus or skin fold, measure along the surface of the skin.
3. Measure a distance from *xiphoid to upper border of pubic hair line in standing position.*
4. *Pinch the skin vertically in the midline (Fig. 5.2)*: Mark the two sides with a marking pen near the tip of the finger. Leave the skin and measure the distance. This may not be possible in obese patient.

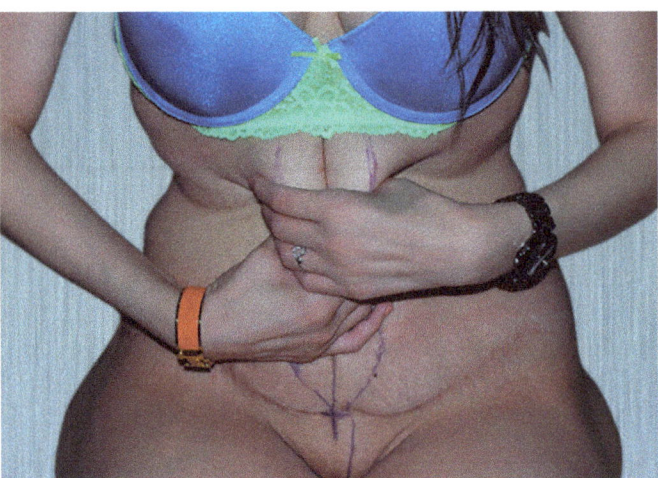

Fig. 5.2: Vertical pinch and marking of excess skin.

Physical Evaluation in Standing Position

Aesthetic Subunits

1. *Upper midline aesthetic units*:
   - Presence or absence of linea alba (midline groove of upper abdomen)
   - Abnormal bulges (hernia and diverification)
   - Umbilicus: shallow, deep, bulges.
2. *Upper rectus aesthetic units*:
   - Apparent asymmetry
   - Skin elasticity, adhesions, creases, and scars
   - Fat bulges/folds
   - Rectus muscle tone
   - Skeletal prominences.
3. *Lower recti aesthetic units*:
   - Apparent unevenness
   - Skin elasticity, adhesions, creases, and scars
   - Fat bulge, folds, panniculus
   - Rectus muscle tone
   - Pubic prominences.
4. *Lateral abdominal aesthetic units*:
   - Symmetry
   - Skin elasticity, adhesions, creases, and scars
   - Fat bulge
   - Muscle tone
   - Bony prominences.
5. *Lumbar aesthetic units*:
   - Symmetry
   - Skin elasticity, adhesions, creases, and scars
   - Fat bulges
   - Muscle bulge.

6. *Posterior midline aesthetic units*:
   - Midline groove and posterior dimples
   - Lumbar pad of fat
   - Skeletal shape: lordosis, kyphosis, etc.

Abdominal Tests

Large amount of intra-abdominal fat, cesarean surgery, multiple pregnancies can cause stretching of linea alba and diverification of rectus muscle. It can also cause stretching of musculofascial layer in the lateral abdominal wall. Thorough examination allows to understand and explain to the patient on expected outcome. Intra-abdominal volume expansion can cause ballooning of abdomen with stretching of muscle and skin.

Abdominal tests are performed to check the tone of the muscle, measure diverification of rectus muscles, and identify any hernias—

1. *Leg raising tests*: It allows to assess the tone of lower abdominal muscle and presence of any weakness or hernia.
2. *Head raising test*: Head raising test is useful to identify and measure diversification of the recti in the upper abdomen and umbilical region. Any abnormal bulges, such as epigastric or umbilical hernia can be detected.
3. *Cough impulse*: Cough impulse is a useful test, if the patient has abnormal bulges. A positive impulse is a sign of herniation.
4. *Abdominal retraction test (Figs. 5.3A and B)*: It is a simple test performed in standing position to assess the tone of abdominal muscles and intra-abdominal volume. Ask the patient to relax the abdomen completely. Note the amount of bulge. Then ask the patient to retract the abdomen as much as possible. If patient is unable to retract at all, it indicates a large intra-abdominal volume. Such patients are not good candidate for any body contouring surgery. If the patient is able to retract as seen in Figure 5.3B, it indicates lack of muscle tone. Such patients get a good result after surgery particularly, if they are encouraged to tone up the abdominal muscles.

Intra-abdominal Volume

Quantification of intra-abdominal volume is difficult clinically in day-to-day practice.

Intra-abdominal volume assessment will help predict the postoperative outcome.

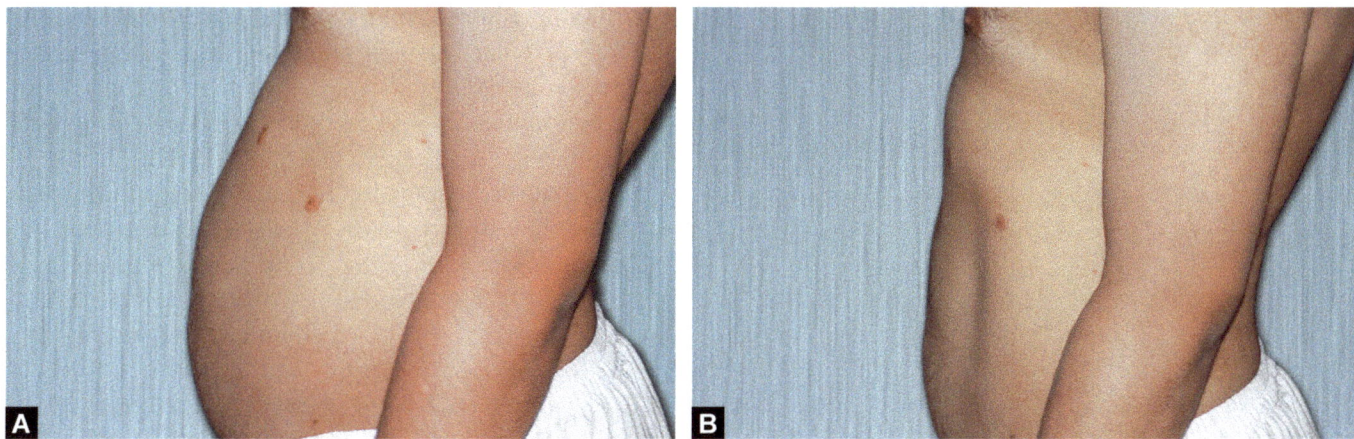

Figs. 5.3A and B: (A) Abdominal bulge with muscle relaxed. (B) Abdominal retraction indicating muscle tone problem of the abdominal wall without significant intra-abdominal volume.

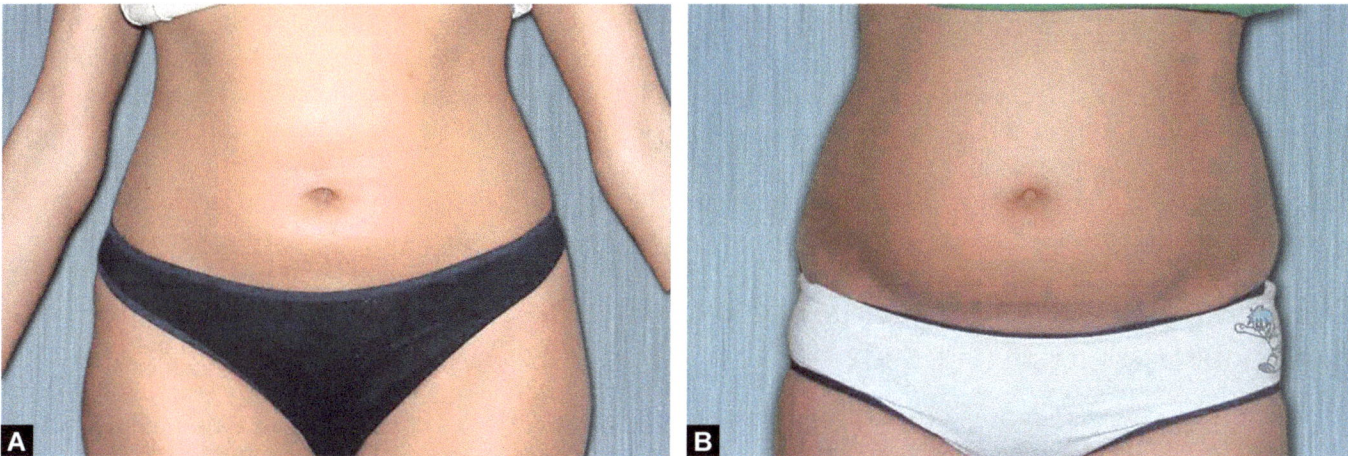

Figs. 5.4A and B: Indications for liposuction (A) A 24-year-old patient with BMI 23 and physically active, and note the deposition of fat limited to the central zone of the abdomen. (B) A 28-year-old patient with BMI 28 and irregular exercise habit. Note the deposition of fat in all the aesthetic subunits of abdomen, centrally and peripherally.

Brauman[5] described a technique to identify intra-abdominal fat and categorized into three types: small, medium, and large.

The patient is asked to protrude his/her abdomen to a maximum:

1. *Supraumbilical (epigastric) protrusions* generally indicate large volume.
2. *Infraumbilical protrusions* (*hypogastric region*) generally denote small volume.
3. *Umbilical protrusions* denote medium volume.

▮ DECISION-MAKING LIPOSUCTION OR ABDOMINOPLASTY

There are three possibilities as given below:

Clear Indications for Liposuction of Abdomen (Figs. 5.4A and B)

1. Young patients, men or women, with excess fat in some or all aesthetic subunits of abdomen.
2. Patients with excess fat and good skin turgor.
3. Male patients with excess fat and folds.
4. Patients with excess fat and skin fold but reluctant to undergo abdominoplasty surgery due to scars or fear of general anesthesia.

There are patients who are clearly suited for abdominal contouring by liposuction alone. The most important determinants for considering liposuction are weight of the patient, skin quality, and amount of extra-abdominal/subcutaneous skin. Patients with average weight or mildly

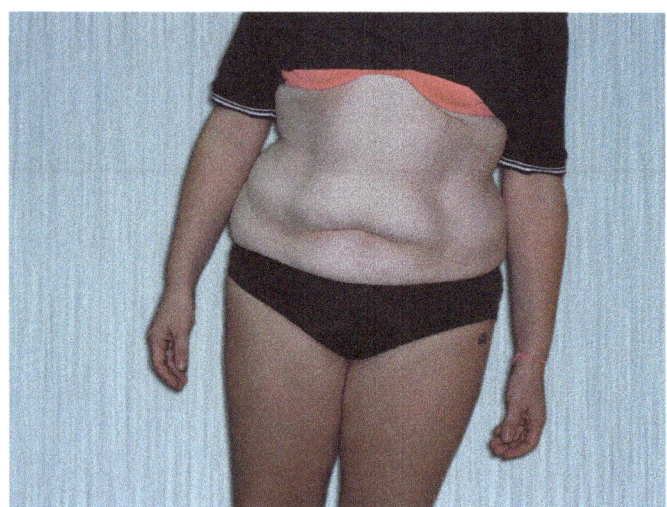

Fig. 5.5: Indications for abdominoplasty. A 36-year-old with BMI 32 and history of excess weight loss. Note excess fat deposits with excess skin in vertical and horizontal direction.

overweight with good skin elasticity and minimal intra-abdominal fat are ideal candidates for liposuction only. It is important to devote time and energy to assess the patient by listening to their desires and examining them as per a standard protocol.

Clear Indications for Abdominoplasty with or without Liposuction (Fig. 5.5)

1. Multiple pregnancy with excess fat, skin, and muscle bulge.
2. Postpregnancy abdominal bulge with extensive striae and muscle diverification.
3. Massive weight loss.
4. Large hanging panniculus.
5. Abdominal wall hernia or pseudohernia.

The above situations are straightforward indications of abdominal contouring with abdominoplasty. Lipoabdominoplasty is indicated when patient desires improvement in all the three elements, i.e removal of excess skin, correction of musculofascial bulge and reduction of extra-abdominal fat. Indications also mean the patient is willing to accept the scars, recovery time and risks involved in the surgery.

Sequential: Liposuction Followed by Second Stage Abdominoplasty if Necessary

1. Younger patients with excess fat and excess skin with doubtful skin stretchability.
2. Patients with large abdomen but reluctant to have scars.

3. Patients with subcutaneous fat, stretch marks, mild muscle bulge/diversification, and minimal to moderate excess skin.
4. Large abdomen with panniculus where the patient wants only fat reduction and flab reduction.
5. Extensive subcutaneous fat in all zones of abdomen along with skin excess and muscle diversification.

On many occasions we come across patients with good quality, but excess skin and a significant amount of subcutaneous fat. In such situations we may not be able to predict the exact outcome and behavior of the skin after liposuction. It is necessary to warn the patient of any residual excess skin or need for abdominoplasty, if the outcome of liposuction is not adequate for the patient. In my experience, patients are happy with liposuction only and are thankful that we did not proceed with abdominoplasty and avoided long scars. However, patient with large amount of fat and excess skin mainly in lower abdomen, I propose a two-stage operation. The first stage is extensive circumferential liposuction and the second stage is of short-scar abdominoplasty or dermolipectomy if after 6 months the skin does not retract enough. The abdomen has excellent retracting capacities as long as the dermis is intact.

In the past, I have done liposuction of the abdomen and flanks to extensively debulk the fat and second-stage abdominoplasty after 1 year (Figs. 5.6A to D).

Gray zone: This is a situation where we are not able to decide whether to do liposuction or abdominoplasty. This happens if the patient is not sure about his/her expectations. The patient may desire a firm, flat, and small tummy despite poor quality of skin and or muscle without undergoing abdominoplasty. Either you refuse surgery on these patients or explain what can be realistically achieved without the scar of abdominoplasty.

■ HOW TO MANAGE THE ABDOMEN IN DIFFERENT PATIENT CATEGORIES?

Type 1: Normal Weight, Firm Skin, Minimal Intra-abdominal Fat (Figs. 5.7A to F)

Type 1 patients are young patients with an average BMI up to 25 and they do not have significant history of weight fluctuation. They have a good shape with an average waist line.

Fat deposit is noticed in aesthetic unit 1 with obliteration of linea alba. There is a thick layer of fat on zones 2–4 over the rectus muscles. Zones 5 and 6 have moderate amount of fat deposits on the pinch test. Zone 6 has

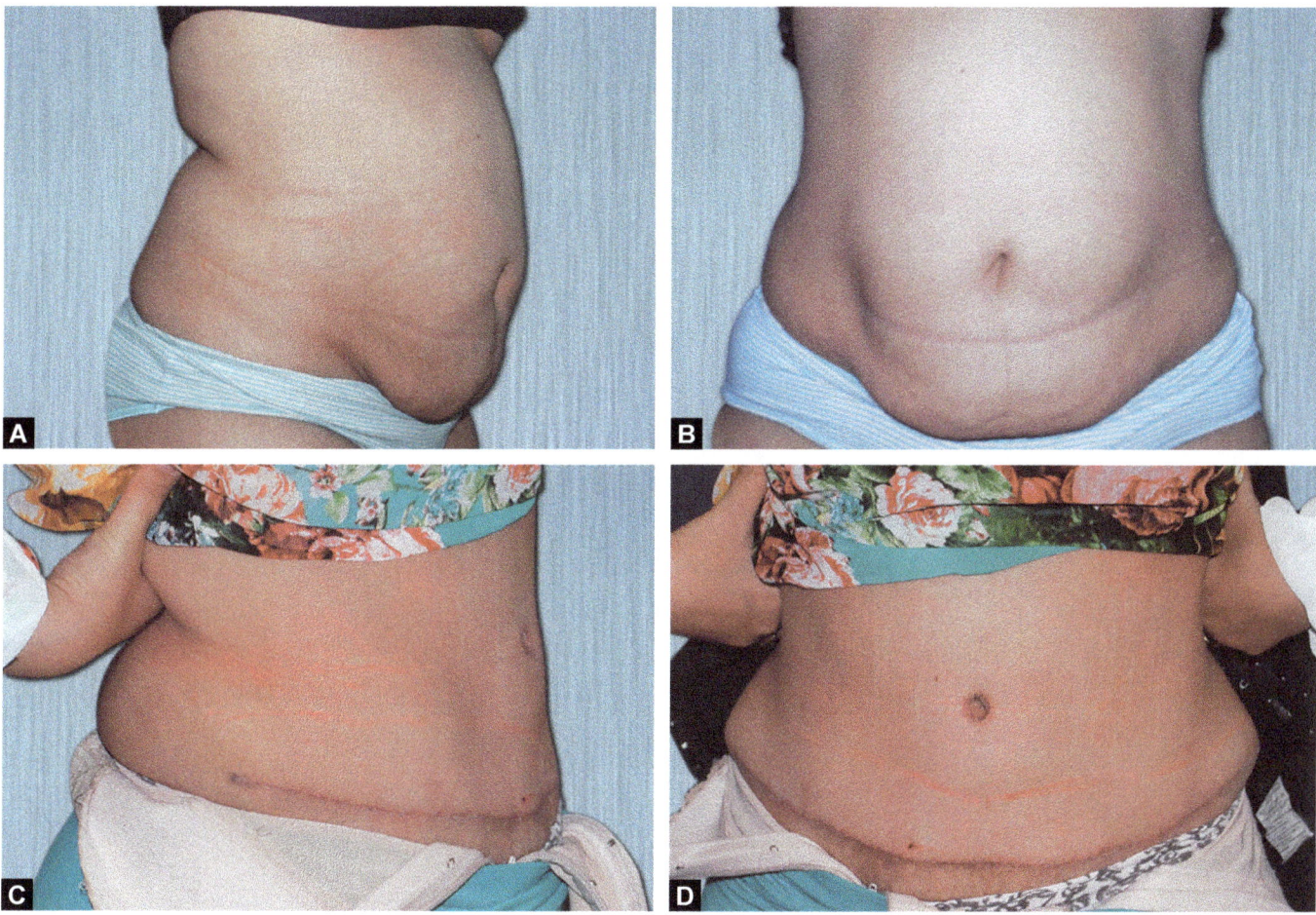

Figs. 5.6A to D: (A and B) Patient had liposuction 1 year ago and has lax skin and bulging abdomen (C and D) After abdominoplasty.

moderate fat deposits causing bulging of the flanks. The skin quality is good and there is a mild anterior abdominal muscle bulge.

Type 1 patient respond well to liposuction alone. So the plan for this patient is to perform a three-dimensional liposuction of all the aesthetic zones under local anesthesia and IV sedation or general anesthesia based on requirement. This is typically done by conventional liposuction technique using 3–4 mm Mercedes cannulas.

Type 2: Disproportionate Abdominal Bulge, Moderate Skin Excess, Moderate Intra-abdominal Fat (Figs. 5.8A to D)

Type 2 patients are young unmarried overweight patients with BMI up to 28. They have a history of weight fluctuation that causes some skin laxity.

There is excess fat in all the aesthetic zones with only mild waist line contour visible. The skin is mildly lax with no stretch marks; mild musculofascial bulge is there indicating mild intra-abdominal fat.

The plan is for three-dimensional liposuction using conventional technique.

Type 2 patient has some risk of skin irregularity and laxity, if liposuction is not properly executed. The key is to undermine the skin to disrupt the fibrous ligaments and perform liposuction all around the trunk. This will allow a uniform contraction and draping of the skin.

Type 3: Fat Bulge, Striae, Mildly Lax Skin, Mild Intra-abdominal Fat, Muscle Bulge (Figs. 5.9A to D)

Type 3 patients are married with history of pregnancy (single or multiple, cesarean, or normal delivery). They are moderately overweight. They have some fat in all the aesthetic zones. There is mild rectus bulge with mild diversification. The skin shows evidence of striae gravidarum, minimal sagging below the lower abdominal creases.

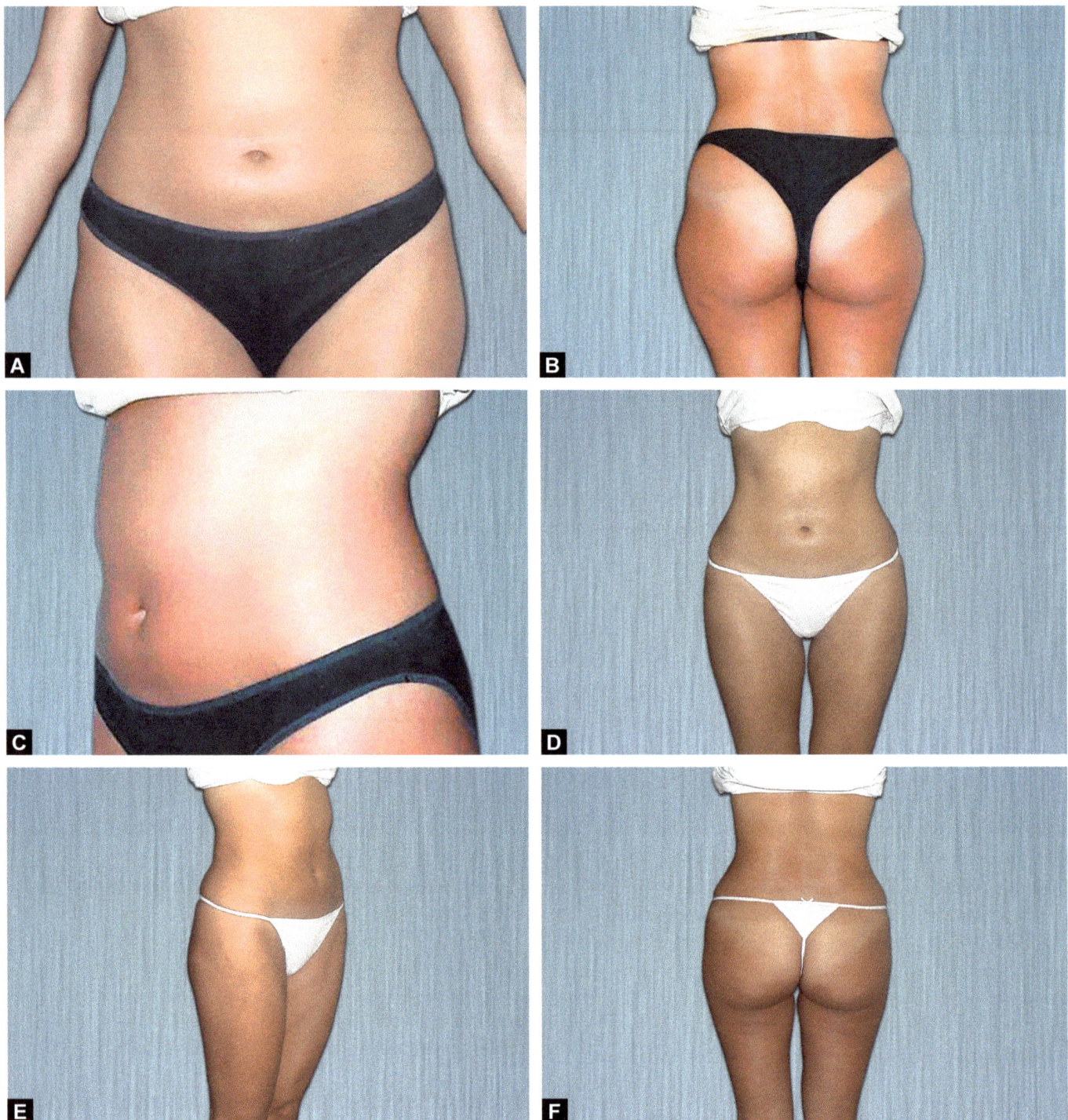

Figs. 5.7A to F: (A to C) Type 1 abdomen in a young patient with good skin elasticity. Fat deposition in zone 1 with obliteration of linea alba; zone 2 upper rectus unit causing bulge in upper abdomen and zone 3 lower recti aesthetic unit causing mild bulge. In posterior view note fat deposition in zone 6 lumbar aesthetic units. (D to F) Postoperative views after liposculptuirng of all the aesthetic subunits.

The patient appears to be a good candidate for lipoabdominoplasty. However, if the patient is reluctant to accept scars then a reasonable alternate is sequential procedure. Liposuction as a first stage and if the result is not as expected, she will be offered abdominoplasty procedure (conventional or short scar).

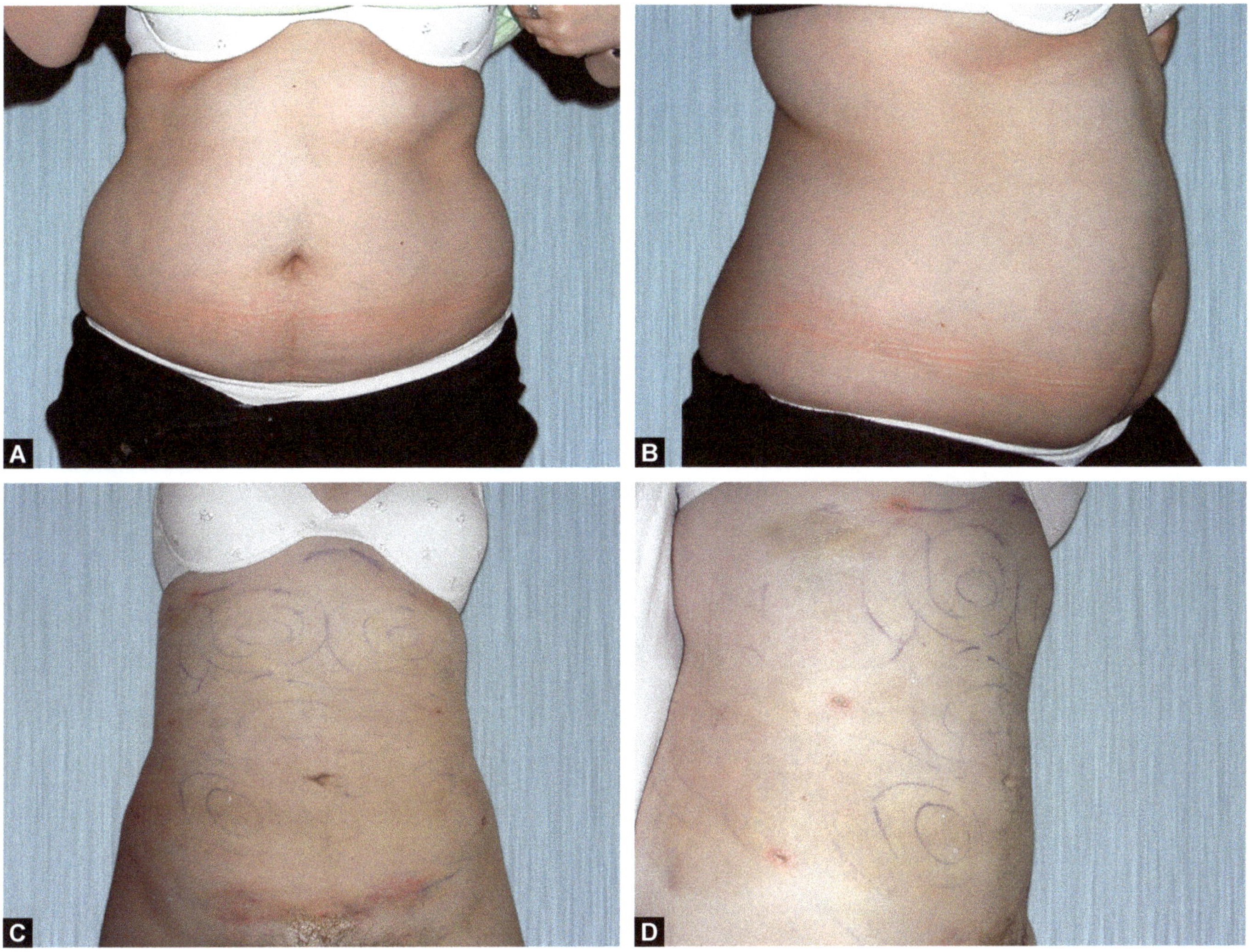

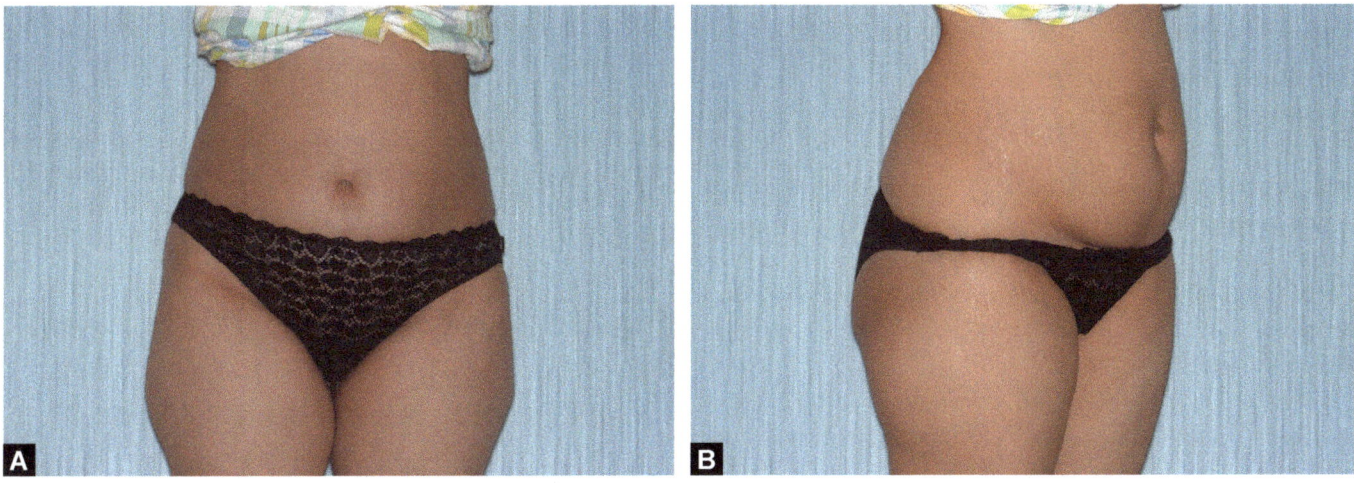

Figs. 5.8A to D: (A and B) Type 2 abdomen with excess extra-abdominal fat and moderate skin laxity. (C and D) First postoperative day after circumferential liposuction, note uniform skin contraction.

Figs. 5.9A and B

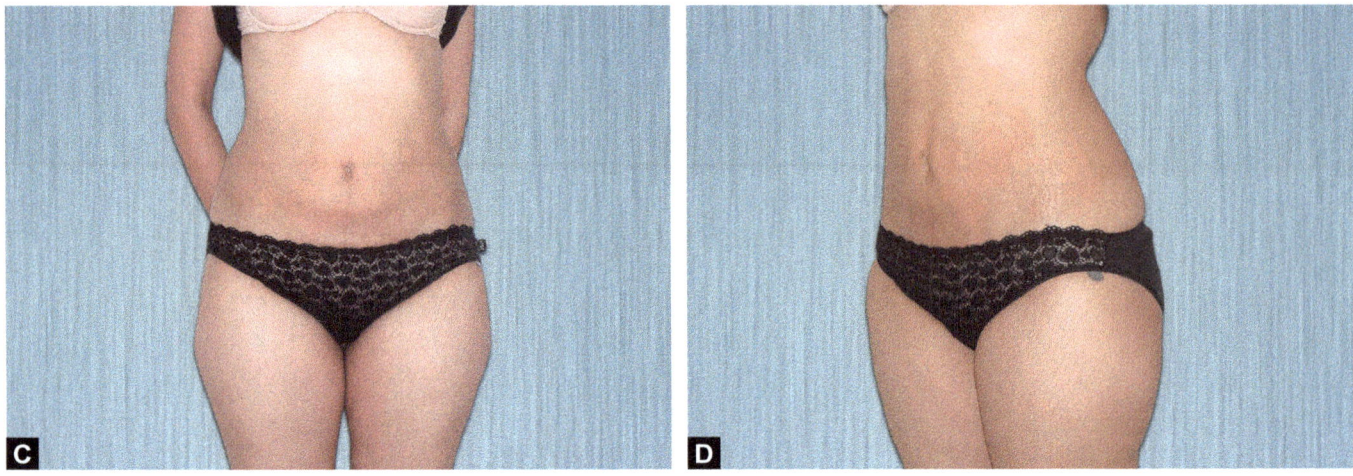

Figs. 5.9A to D: (A and B) Type 3 abdomen in patient with history of pregnancy, stretch marks, excess fat and moderate skin laxity. (C and D) 8 years after liposculpturing of abdomen and flanks.

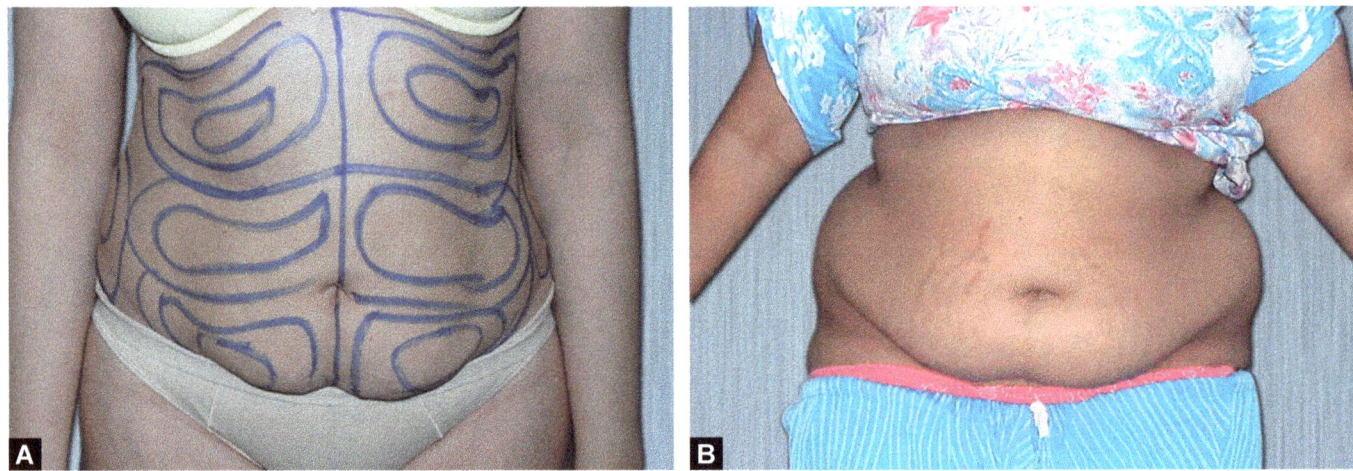

Figs. 5.10A and B: Type 4 abdomen with excess intra-abdominal fat, moderate muscle bulge and mild panniculus.

Type 4: Small to Moderate Panniculus, Muscle Bulge, Moderate Intra-abdominal Fat (Figs. 5.10A and B)

Type 4 patients are overweight to mildly obese with history of pregnancy. They have fat all over the abdomen and flanks. The lower abdomen is hanging below the crease. There is moderate intra-abdominal fat and mild muscle diversification. Overall skin quality is good and it has limited stretch marks.

The possible options are liposuction only, liposuction with lower dermolipectomy, and conventional lipoabdominoplasty. Liposuction will have the risk of lax skin in the upper abdomen above the umbilicus and/or lower

abdominal skin laxity. Liposuction with dermolipectomy will remove the infra-umbilical skin laxity (Fig. 5.11). Lipoabdominoplasty will address all the issues of subcutaneous fat, muscle diversification and bulge, removal of supra- and infraumbilical skin. The potential risks are long scars in the lower abdomen and periumbilical scars and other risks of wound healing, etc.

Type 5: Large Intra- and Extra-abdominal Fat or Large Panniculus with or without Large Diversification (Figs. 5.12A and B)

Type 5 patients are generally obese patients with or without a history of pregnancy. They often have comorbid

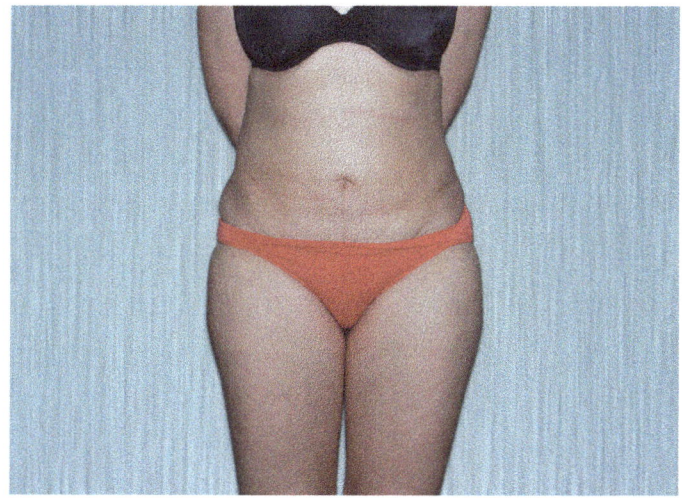

Fig. 5.11: Postoperative photograph after liposuction and miniabdominoplasty of the same patient as in Figure 5.10 A.

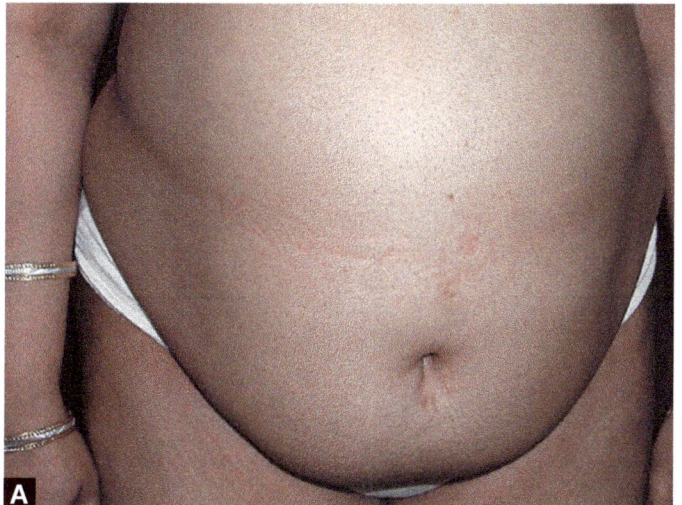

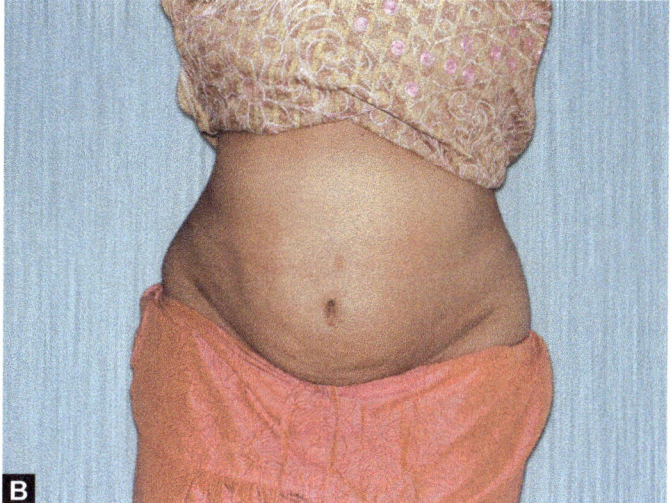

Figs. 5.12A and B: (A) Type 5 abdomen with large intra- and extra-abdominal fat excess, muscle bulging and skin excess. (B) 1 year postoperative view after liposuction of the abdomen, flanks and waistline.

conditions such as diabetes, hypertension, and hypercholesterolemia. On examination they have large subcutaneous volume of fat, intra-abdominal fat, muscle bulge, and absence of waist line.

Obviously, these patients require weight management first. Most often, these patients are under some or other weight management processes either with nutritionist, physician, or endocrinologist. They often complain of joint pain and back pain limiting them from doing exercise. A significant volume reduction is possible by liposuction. The patient needs to understand the purpose and risks of liposuction/liporeduction. Approximately 5–6 L of fat can be safely removed from the abdomen, waistline, and back. This will improve the physical condition of the patient and

motivate her to go on weight management to reduce the intra-abdominal fat. Remember, we discussed how the intra-abdominal fat can easily be mobilized by calorie restriction; primarily, it will not be enough to motivate the patient as the extra-abdominal fat which is more resistant will conceal any intra-abdominal volume loss. After liposuction, the patient will notice even a small amount of intra-abdominal fat loss.

Type 5: P-pathological Abdomen with Abdominal Wall Hernia (Fig. 5.13)

Type 5P is a subclassification of type 5, "P" indicating pathological condition.

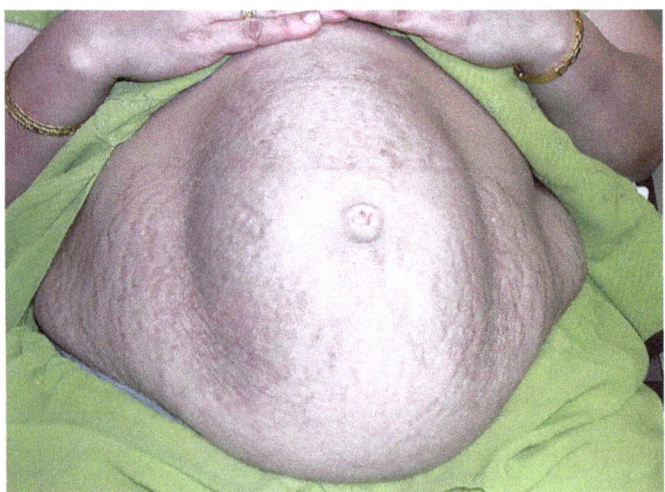

Fig. 5.13: Type 5P abdomen with pathological abdominal wall hernia.

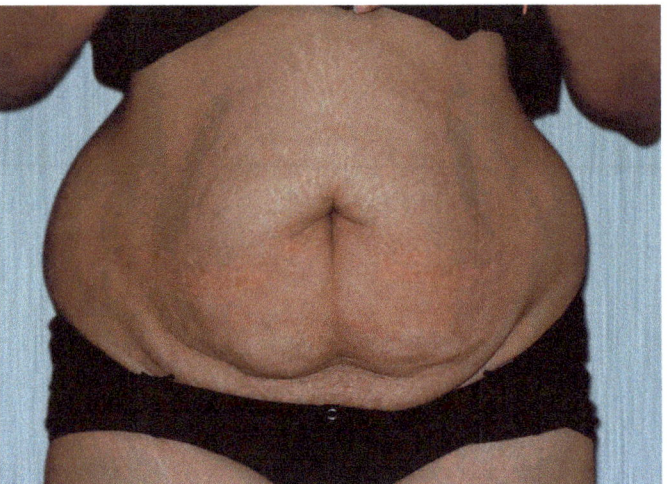

Fig. 5.14: Type 6 abdomen in a patient with multiple pregnancies, excess skin, extensive stretch marks and diversification of recti.

If there is a presence of hernia such as incisional hernia, pseudohernia, large umbilical hernia then it is a strong indication for abdominoplasty and repair of the hernia.

Type 6: Post Weight Loss Abdominal Skin Laxity (Fig. 5.14)

Type 6 patients have a history of either massive weight loss or multiple pregnancies. There is global skin excess (vertical and horizontal) with poor tone of skin and excessive stretch marks. The musculofascial layer is very weak. These patients benefit from abdominoplasty.

REFERENCES

1. Mei Z, Grummer-Strawn LM, Pietrobelli A, et al. Validity of body mass index compared with other body-composition screening indexes for the assessment of body fatness in children and adolescents. Am J Clin Nutr 2002; 75(6):7597-985.
2. Garrow JS, Webster J. Quetelet's index (W/H2) as a measure of fatness. Int J Obes. 1985;9(2):147-53.
3. Prentice AM, Jebb SA. Beyond body mass index. Obes Rev. 2001;2(3):141-7.
4. Gallagher D, Visser M, Sepúlveda D, et al. How useful is BMI for comparison of body fatness across age, sex and ethnic groups? Am J Epidemiol. 1996;143(3):228-39.
5. Brauman D. Diastasis recti: clinical anatomy. Plast Reconstr Surg. 2008;122(5):1564-9.

CHAPTER 6

Concept and Technique of Liposuction

▌ INTRODUCTION

Conventional liposuction or traditional liposuction incorporates deep suction of fat using a high-power suction device and a variety of cannulas that avulse the fat cells and remove them. Wet technique or tumescent technique helps to loosen up the fat cells and remove them uniformly with minimal bleeding. Technically, we are avulsing the fat out of its attachment and septae. There is disruption of fine neurovascular structures causing varying amount of bruising, sensitivity, numbness, etc.

A large-diameter cannula (5–6 mm) removes large quantities of fat rapidly. However, it produces several significant problems like waves, ridges, depressions, and irregularities on the skin surface due to unequal removal of subcutaneous fat. It is very easy to over excise the fat in one area causing depression. If it is not identified immediately and corrected using smaller-diameter cannulas it can cause permanent deformities that are difficult to correct. Using smaller-diameter cannulas (2–4 mm) reduces the incidence of these cosmetic defects.

In the past, the concept was to leave behind subdermal fat pad that was considered necessary to prevent wrinkling and contour irregularities. However, this technique will just remove the fat, thin the abdominal flap, reduce the circumference of abdomen, but it will not enhance the aesthetic units of the abdominal region. Treatment of the superficial layers is necessary to achieve optimal aesthetic results. Conventional superficial liposuction has high risk of contour irregularities, hyperpigmentation, and waviness. There are risks of crumpling of skin if a liposuction is performed in patients with large excess of skin.

A smoother contour is obtained if we use a nontraumatic cannula type such as Mercedes-type or single-hole cannulas. Other cannulas like cobra tip or basket cannulas have more curetting effect on the tissue, it may be desirable to use these cannulas in tough fibrofatty areas like chest or secondary liposuction but a primary abdominal contouring requires gentler cannulas. Intraoperative pain and postoperative pain are more with aggressive cannulas. Remember, even if the patient is under general anesthesia (GA) with tumescent infiltration in the tissues, the anesthesiologist will have to infuse more analgesics during the surgery.

A smaller-diameter cannula with a round tip and a few holes is important to achieve smooth contour with minimum postoperative pain.[1]

Various technologies have been used like ultrasonic-assisted lipoplasty (UAL), radiofrequency-assisted lipoplasty (RFAL), laser-assisted lipoplasty (LAL), and more recently water-jet-assisted lipoplasty, in order to achieve, atraumatic liposuction, skin contraction, and redraping. We will discuss about the details how the technologies help in liposuction in the following chapters.

In the forthcoming section, I will explain to you different terminologies that are used to describe a procedure of liposuction. This is useful because it helps us to set a protocol that is easily understood by our team and patients. There are a variety of terms to educate patients so they understand the concept.

▌ LIPOREDUCTION OR DEBULKING LIPOSUCTION (FIGS. 6.1A TO D)

If a large-volume liposuction is performed in the abdominal region in order to reduce the size of the abdomen without particular attention to the aesthetics it can be termed as liporeduction. The aim is to debulk the abdominal flap and reduce the size of panniculus and circumference of the abdomen.

Limited Liposuction (Figs. 6.2A to D)

This is a term I like to use, when patients want a specific area of liposuction in the abdominal region such as lower abdomen, upper abdomen, flanks, and pubic area. This

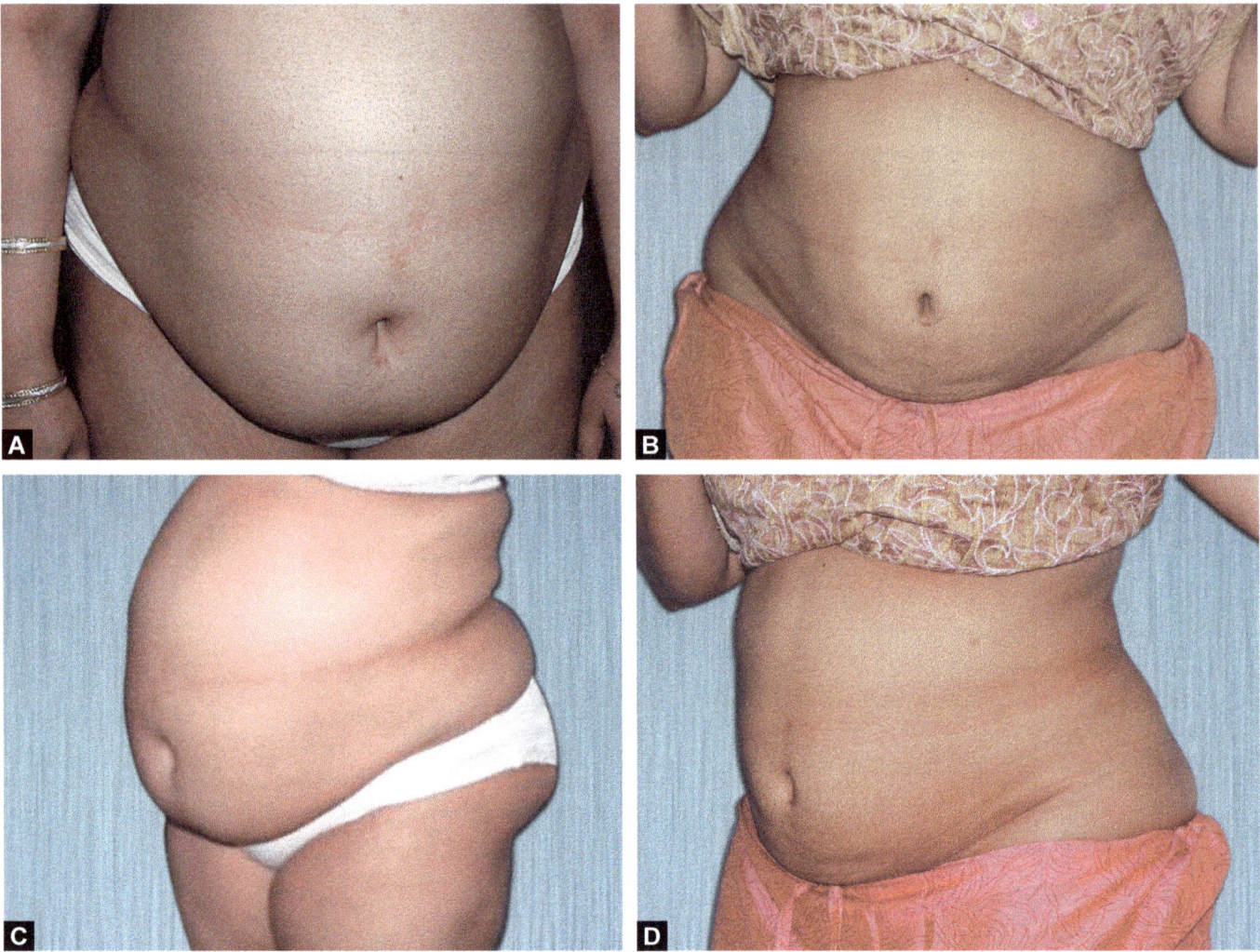

Figs. 6.1A to D: (A and C) A 54-year-old woman with weight 82 kg, body mass index 38. (B and D) Postoperative 1 year after liporeduction.

is also done as a secondary or touch-up liposuction procedure. I rarely recommend primary limited liposuction because although it may satisfy the patient temporarily, in the long run the fat gain is visible in other regions of the abdomen. Patients may come back in future for further liposuction in the other anatomical region of the abdomen.

Abdominal contour surgery could be termed "torso contour surgery" because as Alan Matarasso[2] suggested a long-term result can be achieved by involving all these areas even though the patient may come to you asking for "tummy liposuction" or abdominal liposuction. Rather than liposuction of only one area, such as lower or upper, adequate management of the abdomen might require all of the related aesthetic units of abdomen. Leaving behind other areas has a risk of relative disproportion in the

future. The other important concept is "skin draping." If all the regions of abdomen are treated including the "anchor points" like fibrous connection at the ribs, flexion crease the skin has a better chance of contracting and draping the contours of the underlying muscle. This prevents risks of skin collapse and wrinkling.

Circumferential Liposuction (Figs. 6.3A to D)

This is liposuction[3] all around the abdomen except the spine region in posterior midline "aesthetic unit no. 9." This near circumferential continuous liposuction allows both vertical and horizontal skin contraction and draping. This concept can be applied to abdomen and arms but cannot be applied to thighs because of the risk of skin sagging like "dropped trouser."

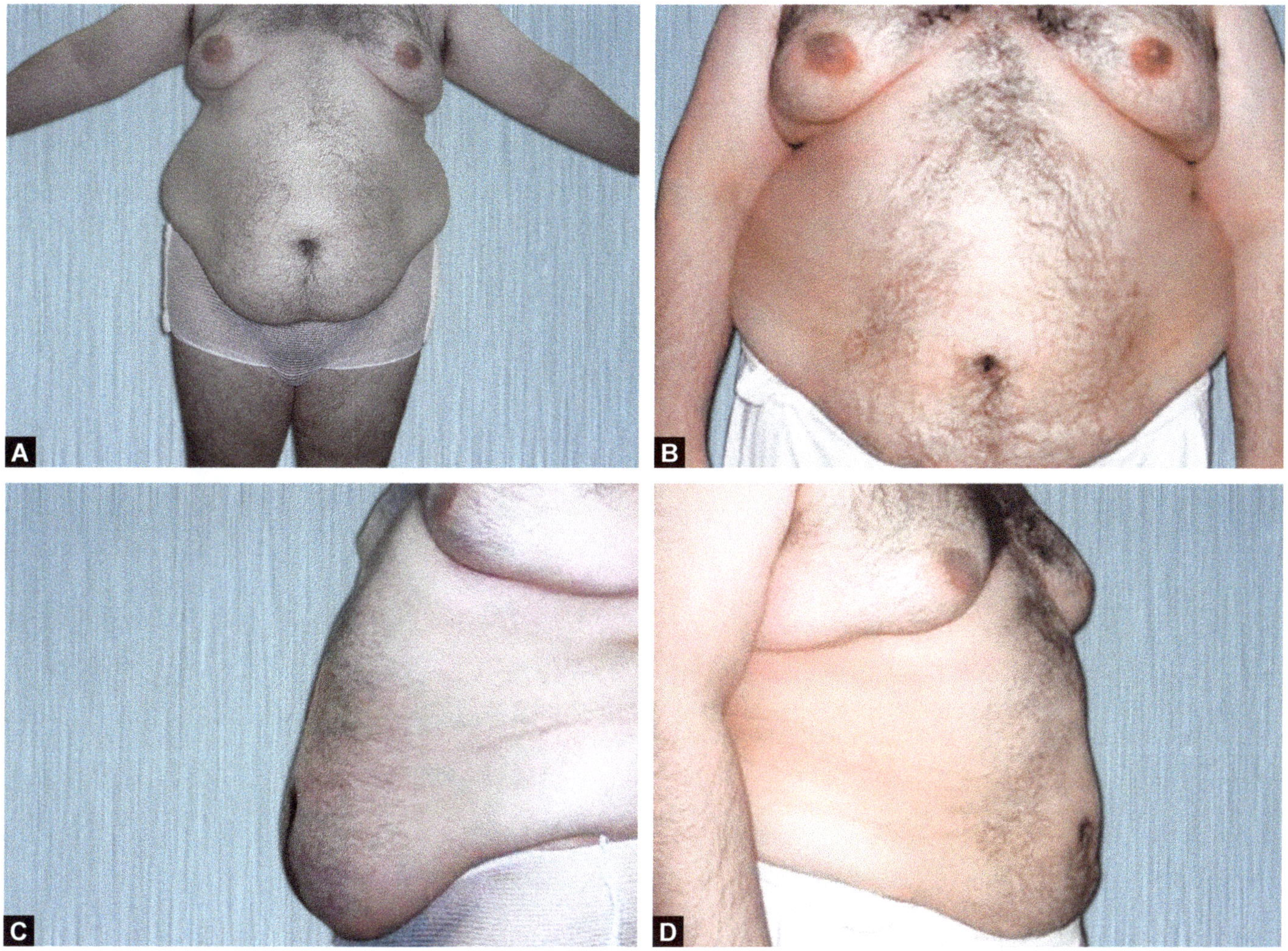

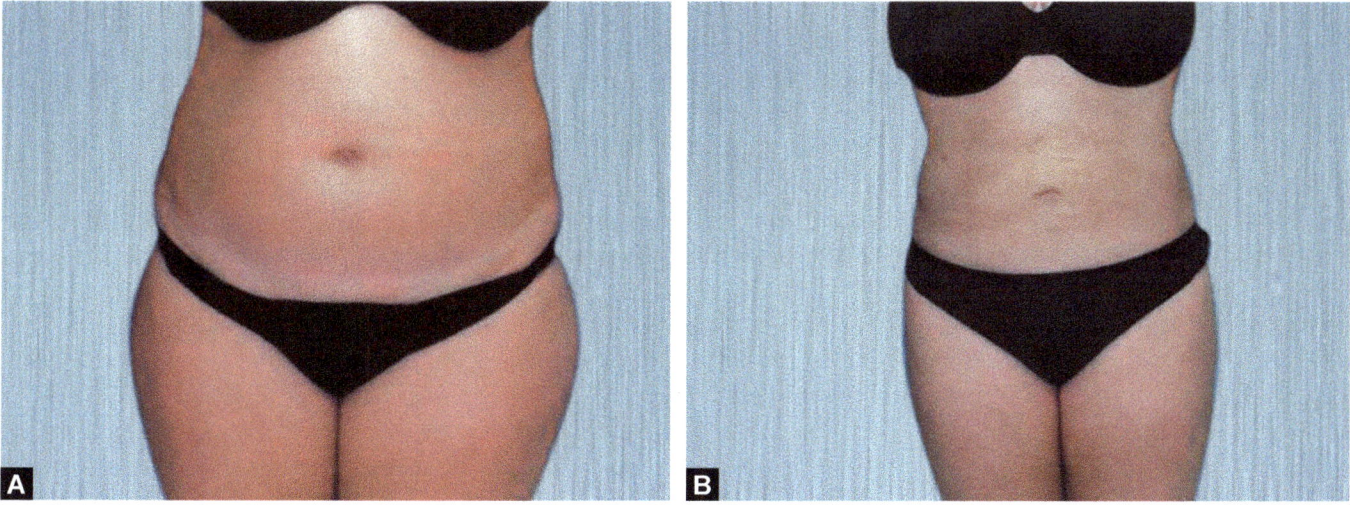

Figs. 6.2A to D: Limited lower abdominal panniculus liposuction for a 28-year-old obese man under local anesthesia. (A and C) Preoperative view, note the lower abdominal pannus. (B and D) Postoperative view, note the reduction in pannus.

Figs. 6.3A and B

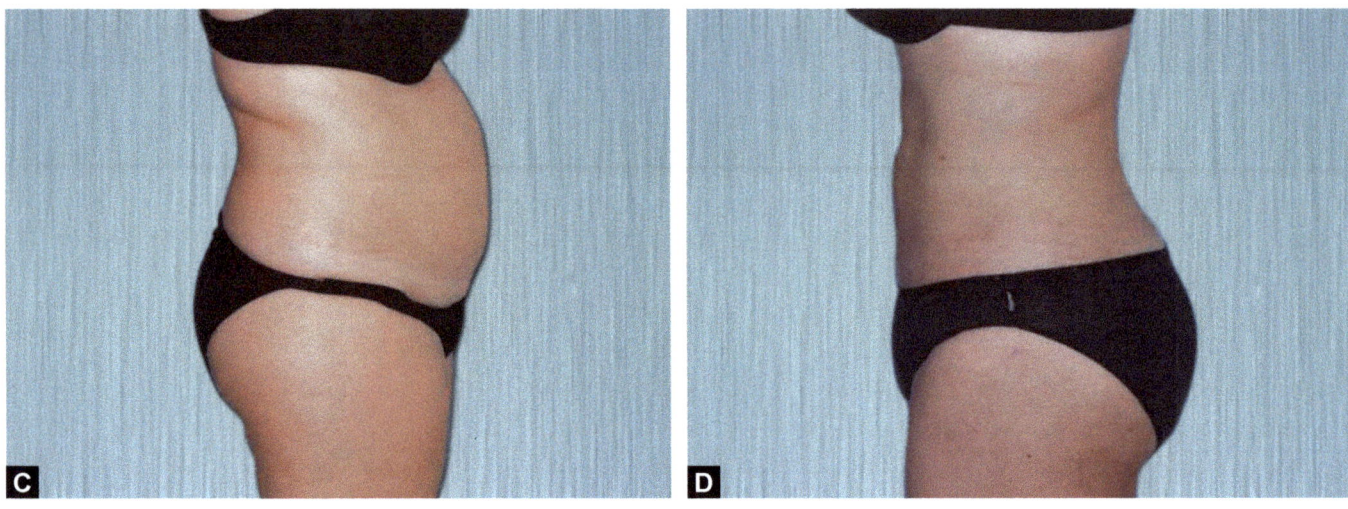

Figs. 6.3A to D: Circumferential liposuction in a 48-year-old woman with body mass index 33.

Liposculpturing

This is a modern term that we use to highlight the importance of aesthetics while we are performing liposuction.[4] The aim is not only to remove fat but also to highlight the body aesthetics, and achieve a harmonious and long-term result.

We know that a redo liposuction is very difficult and results are unpredictable. My philosophy is if you are doing liposuction for an area like abdomen, it should be done thoroughly so that we do not have to go back to the same area again. This is very useful concept because the patients want liposuction in many places at the same time; they do not understand the concept of aesthetics and safety. It is not of great benefit to do "bits and pieces" of liposuction in multiple areas, just to increase the volume of fat extraction. This may please the patient temporarily that he/she has lost a lot of fat, but soon they will be disappointed when they start gaining back in the same areas that has been treated. Physicians performing liposuction of any sort must educate the patients, so they understand the concept.

Liposculpturing is an artistic form of doing liposuction by combining the concept of underlying anatomy, fat distribution pattern, and aesthetics. It also applies to the correct use of instruments and technologies that can help us emulsify the fat atraumatically with better skin contraction and draping. Liposuction in men differs from that in women.

A youthful male abdomen has a triangular shape with a midline depression and well-defined rectus muscles anteriorly. Laterally, the abdomen is more concave with highlighted oblique muscles. The waist line ends at the iliac crest and gives a "V" shape to the back.

The abdominal region in women is more curvaceous. The aesthetic curve is visible in frontal, oblique, and posterior views. The abdomen is not completely flat but it has a gentle convexity below the umbilicus. The waist is higher forming an hour glass that becomes convex in the hip and buttock region. Liposuction with three-dimensional orientations is known as liposculpturing.

HIGH-DEFINITION LIPOSCULPTURING (FIGS. 6.4A TO D)

This concept was introduced by Hoyos in 2003.[4,5] It means removing the fat by liposuction in deep and superficial plane to expose the contour of highly developed musculature of the abdomen. The fat is present in layers, superficial and deep with extension into deep recesses at the borders of the muscles and musculoskeletal junction. Removal of this fat enhances the silhouette of the torso. In men, this technique can be used to remove most of the fat between skin and muscle; this allows better definition of the abdomen. Once they build more muscles by exercise, the "natural six-pacs" are evident.

Extensive superficial liposuction is the key to adequate skin distribution, but with the conventional technique it causes significant postoperative pain, bruising, and discomfort. The overlying skin is hypersensitive and also causes pigmentary changes due to postinflammatory hyperpigmentation. Ultrasound is very useful to emulsify

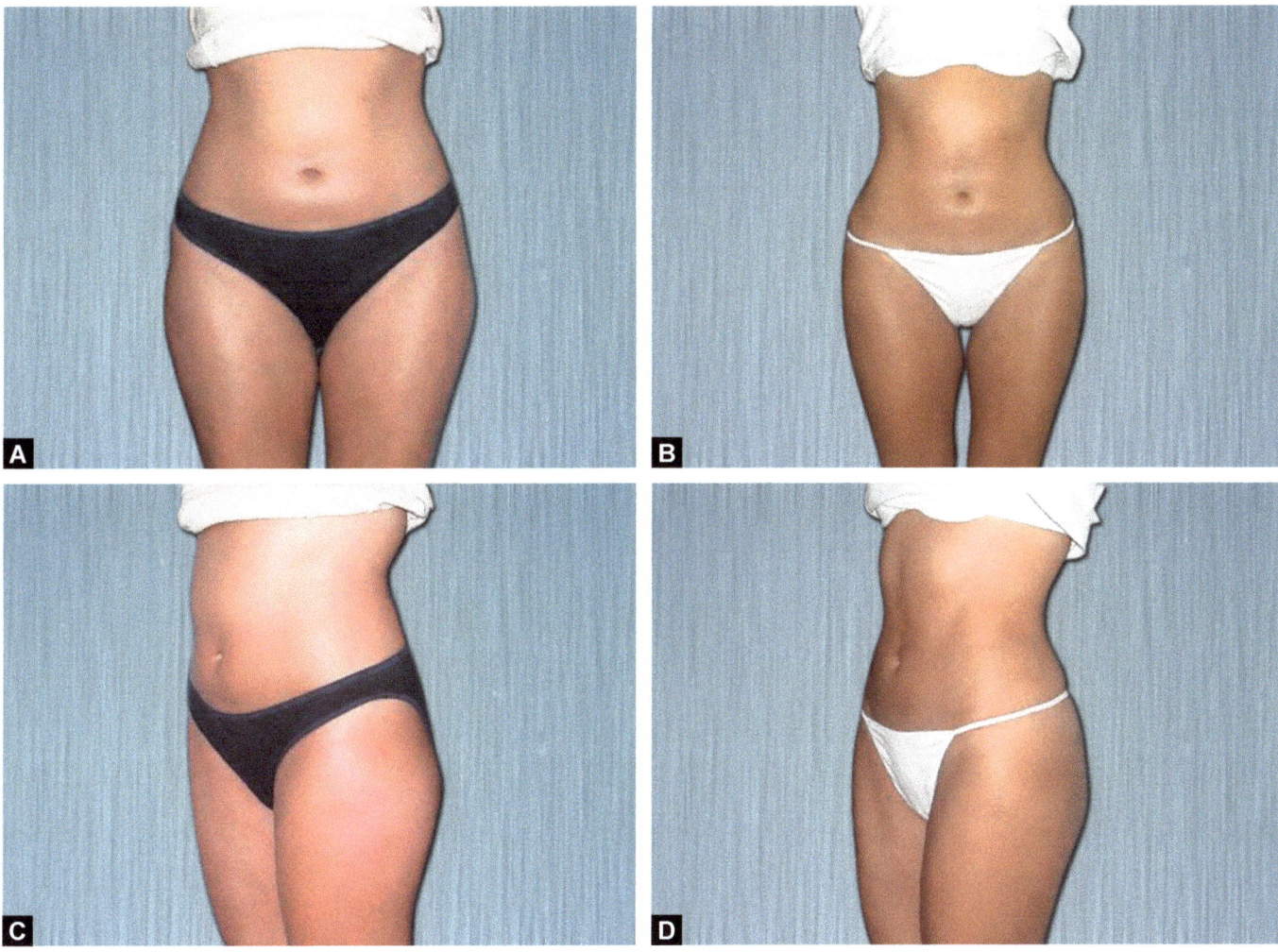

Figs. 6.4A to D: High-definition liposculpturing.

the fat with minimal disruption of fine neurovascular network; the postoperative period is less dramatic and more comfortable. Use of laser-assisted liposuction also allows easier dissection of the skin with minimal postoperative discomfort.

LIPOSUCTION AND LIPODISSECTION

The folds that are formed in upper abdomen, lower abdomen, and bra roll areas are due to fibrous adhesion of the dermis to deep layers (flexion creases). There is a compact layer of fat with dense fibrous septae. The fat accumulates above the crease and eventually skin folds down forming roles or panniculus. These fibrous adhesions need to be addressed during liposuction; extensive dissection in this area allows the skin to drape well and slide below the

adhesions. The dissection can be performed using a basket cannula or an energy device as in LAL and UAL.

Lipodissection with or without simultaneous suction aids in dissection the skin flap by releasing the underlying ligaments. Lipodissection can also be performed during abdominoplasty procedure to advance the flap.

FOUR-DIMENSIONAL LIPOSCULPTURING

This was described as a combination of high-definition liposculpture with lipofilling of abdominal, pectoral, and deltoid muscles that helps us to augment the chest and anterior abdominal muscular definition. Predicting skin retraction is difficult. This could affect the final outcome and may be not as expected. The integration of additional

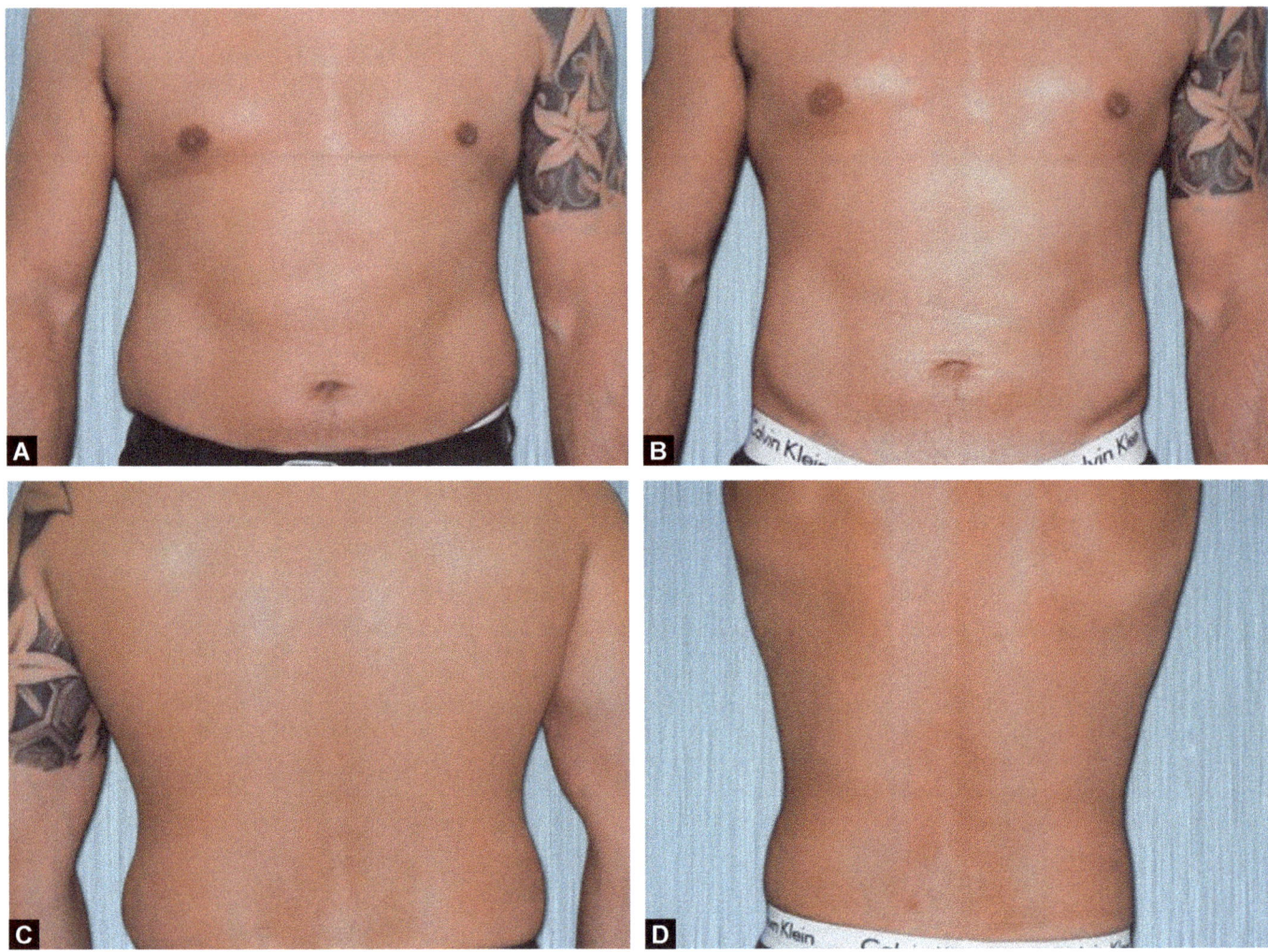

Figs. 6.5A to D: Abdominal etching in men. (A and C) Preoperative views, (B and D) Postoperative views after 3 months.

marking by Hoyos to define the abdominal, pectoral, and deltoid muscles led to the whole new concept of four-dimensional (4D) Liposculpturing. The debate was, if the fat grows as the patient gains weight, then it may appear as abnormal lumps and may look unaesthetic. Hoyos explained markings in different motions of the muscle and showed stable results up to 2 years.[6]

ABDOMINAL ETCHING (FIGS. 6.5A TO D)

This was another term coined by Mentz.[7] He used differential liposuction technique to highlight the detail anatomy of abdominal musculature, specifically the rectus abdominis muscle, between the linea alba and the linea semilunaris, and the tendinous inscriptions (intersectionus tendineae) of the rectus abdominus muscle. However, abdominal etching was designed specifically for male body builders with between 8% and 15% body fat, and was limited to only the anterior abdominal wall.

It has become clear now that the differences are more than semantic. These concepts will help us improve our technique and give the result that is required for an individual patient.

A detailed discussion is important to understand the requirement of the patients and their expectations. The type of procedure is selected on the basis of the anatomy of the body and the abdominal region. A high-definition liposculpturing is not suitable for obese patients or overweight patients with large intra-abominal volume. A 4D liposculpturing is not indicated in patients who do not exercise and control their weight. Similarly, a normal weight, physically fit individual will not be satisfied by limited liposuction.

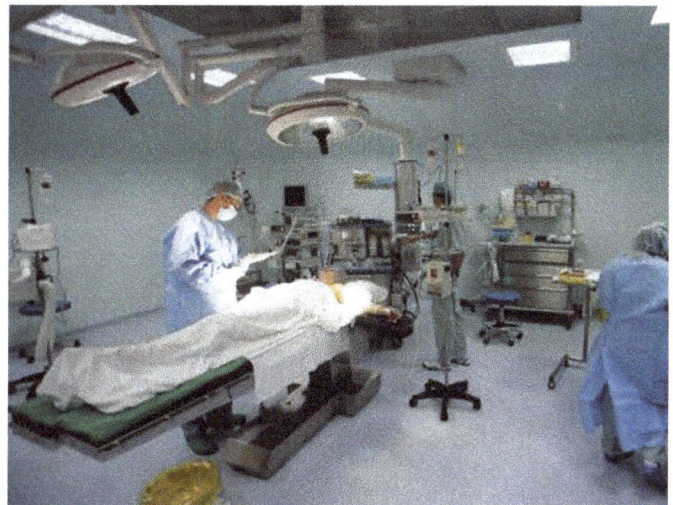

Fig. 6.6: Operating facility in a hospital.

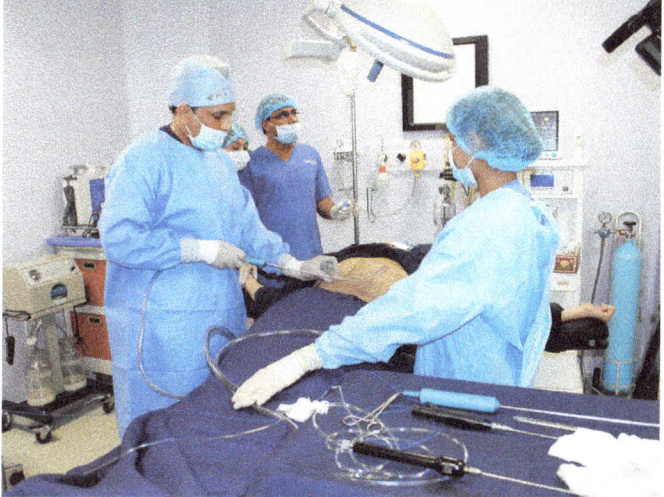

Fig. 6.7: Operating facility in a day care surgery center.

TECHNIQUE OF LIPOSUCTION

The result of liposuction is dependent upon the technique and skills of the surgeon. It appears to be a very simple operation but, believe me, it has a long learning curve. We need to go back to the literature or our own cases and find why there have been complications and dissatisfactory results such as lumpiness, waviness, and disproportion. We have seen how important it is to understand the anatomy, aesthetics, fat distribution pattern, and skin elasticity of the abdominal region. To achieve finesse in our results, we need to perfect our technique, understand the process of liposuction and movements of the cannula to achieve the ultimate goal of the surgery.

MEDICAL FACILITY FOR LIPOSUCTION (FIGS. 6.6 AND 6.7)

Majority of liposuction procedure worldwide is performed in a day care setting as economic consideration plays a major role. In many countries, where the medical laws are not stringently followed, the procedure is done in office setting or small facilities. Regardless of which type of facility is selected or type of anesthesia is planned, the operating room must be equipped with appropriate monitors, resuscitative equipment/medications, patient's safety, and comfort equipment (pneumatic cuffs, patient warmer, fluid warmers, etc.) and trained staff with knowledge of basic and advanced cardiac life support system (basic life support and advanced cardiac life support).

There should be following protocols in place:
1. Emergency protocols.
2. Infection control.
3. Patient transfer protocol to a nearby hospital.
4. Postoperative protocol.
5. Discharge protocol with clear instructions to the relatives.

ANESTHESIA FOR LIPOSUCTION

Two broad categories of anesthesia commonly used for abdominal contouring are as follows:
1. Local anesthesia (LA) with oral/ intravenous (IV) sedation.
2. General anesthesia (GA).

Local Anesthesia with Oral/IV Sedation

Recent guidelines by the American Academy of Cosmetic Surgery recommend a maximum of 45–50 mg/kg.[8] Significant toxicity has been associated with high doses of lidocaine and it is directly related to its serum concentration.
1. *3–4 µg/mL*: Circumoral numbness, light headedness and tinnitus.
2. *8 µg/mL*: Tachycardia, tachypnea, confusion, visual disturbances, muscular twitching and cardiac depression.
3. *10 µg/mL*: Unconsciousness, seizures and cardiorespiratory arrest.

Rapid infiltration in upper part of the abdomen can be excruciatingly painful because of tight adipose compartments. It can cause tachycardia or even vasovagal attack (hypotension, bradycardia, diaphoresis, pallor, and loss of consciousness). I will explain the technique to minimize this pain in subsequent sections.

Pain associated with the pH of lidocaine solution can be reduced by adding 1 mEq of sodium bicarbonate to 10 mL of anesthetic.

Supplemental sedative-analgesic medications (SAMS) are used along with anesthesia infiltration for the following purpose:
1. Reduce anxiety
2. Sedation
3. Analgesia
4. Amnesia

Generally anesthetists use a combination of medications from different categories to achieve a desired level of sedation analgesia. Midazolam (benzodiazepines) is more rapidly metabolized so recovery is rapid and complete.[9] It is typically combined with narcotic analgesics such as fentanyl. Fentanyl has advantages of rapid onset and duration of action of < 60 minutes. Adjunctive analgesics such as ketorolac may be administered if the patient feels pain during the procedure. The major risk of these combinations is respiratory depression that needs continuous monitoring. Some anesthesiologists prefer propofol (alkylphenol group) as sedative hypnotics instead of midazolam. The advantages are that it has less postoperative hangover and has antiemetic property. Major disadvantages are that it is painful to administer and does not have amnestic effect. So the patient remembers the pain of both propofol and the surgery.

The advantages of sedation–analgesia with LA infiltrations are several. It is more acceptable to the patient; recovery is early; and it allows easy movement of the patient intraoperatively; and is more economical. It provides significant postoperative comfort to the patient.[10] There are many reports that indicate lidocaine and sodium bicarbonate in the tumescent fluid have significant antibacterial properties.[11,12] However, this technique requires proper patient selection, and has risks of lidocaine toxicity, respiratory depression, and uncooperative patients. The procedure may remain incomplete or it may have to be converted to GA.

General Anesthesia

The same medications that have been discussed for SAM can also be used for GA along with inhalational agents. The newer inhalation anesthetic agents, sevoflurane and desflurane, are much safer.

The laryngeal mask airway (LMA) is a supraglottic airway device developed by British anesthesiologist Dr Archi Brain. It has been in use since 1988. Less anesthesia is required for insertion and maintenance of the LMA than endotracheal intubation.[13] Paralysis is unnecessary; so it allows quicker recovery and less postoperative nausea and vomiting. I have now switched over to GA using LMA in most of my cases of body contouring if I find the patient is sensitive or has anxiety.

The major advantage of this anesthesia is that the surgeon can focus on the contouring process without worrying about crossing the limit of LA. Secondary liposuction and technology like RFAL/(Vibration Amplification of Sound Energy at Resonance) can be used more extensively without causing pain.

The disadvantages are patient's reluctance to have GA, positioning of patient, hospital setup requirement, and associated cost involved.

Infiltration Anesthesia

I prefer to use following concentrations if the procedure is done under LA and SAMs;
1. Normal Saline: 1 L
2. Lidocaine: 50 mL 2% plain (1,000 mg)
3. Adrenaline: 1.5 mL of 1:1000 (1.5 mg)
4. Soda bicarbonate: 10 mEq

Total Volume

I prefer superwet technique with 1:1 or 1.5:1 proportion. If I plan to remove 1 L fat I would infiltrate 1–1.5 L of infiltration solution.

In tumescent technique, the fluid-to-aspirate ratio is 2:1. I use in selective cases where the fat is more tough and fibrous, the patient is sensitive, the patient with high risk of bruising, etc.

The amount of lidocaine and adrenaline can also be varied depending upon the individual cases. It can vary from 35 mg/kg to 45 mg/kg depending upon the requirement. Studies indicate that levels up to 55 mg/kg may be tolerated safely.[14]

For example, in an 80 kg patient, maximum amount I would use is 80 × 45 = 3,600 mg. Based on the above chart I would infiltrate maximum 3.5 L of solution (1,000 mg in 1 L).

Therefore, I can remove up to 3.5 L of fat (1/1.5:1 proportion). If the estimated removal of fat is > 3.5 L, then I would use larger volume of infiltration with lower lidocaine concentration. Epinephrine is a potent vasoconstrictor that enhances hemostasis, prevents rapid systemic absorption of lidocaine and prolongs the anesthesia. There is not much available in the literature about the dose calculation for tumescence; it has been empirically derived with experience showing that 0.5-1 mg/L (concentration of 1:2,000,000–1:1,000,000) provided consistent vasoconstriction with low incidence of tachycardia.[1] In my practice, if I am using superwet technique I use 1.5 mg/L concentration whereas if I am using tumescent technique, I prefer to reduce the concentration to 1mg/L.

If GA is administered, low-dose lidocaine can still be used in the infiltration. This reduces the dose of general anesthetic medications and in my opinion has better pain control immediate postoperatviely. A detail review of pharmokinetics is described in Shiffman's textbook of Liposuction, Principles and Practice.[13]

TECHNIQUE OF INFILTRATION

After administering IV sedation by the anesthesiologist, adequate LA is injected in the incision sites. Ensure that the injection starts with the deep layer followed by the subdermal layer that is the most sensitive area to pain. If this initial injection is painful the patient becomes anxious and uncooperative. The anesthetist is advised to keep the patient sufficiently awake to prevent his/her sudden withdrawal movement. The incisions are located in the bikini line, umbilicus, and submammary areas (multiple entry points). Sometimes additional incisions at the mid abdomen level are used to safely infiltrate the costal areas (if ribs are prominent), waist line, and bra roll areas. The incisions can be staggered to prevent telltale signs of liposuction. These incisions are avoided in patients with pigmentation or scarring tendencies.

The superficial compartment of fat is more compact and sensitive and hence can be painful. The plane under the Scarpa's fascia in the infraumbilical region or deep plan in supraumbilical region is less compact and sensitive. Start the infiltration in deep plane generously with low flow rate (20 mL/min). Proceed in radial fashion and gradually advance. In the upper abdomen it can be more painful, so proceed slowly in deep layers with low flow rate. The other sensitive areas are subcostal region, umbilical region, and lumbar areas. Slow and gradual advancement with a fine infiltration cannula will minimize the discomfort.[12]

After deep infiltration, proceed in the midlayer and finally in the superficial layer. If you are using the energy device or planning to do extensive superficial liposuction, copious superficial infiltration will prevent pain and burning sensation.

Finally, use the infiltration cannula like liposuction cannula to ensure all layers and areas are anesthetized. A waiting period of 10–15 minutes ensures adequate fluid dispersion in the tissues, prior to liposuction.

Tips for a successful infiltration anesthesia:
1. Proper patient selection: Patients who have anxiety attacks/panic attacks, secondary liposuction or multiple areas are not ideal candidates.
2. Proper explanation to the patients so they are aware of the steps involved and is not taken by surprise.
3. Premedications, IV midazolam, intramuscular pethidine and antiemetic injections are a great combination to minimize the pain during infiltration.
4. Infiltration with a small cannula and low flow rate.
5. Adequate concentration of solution.
6. Adequate fluid infiltration in deep, medium, and superficial planes.

SELECTION OF CANNULAS

Most of my liposuction has been accomplished with 2–4 mm Mercedes Benz-type cannulas. There are many advantages of these microcannulas. They are less painful, easily penetrable, cause less avulsion injury and aspirates small amount of fat hence more precise. They can be slow for large abdomens or difficult to aspirate in secondary liposuction procedures. Basket cannulas, Keel Cobra, and 5 mm cannulas can be more aggressive and rapid in aspiration. But they have more avulsion effect on the tissue.

TECHNIQUE OF LIPOSUCTION

In my opinion, the key to a successful liposuction is nothing but combination of following things:
1. Understanding: Anatomy, pathology, and aesthetics.
2. Technical artistry.
3. Manual labor.

I have realized, after many years of performing liposuction, sculpting is a manual art and no technology can replace that. To achieve a good outcome after abdominal contouring, I would recommend you to follow a guideline. I use this guideline for liposuction of all regions of the body.

GUIDELINE FOR GOOD OUTCOME

APPEAL (Assessment, Patient Expectations, Proportions, Eliminate Dead Space, Adjacent Structures, Laxity and Skin Elasticity)

1. *Assessment*: Identifying location of fat, quality of skin.

A careful assessment of distribution of fat in all the abdominal aesthetic units will help us plan the procedure and anticipate the outcome.

2. *Patient expectation*: Once we have assessed the local condition we can explain the patient what to expect. It is very important that we give a realistic outlook of the procedure and expected outcome. This is essential to have a satisfied patient.

3. *Proportion*: Aesthetics subunits.

A careful assessment of each aesthetic unit on both sides will help understanding the proportion of fat distribution, symmetry, and plan the liposuction procedure, to highlight the aesthetic curves and musculoskeletal silhouettes in female and male abdominal contouring, respectively.

4. *Eliminate dead space*: Plan of garment, foam, duration.

Plan the pressure garment in advance. No single garment is ideal; there is always a challenge to get the ideal garment. It should be conforming and covering all the areas of the abdomen anteriorly and posteriorly. Using foam to supplement the pressure gives a good result. Advise the patients to keep their posture straight, to prevent skin folding. Foam also acts as a splint and prevents flexion creases. There is no literature available to support the duration of pressure garment. It is based on individual experience. I recommend a first-stage customized pressure garment for 4 weeks followed by second-stage normal pressure garment (spanks) for another 4–6 weeks. If there is more excess skin then two garments, a customized pressure garment with supplemental abdominal binder to support the panniculus will improve the result.

5. *Adjacent structures*: Neurovascular, muscles, skeletal.

During the liposuction be always wary of important structures that you do not want to traumatize. Prevent inadvertent injuries to costal region, iliac crest, abdominal muscles, and peritoneal cavity. The cannula movement should be directed up and should be always either visible and/or palpable with your other hand.

6. *Laxity and skin irregularity*: Assessment of tone and elasticity of skin are required for the following:

   a. Type of liposuction—superficial/deep.

Extensive superficial liposuction is known to cause skin redraping and skin contraction. However, it carries a risk of skin wrinkling. Based on the patient's expectation you may or may not want to take that risk.

   b. Technology-assisted lipoplasty for skin contraction.

In the subsequent chapters, a detail description of different technologies is discussed. Based on the availability and expertise you could choose a technology to get more skin tightening. In my experience, RFAL tends to cause more skin contraction than any other technology.

   c. *External skin treatment in the post liposuction period*: Radiofrequency/endermology.

Patients with significant excess skin will benefit from some sort of external skin stimulation that ranges from just mechanical massage to external energy sources (detail description is in subsequent chapters).

Five Pillars of Success in Abdominal Contouring

Safety: Local/general safety.

Constantly think of preventing complications and take preemptive measures in a routine manner for all the surgeries that you perform:

- Bleeding
- Infection
- Seroma/ hematoma
- Skin necrosis
- Neurovascular damage
- Deep structure injuries.

Accuracy: Accurate plane/level of liposuction.

Accuracy in moving your cannula in a systematic fashion will help prevent unevenness and lumpiness. It is almost like elevating a flap for reconstructive purpose. Fanning technique with controlled and measured strokes of movement will ensure accuracy.

Precision: Use of appropriate cannulas, removal of precise amount of fat, monitoring of the skin contour frequently are all essential part of abdominal contouring to prevent step deformities and disproportion.

Balance: The balance between the two sides of abdomen in all the aesthetic units will give us a more symmetrical result. Be very critical during the procedure to judge the two sides of each zone.

Comfort: This is important for both the patient and physician. Keep patient's comfort to the priority. If the procedure is performed under LA then lying in one position for long time in a firm operating room (OR) table can be very uncomfortable. Using a soft mattress/foam on the OR table will help the patient. Keep the environment warm; use warm scrubs and warm fluids to prevent cold and shivering.

A surgeon needs to work very comfortably to prevent fatigue, wrist or forearm injuries (carpal tunnel, tennis elbow). I will describe in more detail the movements that will help perform liposuction safely, effectively, and comfortably.

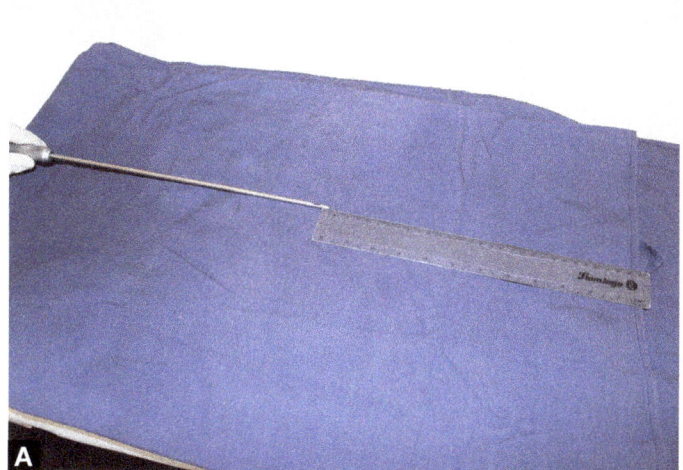
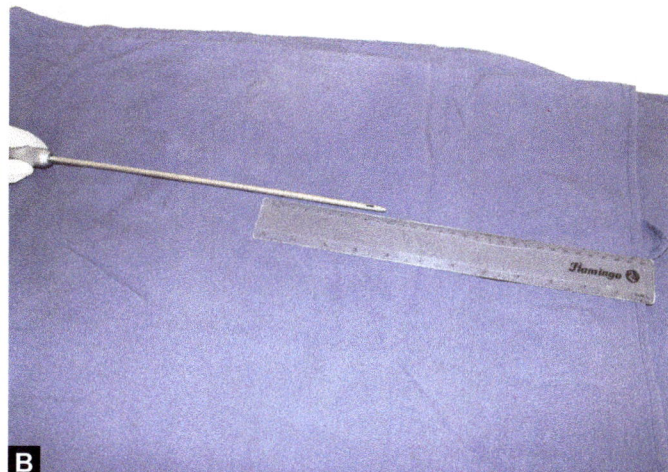
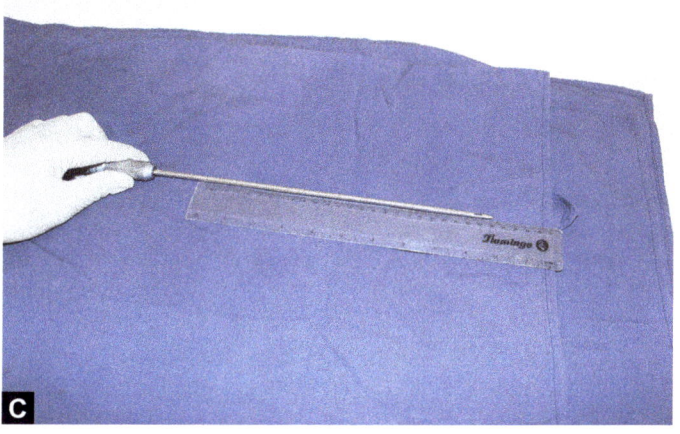

Figs. 6.8A to C: Strokes of liposuction. (A) Entry point, (B) Short stroke of 4–5 cm, and (C) Long strokes of 25–30 cm.

LIPOSUCTION MOVEMENTS/ MANEUVERS (STROKES)

The back and forth movement of cannulas using your arms are called liposuction strokes. The direction, numbers, and distance of each stroke comprise a good technique. The dexterity and hand-eye-brain coordination will ensure the five pillars for a successful outcome: safety, accuracy, precision, balance, and comfort.

Short Strokes Versus Long Strokes

Short strokes are when the movement of the cannula is performed using only wrist or short rapid movement of approximately 4–5 cm distance (Figs. 6.8A to C). It is a safe and controlled movement for beginners and safe in difficult areas like face, chest, subcostal areas, lumbar areas, inner thighs and ankles.

Short strokes ensure that the cannula does not penetrate into deeper tissue inadvertently. It also allows performing fan movements for uniform suction. The disadvantage is one can over excise the fat tissue near the entry port causing depression.

Long strokes involve shoulder movement and it is in the entire length of the cannula approximately 25–30 cm. It is safe in large surface areas as abdomen, flanks, back, anterior thighs, and arms. During long strokes, the tip of the cannula should be visible or palpable at all times, and the direction of the movement should be either parallel to the underlying muscles or below up.

A novice should use slow movement and only a few numbers of strokes using a wider and blunt cannula rather than a thin cannula.

The advantages of this movement are quick extraction of fat, removal of fat from wider areas, and uniform superficial suction. It is also used as pre- and post-tunneling

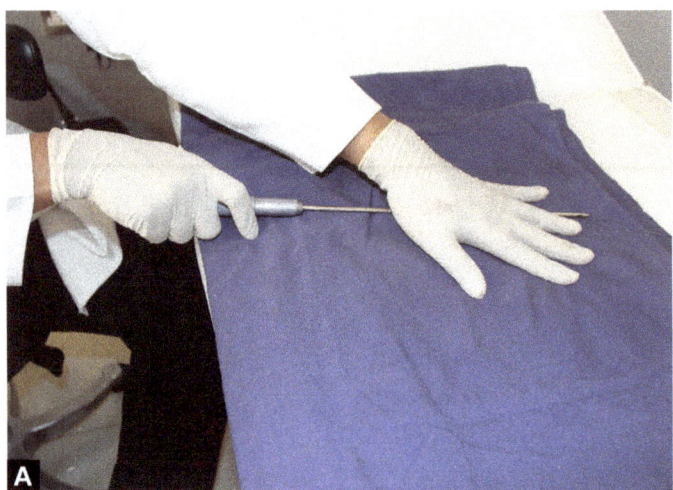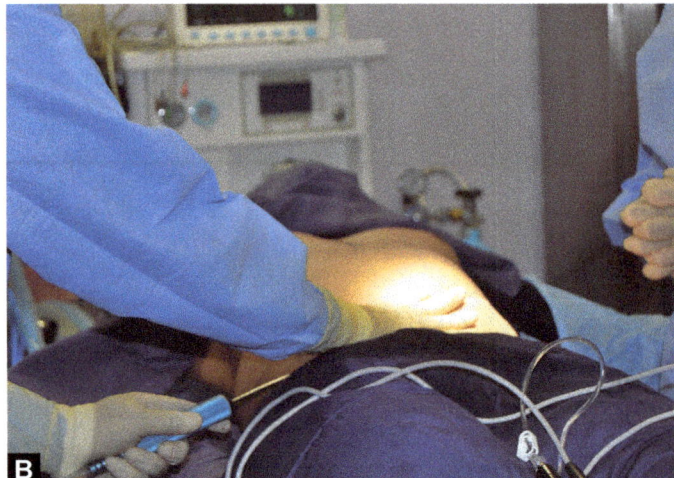

Figs. 6.9A and B: Five finger technique.

without suction to undermine the skin and cause controlled subdermal injury for better skin retraction.

Number of Strokes

For youngsters an important guideline is one... two... three... cannula out! and observe, one... two... three... cannula out! and observe.

Watch for the plane of cannula movement, amount of fat removal, and uniform contour. Once a depression or unevenness occurs, it can progress and become difficult to improve if necessary measures are not taken.

1. *Three strokes and observe*: For small areas and as final stage contouring mainly in upper abdomen, pubic areas and lumbar areas.
2. *Five strokes and observe*: For larger areas such as sides lower abdomen, pararectal areas, and flanks.
3. *Eight strokes and observe*: For large volume reduction in the all abdomen regions.

Fanning Movement

This is the movement when the cannula moves in a radial fashion back and forth. It can be as short or long strokes based on experience and area treated.

A good way to begin is to keep your palm stretched out and move the cannula under each digit, thumb and back, index finger and back, middle finger and back, ring finger and back, and little finger and back and out. Then observe and go back from little finger to thumb (five finger technique; Figs. 6.9A and B). This movement ensures uniform skin undermining and equal fat aspiration with less risk of lumpiness.

Back and Forth Movement/ Reciprocating Movement

It is back and forth movement in one direction (without fanning); it can be short or long strokes and is used for thinning of flap while pinching the skin or grabbing the skin.

It is also useful for tough fibrofatty areas or secondary liposuction, as multiple attempts are required to break into the adipose tissue and dislodge/avulse fatty tissue. Major disadvantage of this maneuver is that, if not careful, it can over excise fat and cause depressions and unevenness.

Tip should always be visible or palpable.

Pinching the Skin Versus Stretching the Skin (Figs. 6.10A and B)

Pinching or grabbing a skin fold and aspirating the core are a good technique to estimate the thinness of the skin, to aspirate deeper fat tissue in a safe manner (because the cannula is literally in your fist), preventing injuries to deeper structures such as ribs, deep vessels in inner arms and inner thighs. Pinching allows the skin to lift away from important deep structures.

Stretching the Skin

Either stretching the skin with the palm of the hand or pulling the skin proximally against the cannula movement allows the skin to become tight; this permits easy and controlled movement of the cannula in radial or reciprocating fashion. This maneuver is good for deep fat removal and uniform contouring.

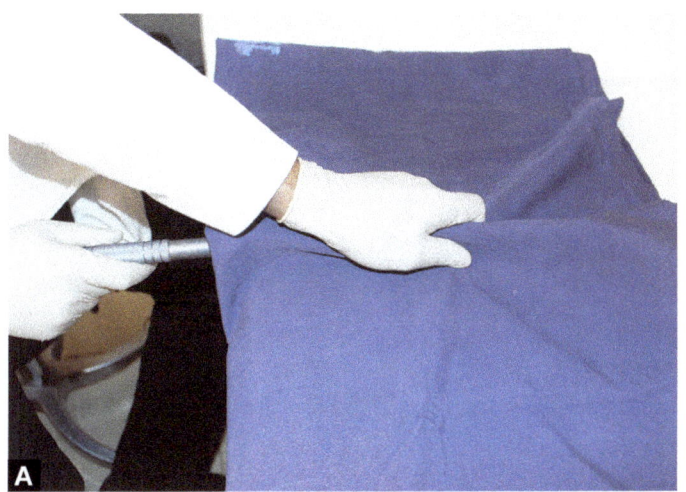

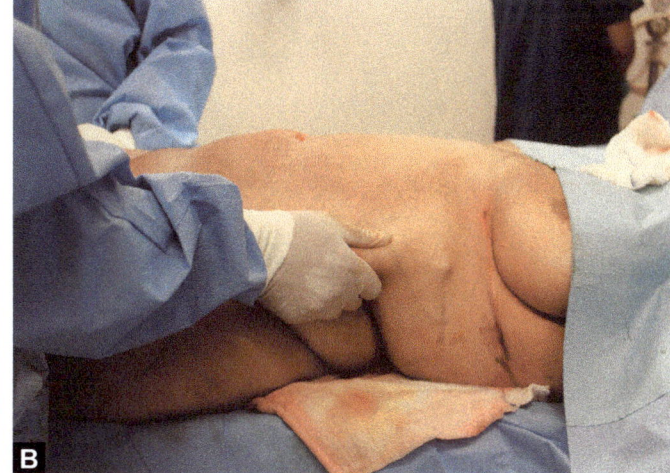

Figs. 6.10A and B: Pinching skin, stretching the skin.

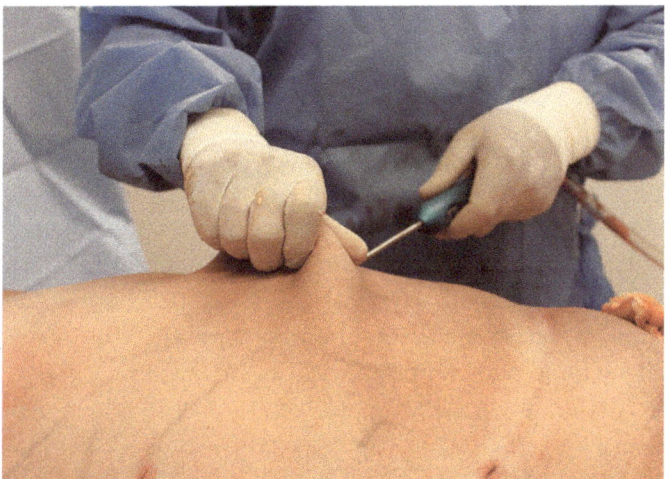

Fig. 6.11: Skin tenting technique.

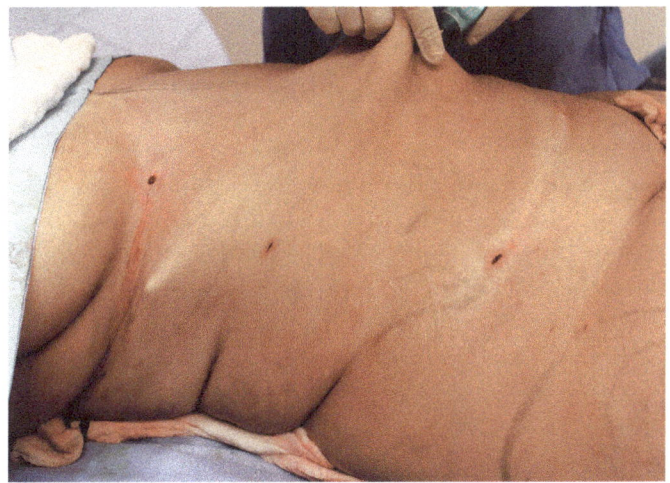

Fig. 6.12: Cannula tip should be visible or felt at all the times.

The disadvantage is that you may not see or feel the tip of the cannula, so it is recommended only by experienced surgeons.

Skin Tenting (Fig. 6.11)

Pinch the skin with thumb and forefingers, and retract away from the muscles then direct the cannula deeper to aspirate deep fat tissue. It is to be performed after the initial superficial and medium liposuction and can be done safely by experienced surgeons.

■ SUPERFICIAL AND DEEP LIPOSUCTION

The procedure starts with a 3 mm cannula for microtunneling and breaking through the fibrous septa. It can be performed with or without suction, when done without suction it is called as pretunneling. This is followed by a 4 mm cannula; first the medium layer is removed. This allows the surgeon to grab the skin and perform the rest of the maneuvers as described earlier. The skin is then pinched and deep liposuction is performed. I use 5 mm cannulas in large volume liposuction and only for a short while.

Fanning and reciprocating movements are done to thin the flap evenly. Finally, the 3 mm cannula is used to perform superficial liposuction.

Always remember that the cannula tip should be directed up and away from the underlying musculoskeletal areas (Fig. 6.12). The tip should be either visible of palpable at all times unless doing a deep liposuction with slow and gentle movements.

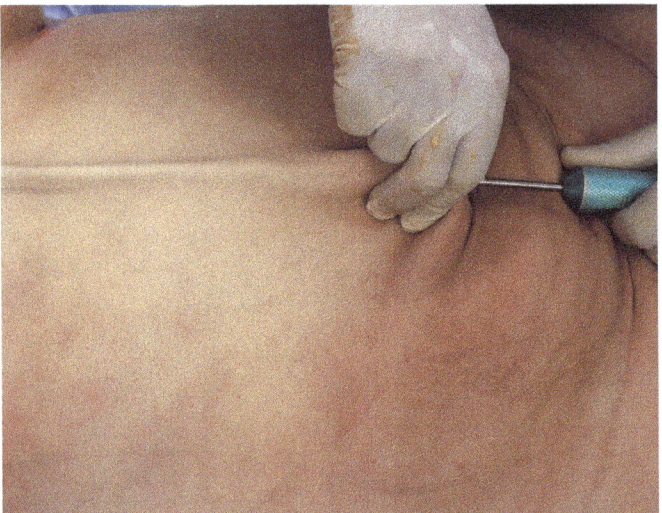

Fig. 6.13: End point of liposuction.

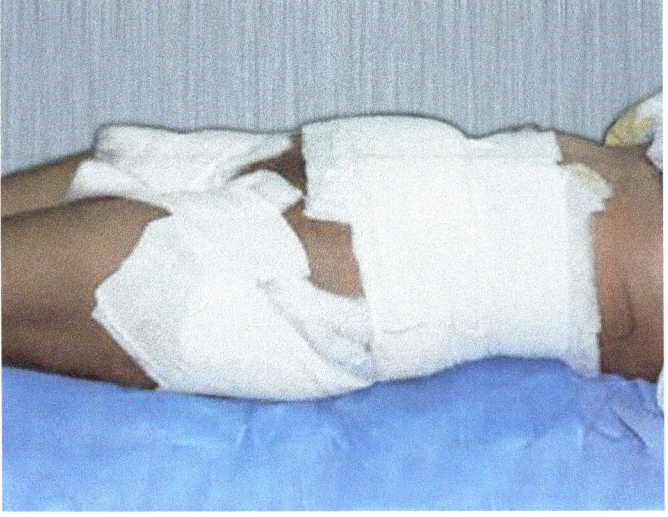

Fig. 6.14: Compressive dressing for first 24 hours allows drainage and does not mess up the garment.

Positioning of the Patient

The procedure is started in supine position with mild hyper-extension of the table to stretch the abdomen. This position will also help us to prevent cannula injury to subcostal region. Once the flap is thinned enough I prefer to flex the table minimally to perform deep liposuction.

After the anterior part of abdomen I proceed with liposuction of lateral and posterior parts in the same supine position. This allows the fat to fall away from deep structures.

Then I turn the patient to the lateral position to complete liposuction of lateral and posterior parts of the abdomen. This position allows observing the contour as you perform liposuction. Tilting the patient in oblique fashion allows more contouring in the lateral abdominal unit and lumbar unit.

▮ END POINT OF LIPOSUCTION

End point in normal weight individual is the final contour that you want to achieve (Fig. 6.13) and is visible immediately after the liposuction cannula is removed. After a few minutes, the contour is diminished due to tumescent fluid. End point in overweight and obese patients is the appearances of reddish aspirate and significant palpable skin flap thinning.

Post-tunneling can be performed using 4 mm Mercedes cannulas or basket cannulas without suction to break the fat lumps and release any tethering.

▮ POSTOPERATIVE DRESSING AND COMPRESSION (FIG. 6.14)

I prefer to keep the incisions open except in few where I have used a port for ultrasonic liposuction. Keeping the port open helps a lot to drain the fluid out and I do that for lipoabdominoplasty patients as well. Closing all the wounds can cause seroma and extensive bruising (collected blood under the flap).

Absorbant pads are applied over the abdomen and flanks and an elastic compression garment is left in place for 24 hours.

Next day the patient is advised to remove the garment and shower to rinse all the stains. I do not recommend the patient to apply ointments or cover the wounds with occlusive dressing as in my view that leads to more inflammation and scarring. A dry and exposed wound heals better with minimal scarring. If there is friction/heat burns at the port site then a cream containing mild steroid can be used. The patient is advised to wear the surgical garment. If there is lot of excess skin, an inner garment with additional binder can provide a good compression. After 4 weeks, the surgical garment is replaced by an elastic wear such as spanks.

A regular follow-up is necessary to ensure they are compliant with the garment and based on the skin changes they can be advised conforming foam. Foam is recommended only for 12 hours a day either day or night time based on patient comfort.

If there is excessive skin, unevenness, lumpiness then they are recommended for external treatment with equipment that has suction and roller mechanism. An additional low-level laser and/or radiofrequency are useful adjunct for healing and skin contraction (covered in the forthcoming chapters).

▌ REFERENCES

1. Shiffman MA, Di Guseppe A. Liposuction Principles and Practice. Berlin, Germany: Springer-Verlag; 2006.
2. Matarasso A, Wallach SG. Abdominal contour surgery; treating all aesthetic units, including the mons pubis. Aesthet Surg J. 2001;21(2):111-9.
3. Cárdenas-Camarena L, Tobar-Losada A, Lacouture AM. Large-volume circumferential liposuction with tumescent technique: a sure and viable procedure. Plast Reconstr Surg. 1999;104(6):1887-99.
4. Hoyos AE. High-definition liposculpture. Presented in the XIII International Course of Plastic Surgery, Bucaramanga, Colombia, 2003.
5. Hoyos AE, Millard JA. VASER-assisted high-definition liposculpture. Aesthetic Surg J. 2007;27:594-604.
6. Alfredo Ernesto Hoyos, MD Introducing VASER 4-Dimensional Liposculpture Plastic Surgery Pulse News, QMP. 2009; 3(4):1-3.
7. Mentz HA III, Gilliland MD, Patronella CK. Abdominal etching: differential liposuction to detail abdominal musculature. Aesthetic Plast Surg. 1993;17:287-90.
8. The American Academy of Cosmetic Surgery: 2000 Guidelines for Liposuction Surgery. Am J Cosm Surg.2000;17(2): 79-84.
9. Philip BK. Supplemental medication for ambulatory procedures under regional anesthesia. Anesth Analg. 1985;64(11): 1117-25.
10. Klein JA. Tumescent technique for regional anesthesia permits lidocaine doses of 35 mg/kg for liposuction. J Dermatol Surg Oncol. 1990;16:248-63.
11. Craig SB, Concannon MJ, McDonald GA, et al. The antibacterial effects of tumescent liposuction fluid. Plast Reconstr Surg. 1999;103:666-70.
12. Thompson KD, Welykyj S, Massa MC. Antibacterial activity of lidocaine in combination with a bicarbonate buffer. J Dermatol Surg Oncol. 1993;19(3):216-20.
13. Pollack CV Jr. The laryngeal mask airway: a comprehensive review for the Emergency Physician. J Emerg Med. 2001;20 (1):53-66.
14. Ostad A, Kageyama N, Moy RL. Tumescent anesthesia with a lidocaine dose of 55 mg/kg is safe for liposuction. Dermatol Surg. 1996;22:921-7.

CHAPTER 7

Technology-Assisted Liposuction

▌ INTRODUCTION

This chapter brings together a medley of technologies that are relevant to our practice of liposculpturing. In selecting these technologies, an in-depth understanding of machineries, mechanism of action, tissue response, and related details are necessary.

The question we have for ourselves is as follows:

What do we want from liposuction?

1. *Easy emulsification of fat*: Emulsified fat is easy to aspirate. If the fatty tissue is improperly emulsified it requires avulsion to remove. Avulsion and high power suction causes brushing, bleeding, severe postoperative pain and may be cause of lumpiness.

2. *Good skin retraction*: To achieve a uniform contour the skin needs to retract uniformly. If the skin does not retract uniformly, it can lead to excess skin folds and creases.

3. *Less brushing and swelling*: Patients get apprehensive when they see excessive brushing and swelling. Bruising can take several days to resolve, it is also associated with significant burning sensation. Any new technology has a learning curve, but it is less steep, if one is well acquainted with conventional form of liposuction.

4. *Less tiring for surgeons*: Conventional liposuction is physically demanding. As young surgeon, it is easy to deal with it. As surgeons age the conventional technique becomes tiring. Ultrasonic or power assisted devices increases the efficiency of the surgeon and is less strenuous.

5. *Easy to learn and perform for surgeons*: Surgeon should get acquainted with conventional liposuction technique before they explore technology assisted liposuction.

6. *Economically viable*: Technologies come for a price. The sophisticated ultrasonic machine is the most expensive of all. You need to build-up your practice to an adequate volume, where it will be economical to invest in some of these technologies. Some of the companies are flexible enough to provide on easy payment plans. This allows the surgeon to use different technologies.

This equates to better outcome for the patients. The surgeon enjoys the liposuction, it is less strenuous for the surgeon, so he or she can focus on aesthetic outcome and safety during the procedure. The postoperative event is less dramatic and this encourages, the patient to talk positively and refer patients to the surgeon. Patients often exaggerate their experience when they share it with their friends. This often scares people away.

▌ BASICS TO UNDERSTAND

Fat Avulsion Versus Emulsification (Figs. 7.1A and B)

The conventional liposuction involves curetting and avulsion of fatty tissue with the use of cannula that has sharp edges, large, and multiple holes. This is aided by high-power vacuum and mechanical movements of the arms. Curettage and avulsion are defined as forcibly removing the tissue or scraping the tissues off their bed. Tumescent technique is very useful to loosen the adipose tissue along with vasoconstriction, thus minimizing the bleeding and removing "pure yellow" fatty tissue (Fig. 7.1A).

Emulsification is the breakdown of large fat globules into smaller, uniformly distributed particles that can easily be removed by low-power vacuum (Fig. 7.1B). This process requires a technology to do so with less of human force. Emulsification rather than avulsion is the paradigm shift that we must get used to while performing liposuction procedure.

Emulsification of the fat allows easy extraction of fat with minimal trauma to adjacent tissues. The end result is more comfortable to the patient with better contouring.

Primary Versus Secondary Skin Laxity (Figs. 7.2 and 7.3)

We need to understand the difference between primary and secondary skin laxity.

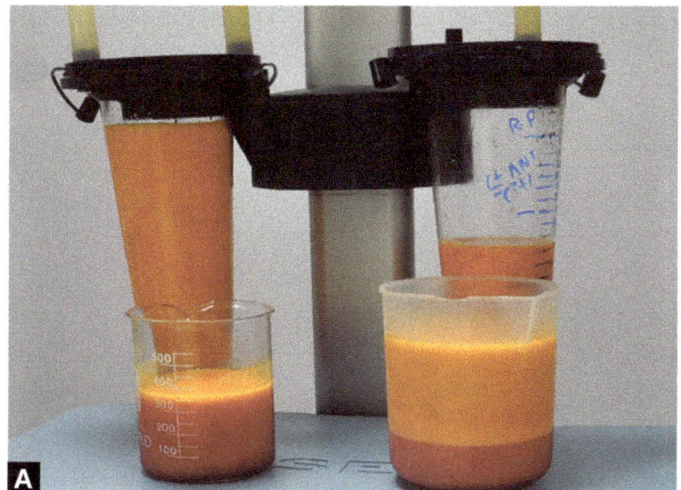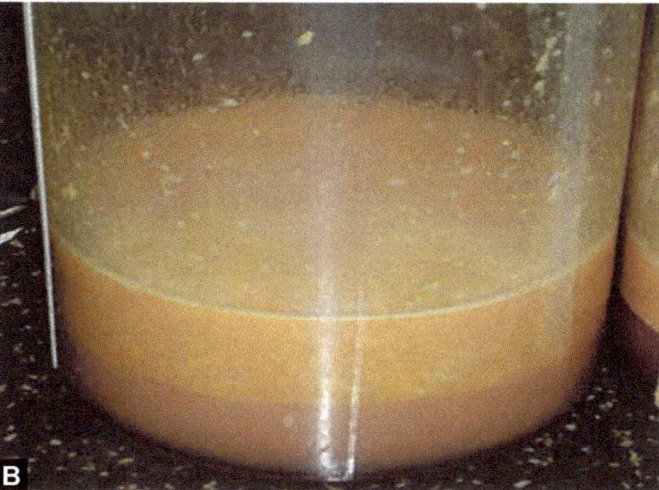

Figs. 7.1A and B: (A) Emulsified fat is uniformly suspended, and (B) Avulsed fat are pieces of fatty and fibrous tissue.

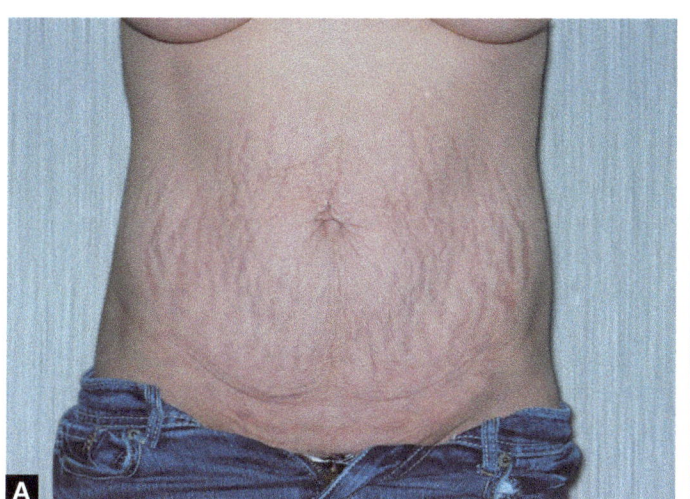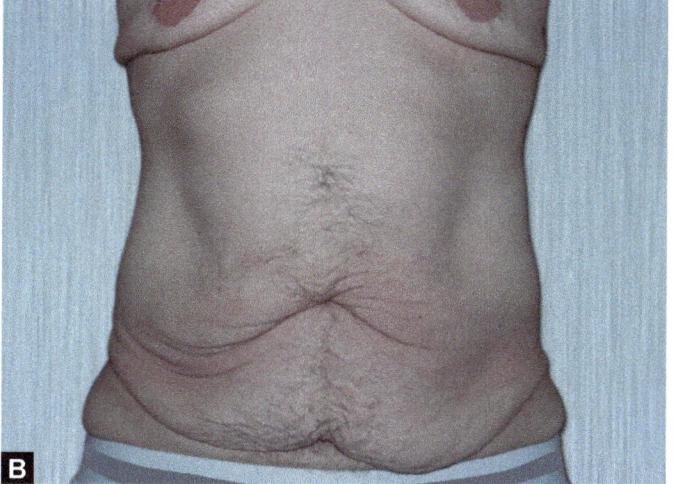

Figs. 7.2A and B: (A) A primary skin laxity due to excessive stretching during pregnancy. Note extensive striae gravidarum indicating lack of elasticity of the skin. (B) Residual lax skin envelop after loss of fatty tissue. This is often seen in massive weight loss patient and is associated with extensive striae and wrinkling of skin.

Primary skin laxity, in my opinion, is present when there is excess of skin with inherent loss of elasticity. This is typically seen in patients with excess weight loss; the quality of skin is poor with extensive striae and wrinkling (Figs. 7.2A and B).

Secondary skin laxity is mainly due to turgidity of tissue. It will either have a large amount of fat cells and fatty tissue (obese patients with panniculus) or there will be some fat cells with more of residual adipose tissue framework. Secondary skin laxity can be improved with the removal of the adipose tissue irrespective of the technology used (Figs. 7.3A and B). The challenge is the primary

skin laxity that cannot be improved with any technology. There are no studies comparing the effect of technology on skin contraction in primary and secondary skin laxity. Most of the papers if you notice will have patients with secondary laxity of varying degrees. Measuring and comparing skin contraction cannot be justified unless it is randomized controlled trial. The question remains, how much of the skin contraction can be achieved by technologies? Let us understand the various technologies, that are available in the market.

Liposuction can be accomplished by following techniques/technologies:

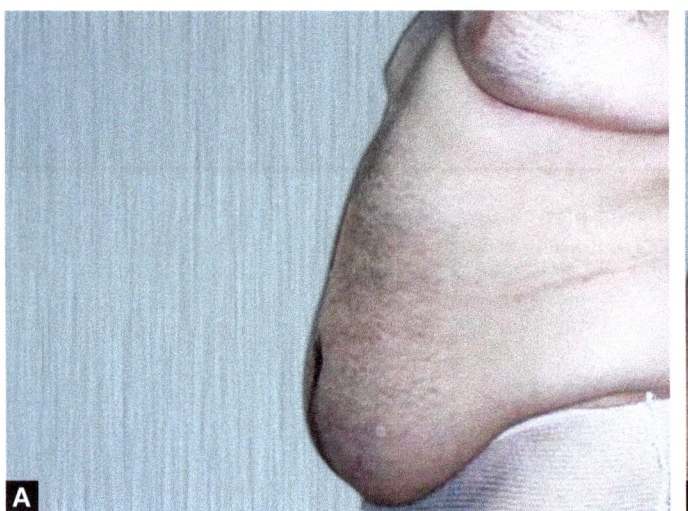 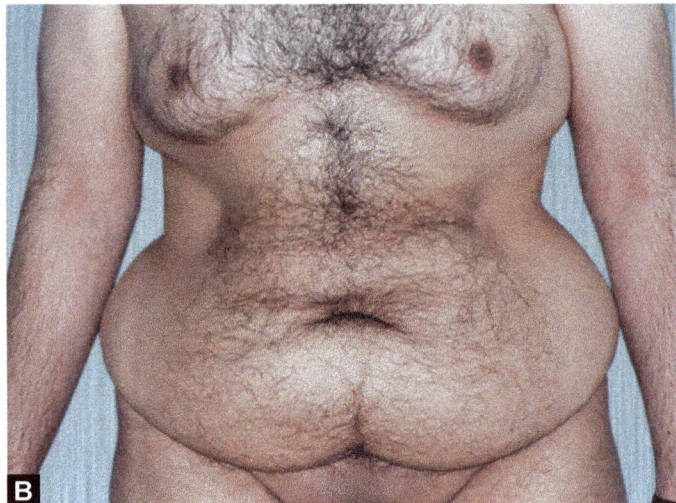

Figs. 7.3A and B: (A) Secondary skin laxity due to underlying adipose tissue in an obese patient. (B) Secondary laxity due to residual adipose tissue in weight loss patient.

1. *Conventional liposuction*:
   a. Suction-assisted lipoplasty/liposuction (SAL)
   b. Syringe liposuction.
2. *Energy based*:
   a. Laser-assisted liposuction (LAL)
   b. Ultrasonic-assisted liposuction (UAL)
   c. Radiofrequency-assisted liposuction (RFAL).
3. *Power-assisted liposuction (PAL)*:
   a. High-power vibration assisted
   b. Low-power vibration
   c. Water-jet-assisted liposuction.

▌ CONVENTIONAL LIPOSUCTION

Suction-Assisted Lipoplasty (SAL)

This is a traditional way of liposuction using standard cannula of size 3–5 mm and high-power suction machine with a pressure of 1 atm (760 mm Hg). The fat is removed by the avulsion method. Tumescent fluid infiltration helps us to emulsify the fat only to some extent.

Large cannulas allow faster removal of fat are more aggressive cannulas with sharp edges, larger holes, multiple holes, basket tip, etc. that allows rapid avulsion of adipose tissue. It also increases the risk of bleeding and adjacent tissue damage. Finer cannulas with blunt tip, less aggressive holes allow fat aspiration at lower speed but are less injurious to the tissues. Larger than 6 mm cannulas are very rarely employed for liposuction and I believe can lead to lot of complications such as seroma, hematoma, thromboembolic phenomenon and lumpiness.

Advantages of SAL

1. *Relatively inexpensive equipment*: The equipments are easily available, the set-up cost is affordable. Most of us starts the journey of liposuction using the conventional method.
2. *Easy maneuverability*: Accurate liposuction and contouring is possible only with manual liposuction. The cannula can be moved freely in all directions and the other hand is used to control the movement of the cannula, support the skin, and assess the depth and accuracy of liposuction. This can be as accurate as sculpting with a hammer and chisel. The hand-eye co-ordination is better allowing better control of the liposuction procedure.
3. No risk of burns except friction burn at the incision port. The port site injury can be minimized by using larger incision than the size of cannula. Other methods are lubricating and infiltrating the port site, and using multiple ports in a sequential manner.
4. Good for beginners to improve hand-eye-brain co-ordination for effective contouring. I recommend the beginners to get thorough with the conventional method. Apart from hand-eye co-ordination, applying your mind throughout the procedure will minimize inadvertent movements that can cause complication or undesired outcome. Hence, I believe in hand-eye-brain co-ordination for all the surgeries.

Once you attain a certain level of confidence with this technique it is easy to use other technologies.

Disadvantages of SAL

1. Physically tiring, particularly in tough fibrous fatty areas. Conventional liposuction using SAL can become tiring and injurious to the surgeon with advancing age. A long liposuction procedure reduces the efficiency of the surgeon to perform more surgery.
2. Overenthusiastic cannula movement can be risky: risks of perforation, muscle injury, etc. Fast and aggressive movement to remove large volume in short-time increases the risk of postoperative morbidly and complications. The cannula tip can change the direction and travel towards less resistant area when it strikes tough fibrous tissue or skeletal structure. Slow and gentle movement is more precise and less injurious to the tissue.
3. It is more traumatic. It is directly proportional to the strength and speed used for suctioning. More aggressive movement can cause more bruising, swelling and pain postoperatively. Extensive superficial liposuction by SAL can cause severe pain and bruising. The results take longer to appear (Figs. 7.4A to F).
4. Risk of lumpiness; groove formation can happen as the cannula avulses fat disproportionately. Again this depends upon the size of the cannula and the speed of cannula movement. There is a natural inclination to move the cannula in least resistant area causing over excision of the adipose tissue. Repeatedly using the cannula in one direction for longer time causes linear depression.
5. Fear factor in patients. Patients have a certain amount of fear factor due to the myths and negative publicity of liposuction procedure. Many patients are scared of a procedure that is considered as "liposuction."

One of the debates of SAL is the amount of skin contraction it can cause. Literature says that there is some degree of skin tightening following SAL due to nonthermal inflammatory process and elastic contraction of skin. DiBernardo[1] reported 10.6% skin surface area reduction obtained with SAL alone. But what is not clear is that, it is inherent or primary skin contraction or reduction in turgidity. Many of us have done large-volume SAL and have experienced significant skin retraction, probably > 10.6% that was reported. I feel it is the loss of internal turgor created by excessive adipose tissue that helps in skin contraction (Figs. 7.5 and 7.6).

Technical Pearls

Suction-assisted lipoplasty (SAL) can be efficiently used for all liposuction procedures. The keys to a successful outcome are finer cannulas, meticulous and gentle cannula movement, understanding the anatomy and tissue behavior and avoiding complications. Having the options of vacuum machine and syringe with few selected cannulas, you can cover most of the indications.

Syringe Liposuction

Pierre Fournier[2] in 1985 performed the liposuction using 5 mL syringe and 19 G needle. Subsequently, he used bigger syringes and abortion cannulas and was encouraged to see less bleeding and less discomfort postoperatively. Later than Tulip model and Toomey tip model were created with 60 mL syringes that had wide bore tips, stoppers to create negative pressure and cannulas of smaller diameters.

Grazer explained the theory of "buffering phenomenon". He explained syringes can be prefilled with saline to act as buffer or shock absorbing system for the fat. This helps to minimize trauma to the fat and it can be used for lipofilling.

The vacuum pressure created by syringe varies between 200 and 450 mm Hg, i.e. much less than SAL. There is less avulsion injury to the tissues.

Advantages of Syringe Technique

1. Relatively inexpensive and transportable.
2. *Better surgical control*: There is less risk of over resection of fat as it cannot be continuously used for long time and needs frequent recharging.
3. Less fatigue to the surgeons.
4. Less friction burn at the incision site.
5. Better quality of result as there are less trauma, avulsion, and bruising. This is due to the fact that the vacuum pressure is less.
6. Easy to recycle the fat for grafting. Hence, it is an excellent tool, when fat grafting is contemplated.

Disadvantages of syringe liposuction are that it can be slower than the machine; negative suction becomes less requiring frequent recharging of the vacuum. However, many surgeons claim to have used it efficiently for large volume liposuction.

I still prefer to use syringe for smaller liposuction limited to upper or lower abdomen or flanks only (Figs. 7.7A to C). If I need more contouring I prefer SAL as it allows me to focus on contouring part without interruption.

Syringe liposuction can also be combined with other methods such as SAL for fat grafting and contour correction purposes. Many surgeons prefer to harvest and store

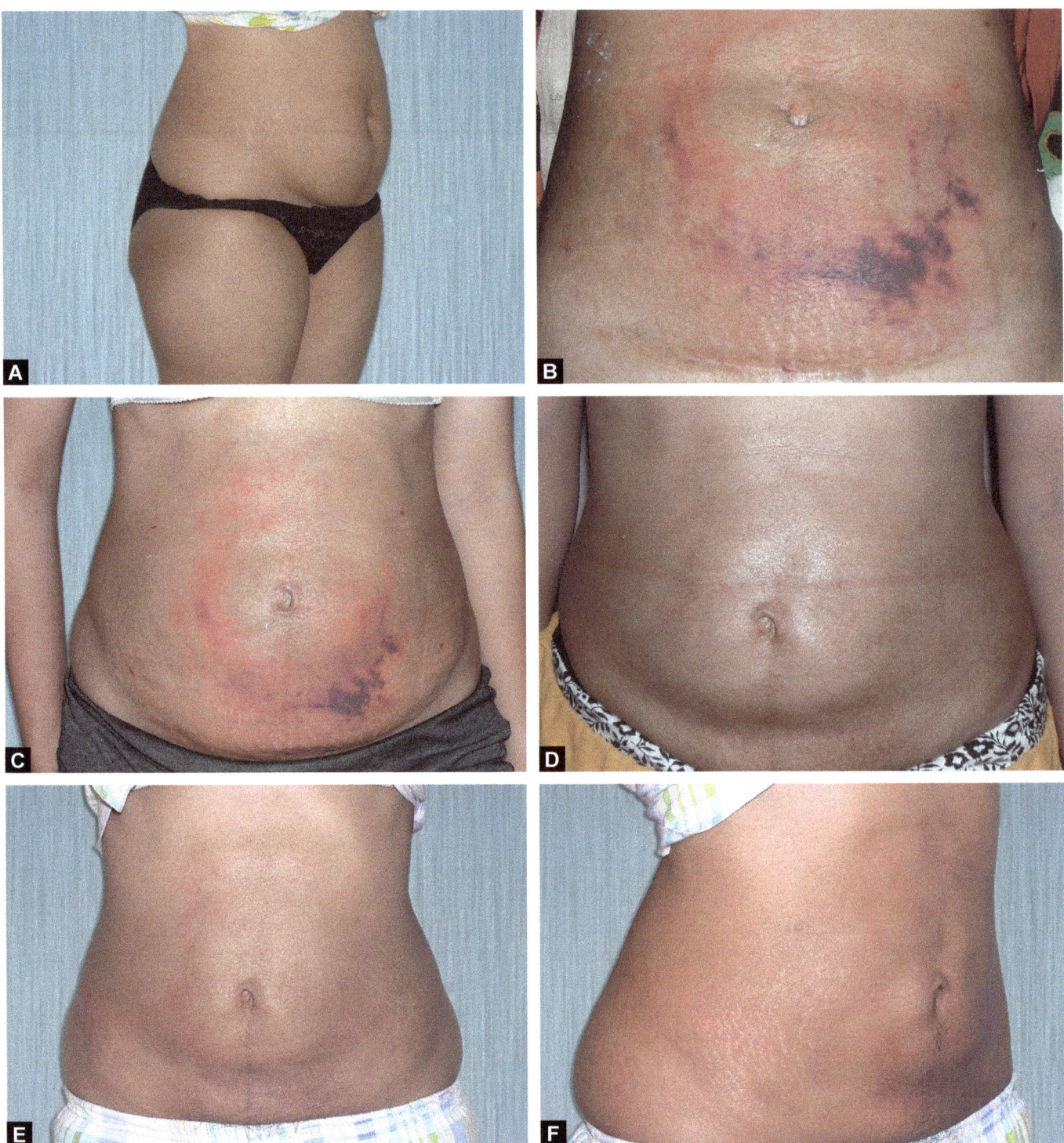

Figs. 7.4A to F: (A) Patient with 2 cesarean section refusing abdominoplasty, (B) Day 1 after SAL with extensive superficial and deep liposuction, (C) Day 5, (D) 3 months postoperative, and (E and F) 6 months postoperative.

some fat using syringe technique to correct any potential depressions that may occur after liposuction. In my opinion gynecomastia surgery often requires contour correction at the end of the procedure. So, if I am doing a combined abdomen and chest contouring in men I would always keep some reserved fat for grafting at the end.

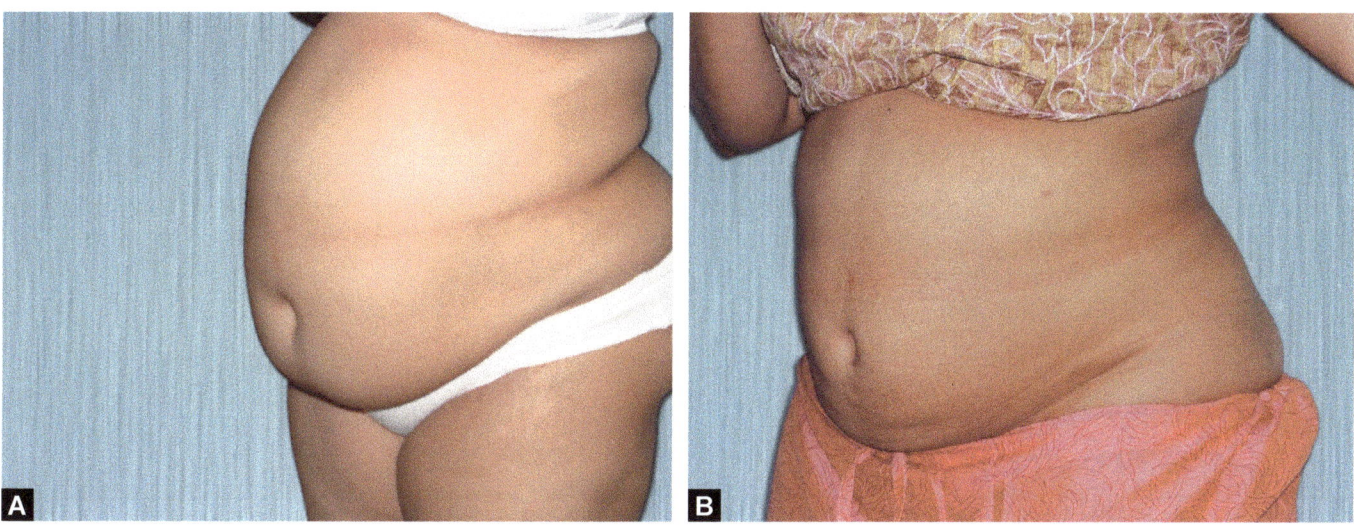

Figs. 7.5A and B: Amount of skin contraction after suction-assisted lipoplasty.

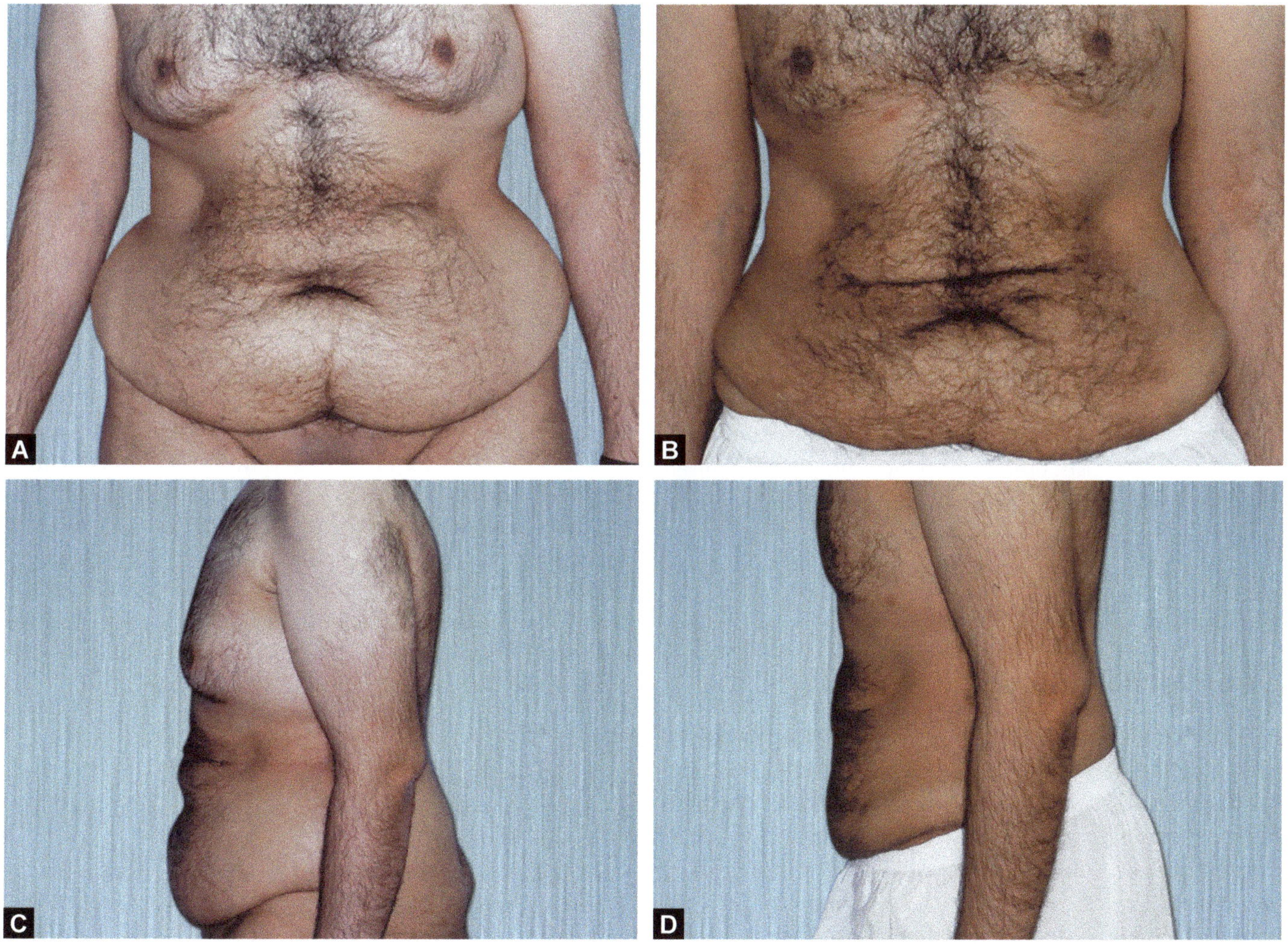

Figs. 7.6A to D: Postmassive weight loss patient after suction-assisted-lipoplasty: 1-month postoperative. Note the skin contraction and reduction of pannus.

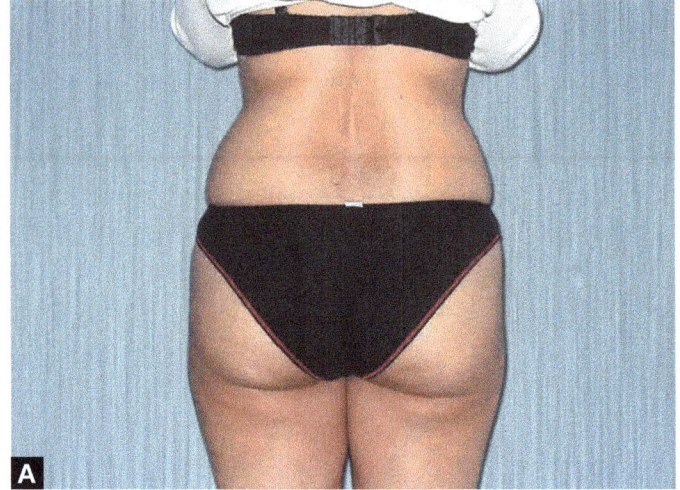

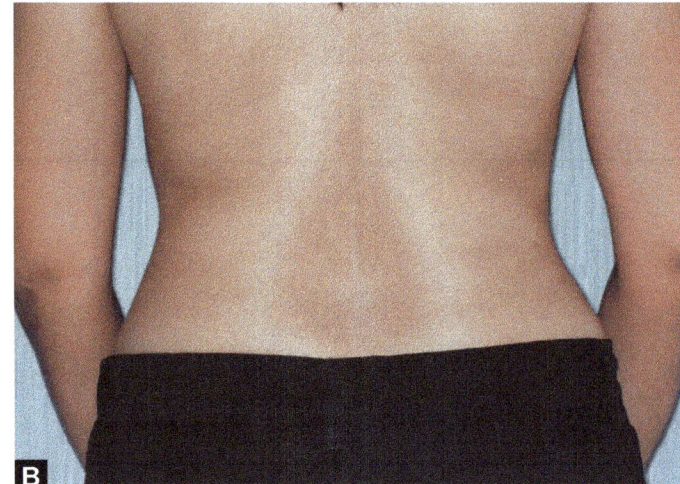

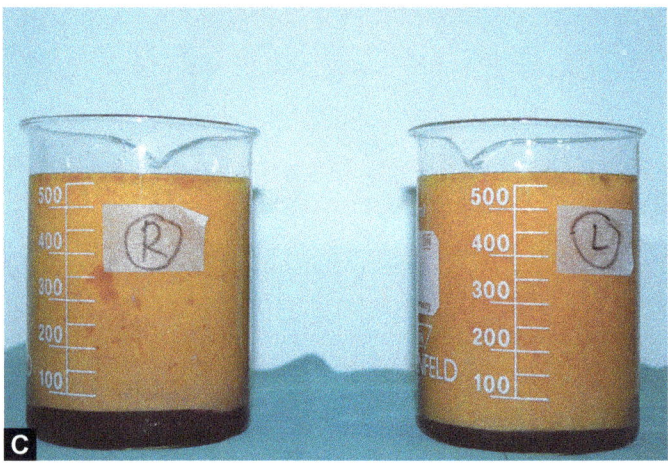

Figs. 7.7A to C: Waist sculpting with syringe liposuction: smooth contouring and the fat showed in the container with minimal blood.

Saylan[2] described a technique to correct postlipoplasty irregularities using syringe that he called "liposhifting." He performs liposuction maneuver without suctioning the fat out and shifts the avulsed fat to correct depressions. I find it very useful in my practice too.

ENERGY BASED

Laser-Assisted Liposuction

Laser was not an advancement procedure for liposuction. It was an increased application of laser and was mostly used by dermatologist as they wanted to get into the field of liposuction by introducing the concept of minimal invasive liposuction. When it started in 1998 it was used as lipolysis device to percutaneously break the fat cells and leave it in, expecting the body to metabolize and remove it. However, it was a failure as patients came back disappointed.[3]

The first laser was neodymium:yttrium-aluminum-garnet (Nd:YAG) 1,064 nm with 6 W energy. Very soon it was realized that the fat needs to be aspirated after adequate lipolysis.

Laser-assisted liposuction was described as a surgical procedure designed to achieve traditional adipocyte removal along with skin tightening from the thermal effect of the laser in the dermis. In laser lipolysis, there is selective photothermolysis of the targets (known as chromophores) that are fat and water.

Three major laser wavelengths that have been used for LAL are as follows:
1. 1,064 nm Nd:YAG.
2. 980 nm diode (continuous wave emission and high-power setting).
3. 1,064 nm/1,320 nm Nd:YAG lasers (selective for neocollagenesis, and therefore possibly skin tightening and hemostasis). In this combination laser fat is targeted by the 1,064 nm wavelength, and water bound in collagen is targeted by the 1,320 nm wavelength.

The Nd:YAG Laser

The Nd: YAG laser (pulsed laser with 200 μs pulses) operates through a twofold mechanism known as selective photothermolysis: photomechanical and photothermal.

The photomechanical effect produces mechanical destruction of the fat cell, and the photothermal acts selectively on the proteins in the fat cell membrane producing necrosis by denaturalization of proteins. The photothermal effect is the destruction of the fat cells that involves rapid thermal expansion and causes violent cavitation from shock waves. When lipids absorb laser energy, the light is turned into caloric energy, causing a sudden rise in the temperature inside the fat cell and ending in its rupture. This emulsifies the fat.

Goldman[4] published that LAL was designed to enhance outcomes of standard liposuction. He showed histological evidence of coagulation of small blood vessels, rupture of adipocytes, reorganization of the reticular dermis, and coagulation of collagen in fat tissue. Kim and Geronemus[5] showed that LAL with the Nd:YAG laser was associated with dermal tightening, rapid recovery, and magnetic resonance imaging-proven reduction in fat volume.

Diode Laser (Continuous Wave and High-Power Output 25 W)

Diode laser is used in a continuous modality using high power that causes disruption of fat cells, thermal coagulation, and remodeling of collagen tissue.

In a study published in 2008 Jean Pascal Reynaud[6] analyzed the application of 980 nm diode laser in 534 patients.

The technique was standard using tumescent anesthesia; a 1 mm diameter microcannula housing a 600 μm optical fiber (larger fiber size as more energy is delivered) was inserted into the subcutaneous fat. The cannula was moved back and forth in a predetermined manner to get a homogeneous distribution of energy at the treated area. Laser settings (power and cumulative energy) were selected in relation to individual body areas: 6 W (chin, arm, and knee), 10 W (abdomen back), and 15 W (thigh, hips, and buttock). It is interesting to see the amount of energy required for adequate emulsification of fat as they uses energy ranging from a minimum of 2,200 J (knee) to a maximum of 51,000 J (abdomen). They reported immediate contour correction and skin retraction without complications such a scarring, infection, burns, or hypopigmentation.

What is noteworthy is the amount of energy required to achieve sufficient lipolysis throughout the layers of fat and this in my experience increases the operating time significantly.

Sequential Laser

The sequential laser system employs both individual and sequential emission of 1,064 nm and 1,320 nm wavelengths (600 μm fibre). Di Bernardo[7] described that the deep fat areas were treated with a 1,064 nm wavelength source (20 W) and a 1,320 nm wavelength source (10 W). Subsequently, in the second step, the superficial subdermal layer (0.5 cm below the epidermis) was treated with a 1,064 nm wavelength source (10 W) and a 1,320 nm wavelength source (8 W). The amount of energy used was in the range of 1,000–2,000 J per 5 × 5 cm^2 region. This study provided objective data showing that LAL with combination of 1,064 and 1,320 nm followed by aspiration provides greater skin shrinkage and skin tightening than liposuction alone.

Both the 1,064 nm and 1,320 nm wavelength energies are absorbed by adipose tissue and converted to heat causing rupture of the fat cells. The laser-induced heating also stimulates activity of dermal and fat cell collagen. The 1,064 nm wavelength energy is absorbed by both oxyhemoglobin and methemoglobin, which is responsible for coagulation of small blood vessels in the fat tissue. Since absorption of 1,320 nm energy by hemoglobin results in methemoglobin formation and methemoglobin absorbs 1,064 nm energy three-times as strongly as it absorbs 1,320 nm energy, the synergistic 1,064 nm/1,320 nm unit further enhances hemostasis.

DiBernardo further reported a mean area soft tissue contraction of 17.2% with LAL followed by SAL compared with a 10.6% skin surface area reduction obtained with SAL alone.

The contraction of skin is related to the subdermal temperature achieved by any energy source.

Sasaki showed that increasing surface temperatures (40°C–42°C) demonstrated changes in reticular collagen or using combined wavelength along with SAL resulted in better skin tightening.[8]

However, caution should be used when exceeding external skin temperatures of 40°C to avoid unwanted thermal burns. It needs a monitoring device to continuously monitor the temperature of the overlying skin.

1,470 nm Laser

The wavelength of 1,470 nm has high absorption coefficients for water and fat, > 1,320 nm or 1,064 nm. It causes much faster fat emulsification using low power with a very limited thermal damage on peripheral tissues. There is significantly less risk of burns but the flip side is it may not cause adequate skin contraction.

Personally, I prefer to use 1,470 nm wavelength because it is faster and has better skin undermining capabilities.

Advantages of LAL

1. It is easily accepted by the patient as it sounds less dramatic.
2. It can be done as an office-based procedure in a standard treatment room.

    Let me explain to you in details. Patients are scared of surgeon, surgery, operation theater, and general anesthesia. All these intimidate them and make them nervous. This is a reason why patients are attracted to dermatologist/cosmetologist because they make it sound too easy for them. I am not saying you do not follow the norms of operative procedures. But, laser is supposed to be minimally invasive with less risk of trauma, infection, etc. Most of these procedures can be done under local anesthesia and the patient enters the procedure room awake. The aesthetics of the room plays a significant role to calm them down. The minimal anesthesia, less postanesthesia nausea/vomiting and minimal discomfort add to their comfort level. They go through a pleasant experience. This makes it easy for them to narrate and spread word of mouth "publicity." Patients who undergo a lot of intra and postoperative trauma, swelling, bruising, etc. will make it sound even more dramatic to their friends discouraging them to even think about it.
3. It has good skin undermining capabilities so certainly helps improve cellulites and superficial irregularities.
4. It is less traumatic provided enough energy is deployed to allow fat emulsification.
5. It is easy to carry the machine.
6. A major advantage is the public awareness due to "marketing and media." It has certainly increased the range of patients I see in my practice. Earlier I had patient with very large abdomen for liposuction because I had only one option, but now I see a range of patients with small, medium and large bulges (Figs. 7.8 to 7.10).

Disadvantages of LAL

1. It is expensive equipment.
2. The delicate laser fibers can get damaged and are consumable.
3. It is not suitable for large-volume liposuction as it can be very time consuming.
4. Liposuction is a separate procedure that adds to the time.
5. Some lasers require skin temperature monitoring and have risk of skin burns.
6. Risks of deep tissue penetration or skin perforation, if it is used forcefully.

Technical Pearls

Having an option of laser-assisted liposuction increases your patient flow and indications. Choosing the right wavelength is a personal choice. Using the technology to the best of your advantage requires understanding and learning.

Laser-assisted lipoplasty demands care during the procedure. A slow movement to deliver adequate energy and prevent collateral damage, controlled accumulated energy, grid marking to distribute the energy uniformly, and appropriate case selection are keys to a successful outcome.

Despite the effectiveness of different laser wavelengths to selectively target adipocytes and reticular collagen they do not have distinct advantages over other methods. There are no randomized controlled studies comparing LAL with traditional liposuction or any other method.[9]

Ultrasonic-Assisted Lipoplasty

Mechanism

Ultrasound is the process that turns electric energy into mechanical vibrations (high-frequency sonic waves) that cause thermal effects and micromechanical effects (acoustic) or cavitational effects in contracting and expanding circles through a hand piece containing piezoelectric crystals. These mechanical oscillations pass through a titanium cannula that emits the waves from its tip. This causes implosion of fatty tissue and fat liquefaction.[10]

There are three main physiological effects of the ultrasound.

1. The micromechanical effect is the injury produced directly by the unidirectional action of the ultrasonic waves through the molecules. It has minimal effects.
2. The cavitational effects produce cell fragmentation and diffusion of the lipidic matrix.

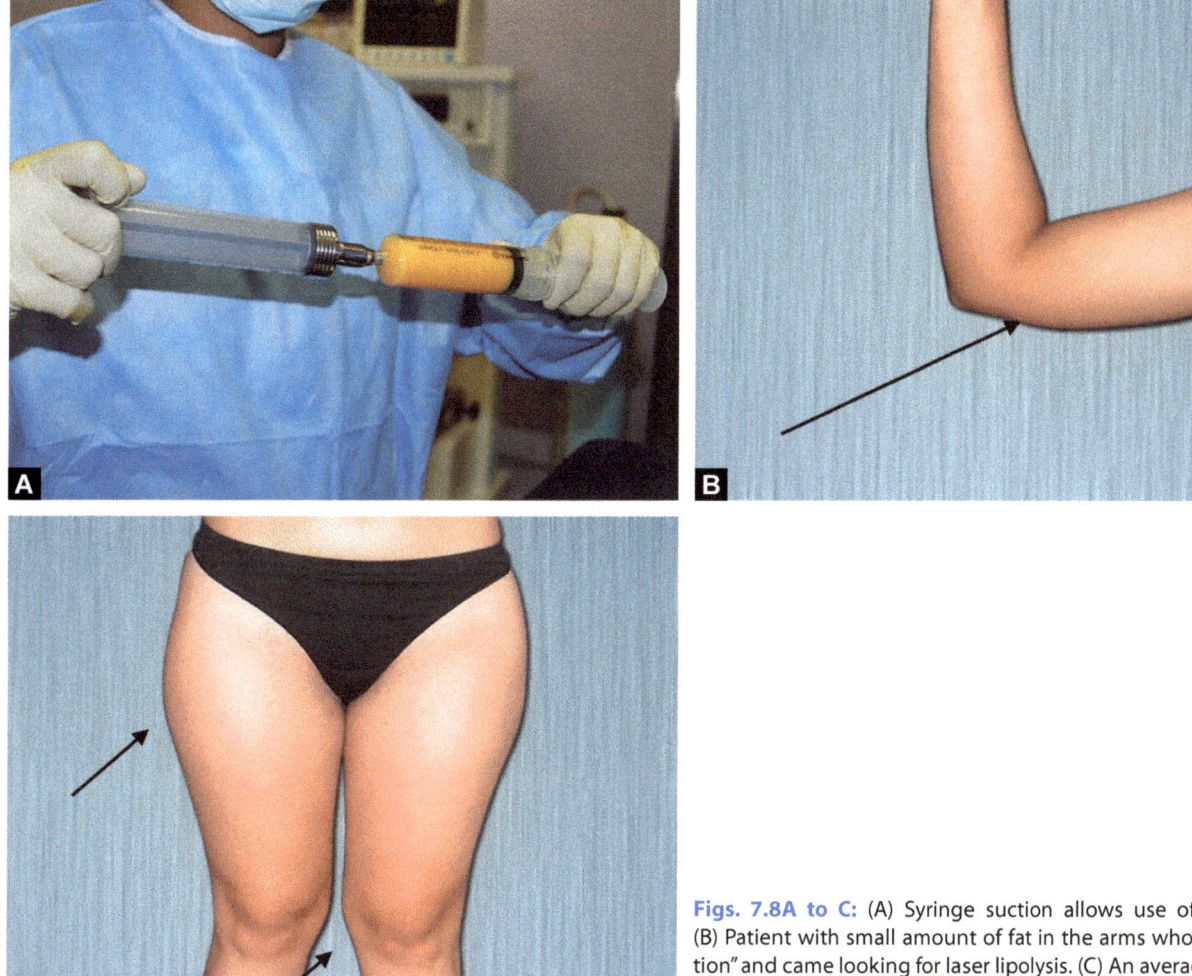

Figs. 7.8A to C: (A) Syringe suction allows use of fat for grafting. (B) Patient with small amount of fat in the arms who refused "liposuction" and came looking for laser lipolysis. (C) An average weight patient with small saddle bags and knee bulges opting for LAL.

Figs. 7.9A and B: Laser lipoplasty in a female patient with small fat in the central abdomen. (A) She wanted small or no scars without any downtime. Laser was performed using 2 mm incision and a 2/3 mm cannula was used with syringe vacuum. (B) Postoperative view after 1 week.

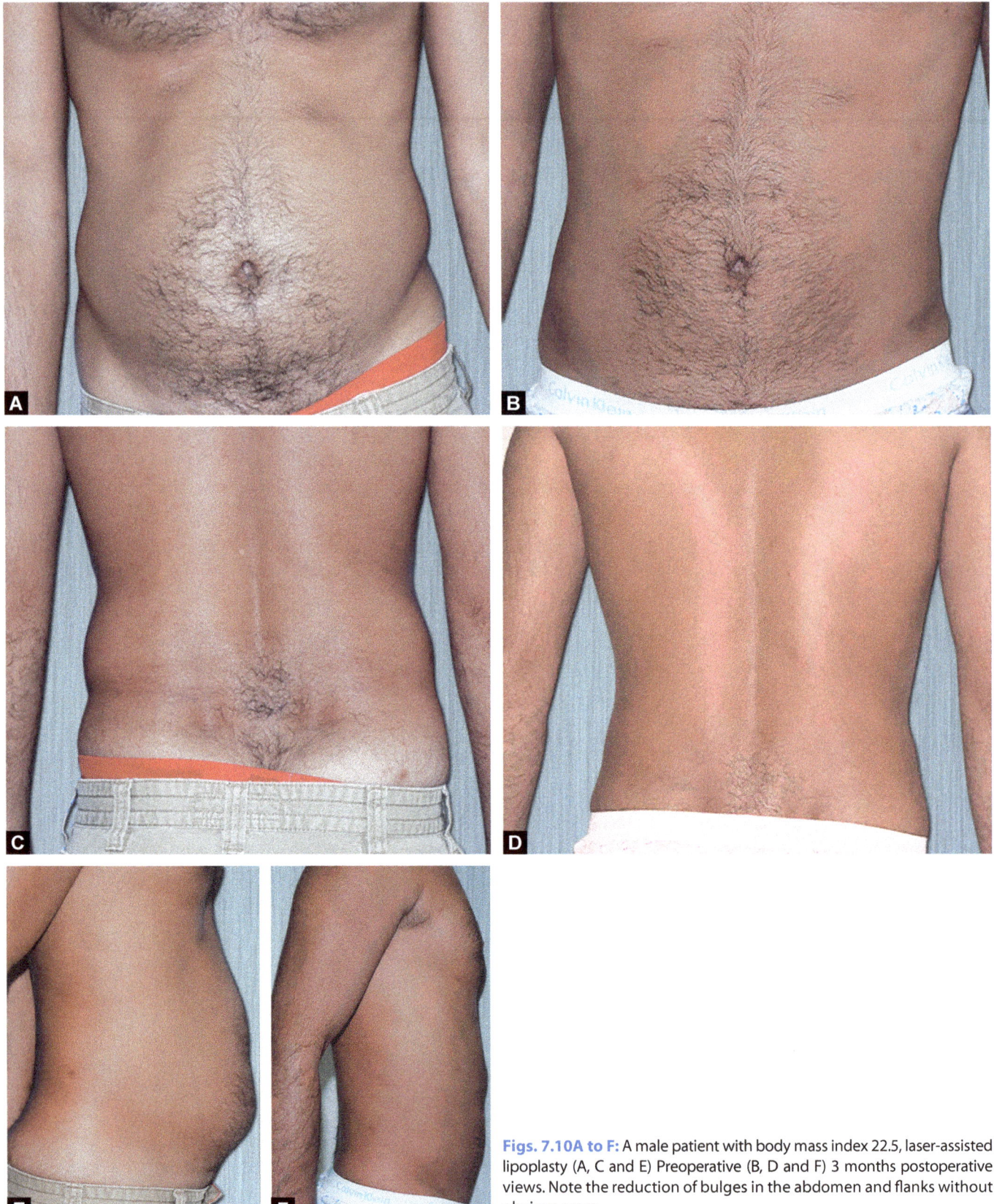

Figs. 7.10A to F: A male patient with body mass index 22.5, laser-assisted lipoplasty (A, C and E) Preoperative (B, D and F) 3 months postoperative views. Note the reduction of bulges in the abdomen and flanks without obvious scars.

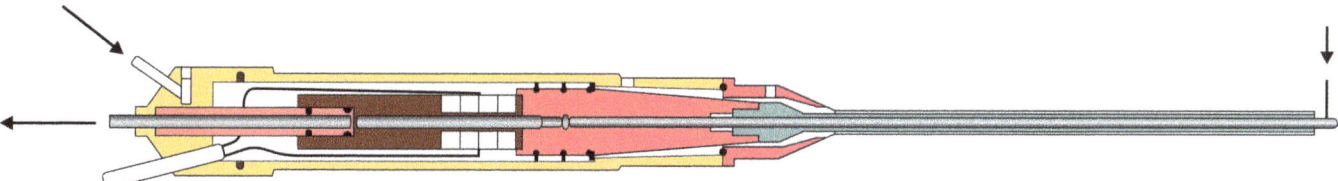

Fig. 7.11: Second-generation ultrasonic-assisted liposuction.

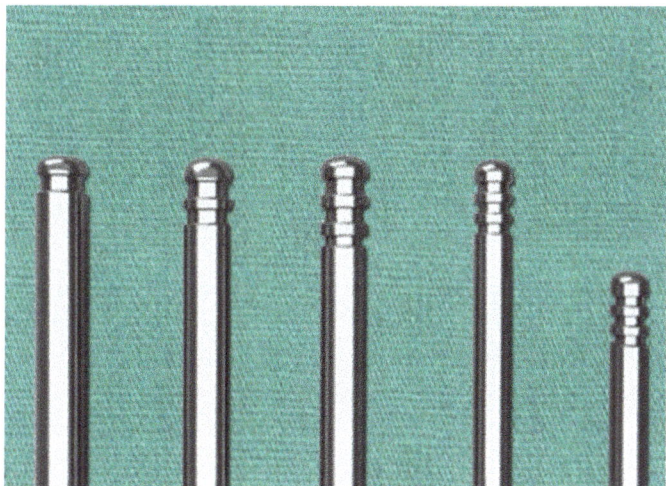

Figs. 7.12: Ultrasonic-assisted liposuction probes.

3. The thermal effect is caused by acoustic waves, cannula friction, and the conversion of the ultrasonic waves into heat as they pass tissue. The heat must be dissipated by tissue infiltration.[10]

The principle of ultrasound was interesting; it is supposed to break down the fat and making it easy to remove. However, the technological limitations of UAL resulted in a high incidence of complications, such as burns, skin necrosis, and scarring.[11]

There were many of improvement in the design of UAL device, including changes in the design of the tips and the development of hollow UAL-integrated probes rather than solid probes, the energy applied to the tissues was still too high for safe use for extended period of time or in proximity to the skin. The second-generation UAL devices had a high heat release to the tissues caused by the high levels of power necessary to make them work efficiently.[11] The hollow probes have a few disadvantages; first, it had less energy inadequate to cause effective emulsification and simultaneous aspiration removes the protective wetting solution increasing the risks to adjacent tissues (Fig. 7.11).

Vibration Amplification of Sound Energy at Resonance (VASER) Lipoplasty

This is the 4th generation UAL technology that has overcome some of the previous problems. The energy applied to the tissues is approximately one quarter that of previous devices and offers both continuous mode and pulsed mode (reduces heat generation).

Vibration amplification of sound energy at resonance uses solid titanium probes with unique rings/grooves; the ring dissipates the energy in all direction (Fig. 7.12). More the number of rings, more is the vibratory energy distributed to the sides of probes and less is the energy emitted through the tip of the probe. A fibrous area that requires high concentrated energy at the tip can be treated with solid probes without any rings. There are thinner probes with three or more rings that can be employed for superficial purpose using pulsed mode. This minimizes the risk of subdermal burns. The bottom line is, the more grooves/rings the more is the emulsification but less is the penetration of fibrous tissue. Smaller diameter penetrates better in fibrous tissue.

The technical specifications of the machine and probes expanded applications of VASER lipoplasty to include treatment of the male and female breast, face and neck; fibrous body areas (trunk and back), and combined excisional body contouring procedures of all types.[12] It is also considered a useful technology to address superficial fat.

The concept of high-definition liposuction as proposed by Hoyos[13] initially used the conventional method to achieve superficial and deep liposuction with excellent results. But the patient experienced very painful and traumatic recovery with burning sensation in the skin for a long time. High-density adipose tissue with excessive fibrous septa was associated with more bleeding due to the avulsion mechanism of conventional liposuction. The VASER enabled emulsification of fat in all the layers and removal of fat using low-power suction (250–400 mm Hg).

This reduces the avulsion trauma of the tissues and the postoperative recovery is better. There is less bruising, sensitivity and better skin draping.

It does require a long learning curve but the ultimate outcome is far superior to that in the past.

Infiltration

Ultrasound requires wetting solution and it cannot function effectively in dry environment and has high risk of burns. Gingrass and Kenkel showed temperature elevations as high as 50°C in experimental models when subcutaneous tissue infiltration was not utilized.[14]

The debate is about the ratio of infiltration and aspiration. In typical tumescent technique with 2:1 infiltration aspiration ratio and the use of VASER-port-closure technique, the incidence of seroma is higher as reported in many publications and personal communications with many surgeons. A wetting solution with 1:1 infiltration aspiration ratio minimizes this risk as I would think.

The technique of infiltration requires a uniform distribution of fluid in superficial, medium, and deep layers of fat. This permits uniform distribution of ultrasonic energy.

Ultrasonic Treatment and Emulsification

Incisions are located in umbilical area (3, 9 and 12 o'clock position) and are 2–4 mm in size depending upon the cannula sizes. Other incisions are located in the groin crease and sub mammary crease. I have stopped using port to minimize the size of incisions; I infiltrate the port site to minimize burn injury. A moist gauze or pack ensures that the port and surrounding skin are protected.

Procedure starts with 60% energy, pulsed mode using three ring cannula of 2.9 mm or 3.7 mm in size. This will give the feel of the texture of fat. Pulsed mode allows safe dissection at superficial level by breaking the superficial cutaneous ligaments.

After few minutes of VASER application using pulsed mode it is switched to continuous mode with higher power going upto 80%. Areas with tough fibrofatty tissue will require no ring or single ring cannula and 100% energy level. This energy level has higher risk of burns either at the tip of cannula if it jabs the skin, at the incision port or where the probe comes in contact with skin proximal to the port.

At the end ultrasound is applied with small and multiring cannula in pulsed mode for superficial emulsification. Differential emulsification is performed in different aesthetic zones of the abdomen. Superficial emulsification may require additional infiltration and precise probe

movement to elevate the skin and disrupt the underlying fibrous connection. This allows better skin contraction and draping. This will also minimize the risk of postinflammatory hyper pigmentation that may be seen with conventional superficial liposuction. Zocchi reports that superficial UAL has 40% more skin retraction than other methods.[15,16] Throughout the superficial movement ensure that the skin temperature does not elevate and there is no dermal penetration with the probe.

The duration of ultrasound application varies in the literature, 1 minute for every 100 or 200 mL of infused soltion.[13] I think it depends upon the amount and density of fat. End point is loss of resistance to the probe. Average time required to do ultrasonic treatment in the abdominal region varies from 10 minutes to 25 minutes.

Postemulsification Liposuction

After the emulsification 3-mm and 4-mm cannulas are employed in a low vacuum pressure setting to remove the fat. The movement of cannula is less aggressive than conventional method but the technique remains the same. After uniformly extracting fat from deep and medium layers, the attention is focused to the "key" aesthetic units of abdomen. A 3 mm cannula is used through 12 o'clock incision of the umbilicus to thin the linea alba area. This is followed by addressing each tendinous insertion of upper rectus aesthetic units. Occasionally you could use small midline incisions to accomplish it. This is mostly performed for male abdomen to enhance the "six-pacs" appearance.

Lateral border of rectus muscle is then differentially suctioned. A thorough liposuction of subcostal areas, and lateral inguinal areas helps us to define abdomen and gives a more sculpted appearance. The technique is similar in men and women except understanding the aesthetic anatomy and expectation of the patient is important to modify the procedure.

Finally superficial liposuction is accomplished until the end point.

Postoperative Compression and Dressing

The incision ports are left open except if the incision appears larger and gaping. We never suture all the wounds, most of the wounds are left open to drain. No drains are used in our practice. A compressive dressing is applied in the first 24-hour period and patients are encouraged to move in the bed and ambulate adequately. In almost all

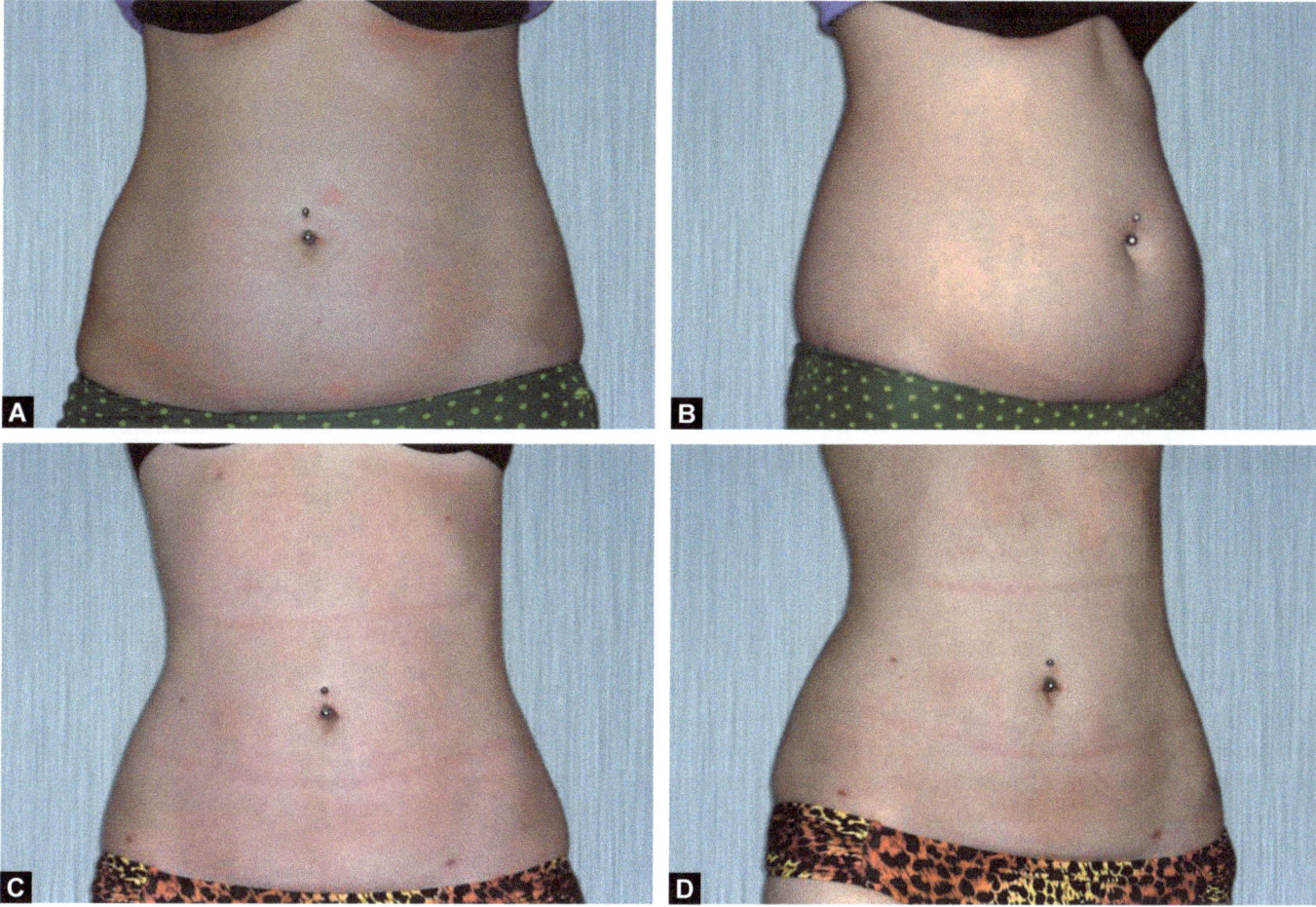

Figs. 7.13A to D: (A and B) Preoperative views (C and D) 1 week postoperative after UAL.

the patients, the drainage stops after 24–36 hours. After that the patients wear a compression garment. We do recommend use of foam under the garment 12 hours a day or night.

The foam has several advantages: additional conforming pressure and splinting of the skin to prevent skin rolling and flexion creases.

Advantages of UAL

1. Easy emulsification of fat and aspiration cause fewer traumas to the tissues.
2. Postoperative healing and recovery is better than conventional liposuction. The results are visible in the first few months (Figs. 7.13A to D).
3. It reduces manual effort of the surgeon particularly in large-volume liposuction.
4. It can be effectively used for secondary or redo liposuction.

5. It has opened newer avenues for high-definition liposuction, and creation of six packs.
6. It has marketing and media advantages.

Disadvantages of UAL

1. Cost of equipment is prohibitive, the cannulas and hand piece are expensive if requires replacement.
2. Heavy equipment cannot be transported.
3. Risks of burns are higher than conventional liposuction.
4. Use of port to the entry site, larger incision that requires closure. It increases the risk of seroma.
5. Long learning curve.

Complications of UAL

It is worth discussing the complications related to UAL in this section. The most common complications are seromas,

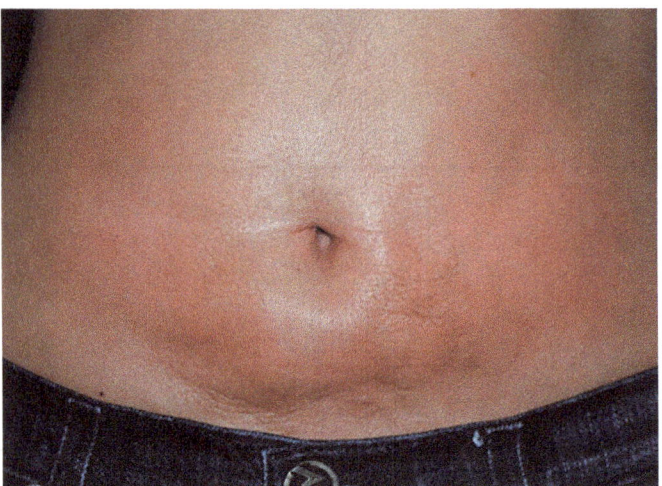

Fig. 7.14: Ultrasonic-assisted liposuction complications: Peau d'orange.

prolonged dysesthesias, burns, induration, contour irregularities, cellulitis, and prolonged swelling.

The seroma incidence reported is 6.5% with VASER and 21.8% with earlier generation UAL.[12] There are some factors[11,14] that have been attributed to it such as tumescent technique as compared to superwet technique, excessive superficial UAL, incision closures, and inadequate number of incisions. In my personal series of more than 250 UAL procedures, I did not experience any seromas.

Many surgeons are now using drains that are left for days. I have my reservation for this approach.

Port skin burns were reported to be 2.94%. It is recommended to use a plastic port to prevent burns.

In my practice, I do not use port at all now; I use at least 10 small incisions at various parts of the abdomen and flanks. Only 3–4 incisions are used for ultrasonic emulsification. I use few small incisions for fat aspiration with 2 mm and 3 mm cannulas only. Using adequate infiltration, applying wet gauge, and avoiding prolonged use of the incision site have been a key to prevent the burns.

Induration and Peau d'orange (Fig. 7.14) appearance can happen if the dermis is penetrated with ultrasonic probe.

Skin necrosis is a very rare complication, but can happen if there is large seroma, excessively tight-fitting garment or over excessive use of ultrasonic energy.

Technical Pearls

In the beginning of your career with UAL, I recommend to start with 70% power and pulsed mode. With experience, the power can be increased to 80 and 90%. In most of the patients, you do not need to go up to 100%, unless it is a secondary liposuction procedure. Using three ring cannula in the beginning will also prevent risks. Always begin with the standard ratio of 1 minute per 100 mL aspiration. You can increase the time of ultrasonic energy based on your experience and requirement of the patient.

There are following purposes of the ultrasonic usage:

1. Skin undermining in the upper abdomen, lower abdomen, waist areas and lumbar areas. This technique allows uniform aspiration of fat and contraction of skin.
2. Emulsification of deep fat particularly above the Scarpa's fascia in the lower abdomen where the fat is more compact. It is also useful for emulsification in upper abdomen, waistline and flanks where the fat is more compact. In my opinion using the ultrasonic device for subscarpal fat is unnecessary and can be a cause of seroma.
3. Subdermal heating to achieve skin contraction. This part is technically more demanding. Excessive heating can cause dermal burns and Peau d'orange appearance of the skin.
4. Creation of "six-pacs" in men by additional use of ultrasonic energy at the linea alba and tendinous intersection for muscular enhancement.

Radiofrequency-Assisted Liposculpturing

This was introduced in 2008 (Invasix, Yokneam, Israel) and it was promoted as BodyLite and BodyTite.

Technology

It consists of a device that has two electrodes, internal and external, connected to a console. Internal electrode is a Teflon-coated cannula that is inserted under the skin. The external electrode is applied to the skin surface.

The electrodes are connected to a radiofrequency (RF)-generating console. The console has settings and display to monitor and control the temperature and adjust power (watts).

The console generates RF and drives an applicator connected to the cannula (with RF emitted from the tip) and the external electrode moves along the surface of the skin. The external electrode receives the ablative RF energy from the internal electrode, and reflects the heat energy in the form of nonablative transepidermal energy for dermal stimulation superficially. The Teflon-coated cannula performs synchronous coagulation and aspiration of the coagulated adipose tissue. The external electrode

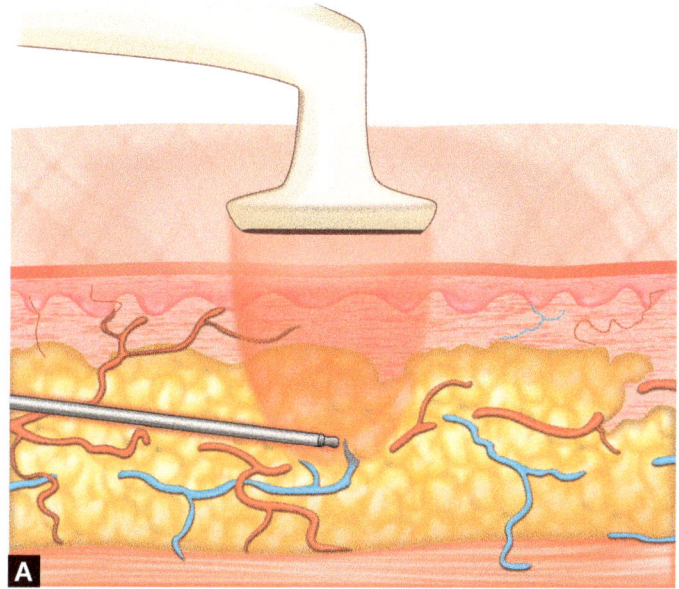

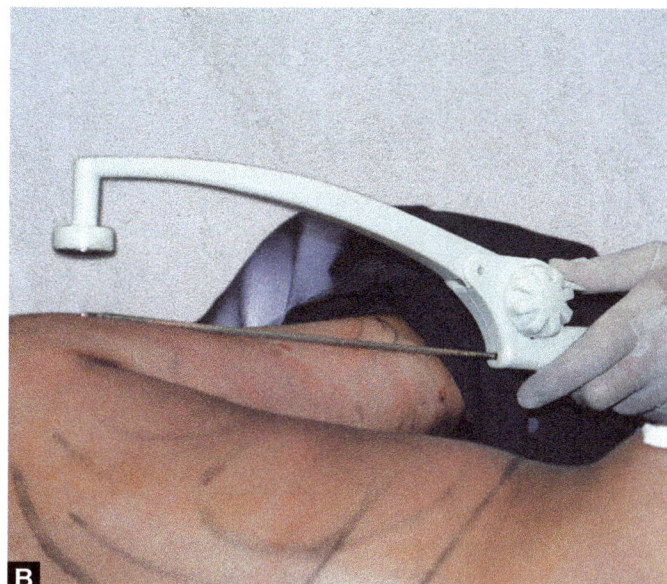

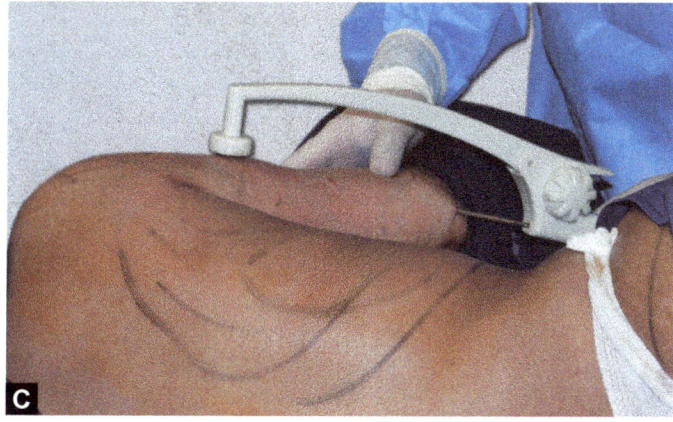

Figs. 7.15A to C: (A) Radiofrequency assisted liposuction (RFAL) mechanism of action, (B) RFAL hand piece with internal and external probe and lever to control the thickness, (C) Cannula in vivo in the arm and the external probe overlying the tip of the cannula.

has temperature thermistors and internal impedance monitoring sensors linked to an online feedback "cutoff" capability in the console. Once a set temperature of 35°C–40°C is achieved the generator stops emitting RF energy, this allows the surgeon to achieve and maintain therapeutic end points and minimizes the risk of thermal injury (Figs. 7.15A to C).

Principle of RFAL

Radiofrequency-assisted liposuction works in the principle of fat liquefaction by RF emission, simultaneous aspiration, and tissue heating for dermal contraction. The technology has significant advantage of generating heat energy that helps in skin contraction and is, therefore, suitable in patients with poor skin tone.

The skin-tightening mechanism is based on the principles explained by Yoshimura.[17] He published that the skin tightening and soft tissue contraction induced by RFAL is due to its effect on the fibroseptal network (FSN) (Figs. 7.16A and B). He showed that > 80% of cells in the region reside in the FSN. Thermal stimulation of the FSN by RF heating has been shown to cause skin surface contraction of up to 45%. The contraction achieved was measured in a study using Vectra computerized measurement system (Canfield Scientific, Inc., Fairfield, NJ, USA) and averaged 34.5% at 1-year post-treatment.[18,19]

Technique of RFAL

Infiltration: This is similar to any other technique of liposuction. The difference is that RFAL works best after the fat and fluid are suctioned out. More the tumescence, more time is required to achieve desired subdermal temperature. This is in contrast to UAL which requires larger volume of infiltration fluid for effective emulsification.

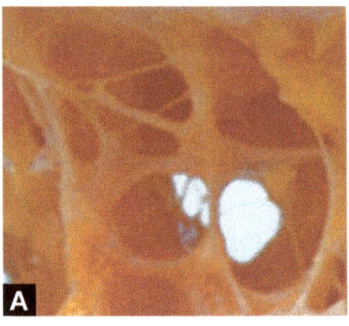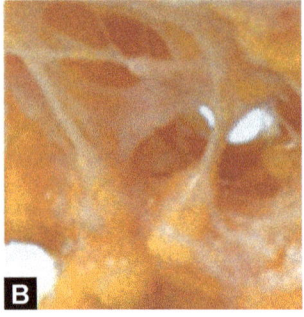

Figs. 7.16A and B: Fibroseptal network. (A) Abdominal tissue treated with suction-assisted liposuction (SAL) alone. (B) Appearance of the same tissue following treatment with radiofrequency heating using the BodyTite device (Invasix, Yokneam, Israel). Note shrinkage of the open regions in all dimensions. Vertical shortening plus contraction in the horizontal and oblique planes is apparent.
Source: Duncan DI. Nonexcisional tissue tightening: creating skin surface area reduction during abdominal liposuction by adding radiofrequency heating. Aesth Surg J. 2013;33(8):1154-66. By permission of Oxford University Press.

SAL and RFAL

The infiltration is followed by conventional SAL. At least 50–60% of the SAL is performed before RFAL cannula is used to heat the tissue. The setting is kept at 35°C–40°C of maximum external heating and power of maximum 40 W. Some centers prefer to start immediately with RFAL after infiltration; I have stopped doing that as the suction is very slow and heating is ineffective. Removing some of the fat and fluid reduces the tissue impedance and allows faster and better heating of the surround tissue and overlying dermal collagen.[19]

If there is improper coupling of the two electrodes, the equipment gives an audible tone and stops working. Maximum temperature setting is 40°C and once temperature is reached, it warns by signaling with different frequencies of audible tone and finally stops automatically. This procedure is carried out slowly so that the desired temperature is reached early, fast movement does not allow enough heat generation.

In vivo studies on soft tissue contraction showed that RFAL-induced temperatures of 69°C applied to the septofascial network can result in a mean 33% contraction, compared with less impressive contraction when the RF thermal stimulus was applied to the dermis or directly to the fat.[19,20]

To achieve an adequate skin contraction in three dimensions, multiple levels of thermal stimulation, from deep to superficial, should be performed.

In situations where excessive skin tightening is required and patient refuses excisional surgery the RFAL can be used in more than one stage to achieve significant skin contraction.

Postoperative Dressings

These are similar to other techniques. However, a word of caution, ensure that there is no evidence of burns or excessive redness. If it is identified it needs to be treated in an appropriate manner. In dark skin even superficial burns due to RFAL, UAL, or LAL can lead to hyperpigmentation at the least.

Complications of RFAL

Seroma: Excessive heating or uncontrolled thermal stimulation at the deep fascial level can increase the risk of seroma, so it is important to keep the RFAL cannula moving continuously as in UAL.

Burns: Superficial heating can cause burn injury to the skin. If there is evidence of excessive redness, then the skin should be cooled with ice cold saline before dressing is applied. If a significant section of skin surface area reduction is needed, two shorter sessions of superficial heating with a maximum external skin temperature of 38°C is safer and will reduce the risk of thermal skin injury.

Disadvantages of RFAL

The cost of the equipment is prohibitive. It is a slow procedure and the skin contraction is directly proportional to amount of time, the probes are used to elevate the skin temperature at multiple levels. There are not enough clinical studies to date, to set a standard protocol to achieve satisfactory result.

Technical Pearls

If you have an opportunity to use RFAL, it is best used after conventional liposuction. The RFAL probe can be used selectively in areas that require maximum skin contraction. The key is to apply radiofrequency energy while withdrawing the cannula. You need to be willing to spend enough time for adequate temperature rise to cause skin contraction.

Power-Assisted Liposuction

There are some nonenergy-based technologies available to help/assist liposuction. These technologies work on the principle of external mechanical power that drives the cannula to move back and forth along with the surgeon's movement. It reduces the surgeon's effort. Historically it was started by Fischer who used CelluTome that contained blades with moving components. Charles Gross used "liposhaver"; William Coleman further improved the designs. But all of the above were traumatic and caused excessive bleeding. Later, it was realized that an oscillating system was more effective that moved the normal cannulas.[21]

High-Power Vibratory Machine: Vibro Liposuction (Euromi, Belgium)

It works with a pneumatic engine triggered by compressed air that endows the cannula with a triple movement: fluctuation, rotation, and vibration.

As a result of these three movements, a helical trajectory is generated, which will emulsify the fat tissue. This tissue will at the same time be aspired by the cannula. The surgeon is required to cautiously and slowly guide the cannula in the layers of the fat.

Advantages

1. It penetrates through the tissue easily therefore less exertional for the surgeon.
2. It allows the removal of larger volume of fat due to less physical effort required.
3. It helps in redo liposuction as the probe can be guided through the tough fibrofatty tissue.
4. Simultaneous suction is possible which is its greatest advantage.
5. Postoperative bruising and pain are less because of less traumatic avulsion as compared to manual liposuction.

Disadvantages

1. It is more expensive than the conventional liposuction set-up.
2. It requires pneumatic motor with at least 6 hp.
3. The vibration causes discomfort to the operator and can cause wrist injury if not used carefully.
4. Vibration reduces the control and perception of the cannula movements and there are anecdotal incidences of deep perforation.
5. It can cause over resection of fat, if it remains in one area as the cannula is continuously moving.
6. It is a noisy apparatus.

7. It cannot be transported as it is a bulky machine and requires pneumatic setup in the OR.
8. It requires focus throughout the use of vibration machine. One still need to do manual liposuction for precision, superficial liposuction, and liposuction in difficult areas of abdomen such as the costal region.

Technical Pearls

In my experience, at some stage of liposuction work you need to depend upon some technology that will reduce your fatigue and increase your efficiency.

Timothy Flynn published that there is an overall 30% increase in the extraction rate in the powered versus the non-powered mode. He mentioned an experienced surgeon can have 45% more fat extracted by PAL than conventional SAL.[22]

If you want to be in the forefront of technologies, you need to have a good relationship with your vendors. Encourage them to lend machines for trial. If you get an opportunity to use this machine, learn the tricks to effectively use it and minimize risks and complications.

Vibrolipo requires a particular method to hold the hand piece between your thumb and fore fingers rather than gripping it all around. This minimizes vibration damages to your hands. A slow movement with constant control of the tip of the machine prevents inadvertent penetration of muscles. A continuous gentle movement allows uniform liposuction in a short period of time. At the end, do spend some time using manual liposuction and finer cannulas to feather and perform superficial liposuction if required.

Low-Power Vibration (Microaire PAL, Virginia, USA)

It works on the same principle as VibroLipo but with 2 mm reciprocating stroke at 4,000 cycles per minute as compared to Vibrolipo with 6 mm cannula movement and above 5,500 cycles per minute. This is an electrical-driven technology.

Advantages

1. It is more efficient than manual liposuction and reduces the surgeons effort.
2. It is less traumatic than manual liposuction.
3. Simultaneous suction is possible.
4. It is a small machine and easy to carry to different hospitals.

Disadvantages

1. It is more expensive than conventional liposuction set-up.
2. It is slower and can be time consuming.

Water-Jet-Assisted Liposuction

This method uses pressurized fluid to dislodge the fat cells and then suction out using specially designed cannulas.

Technique

After the incision in the skin and introduction of cannula water jet is infused in the fatty tissue the pressure of which is controlled by a foot paddle. The fluid used is similar to the tumescent solution.

The high-pressure jet fragments the fat that is simultaneously suctioned out. The cannula is moved slowly in a fan-shaped manner to uniformly dislodge the fat cells. The pressure of the jet can be adjusted to feather the margins of the area treated.

Ahmed Ziah Taufig[21,23] published that this method has several advantages. It is a single-step procedure where infiltration and suction are performed at the same time and as the fluid is immediately aspirated out there is less lidocaine retained in the tissue minimizing the lidocaine toxicity. There is minimal postoperative leakage and risk of seroma.

This is a fairly new technology and has many questions unanswered.

▌ REFERENCES

1. DiBernardo BE. Randomized, blinded split abdomen study evaluating skin shrinkage and skin tightening in laser assisted liposuction versus liposuction control. Aesthet Surg J. 2010; 30:593-602.
2. Fischer G. History of my procedure, the harpstring technique and the sterile fat safety box. In: Fournier, P (Ed). Liposculpture: The Syringe Technique. Paris: Arnette; 1991. pp. 9-17.
3. Saylan Z. Liposhifting: treatment of postliposuction irregularities. Int J Cosm Surg. 1999;7(1):71-3.
4. Prado A, Andrades P, Danilla S, et al. A prospective, randomized, double-blind, controlled clinical trial comparing laser-assisted lipoplasty with suction-assisted lipoplasty. Plast Reconstr Surg. 2006;118(4):1032-45.
5. Goldman A, Gotkin RH. Laser-assisted liposuction. Clin Plast Surg. 2009;36:241-53, vii; discussion 255-60.
6. Kim KH, Geronemus RG. Laser lipolysis using a novel 1,064 nm Nd:YAG laser. Dermatol Surg. 2006;32:241-8; discussion 247.
7. Reynaud JP, Skibinski M, Wassmer B, et al. Lipolysis using a 980-nm diode laser: a retrospective analysis of 534 procedures. Aesth Plast Surg. 2009;33:28-36.
8. Di Bernardo BE, Reyes J, Chen B. Evaluation of tissue thermal effects from 1064/1320-nm laser-assisted lipolysis and their clinical implications. J Cosm Laser Ther. 2009;11:62-9.
9. Sasaki GH. Quantification of human abdominal tissue tightening and contraction after component treatments with 1064-nm/1320-nm laser-assisted lipolysis: clinical implications. Aesthet Surg J. 2010;30:239-45.
10. Fakhouri TM, El Tal AK, Abrou AE, et al. Laser-assisted lipolysis: a review. Dermatol Surg. 2012;38:155-69.
11. Graf R1, Auersvald A, Damasio RC. Ultrasound-assisted liposuction: an analysis of 348 cases. Aesth Plast Surg. 2003; 27:146-53.
12. Jewell ML, Fodor PB, Souza Pinto EB, et al. Clinical application of VASER-assisted lipoplasty: a pilot clinical study. Aesth Surg J. 2002;22(2):131-46.
13. Hoyos AE. High definition liposculpture. Presented in the XIII International Course of Plastic Surgery, Bucaramanga, Colombia, 2003.
14. de Souza Pinto EB1, Abdala PC, Maciel CM, et al. Liposuction and VASER, Clin Plastic Surg. 2006;33:107-15.
15. Gingrass M, Kenkel J. Comparing ultrasound-assisted lipoplasty with suction-assisted lipoplasty. Clin Plast Surg. 1999; 26:283.
16. Zocchi ML. Ultrasonic-assisted lipoplasty. Technical refinements and clinical evaluations. Clin Plast Surg. 1996;23:575.
17. Duncan DI. Nonexcisional tissue tightening: creating skin surface area reduction during abdominal liposuction by adding radiofrequency heating. Aesth Surg J. 2013;33(8): 1154-66.
18. Paul M, Blugerman G, Kreindel M, et al. Three-dimensional radiofrequency tissue tightening: a proposed mechanism and applications for body contouring. Aesthetic Plast Surg. 2011; 35(1):87-95.
19. Hurwitz D, Smith D Treatment of overweight patients by radiofrequency-assisted liposuction (RFAL) for aesthetic reshaping and skin tightening. Aesthetic Plast Surg. 2012; 36(1):62-71.
20. Paul M, Mulholland SR A new approach for adipose tissue treatment and body contouring using radiofrequency-assisted liposuction. Aesthetic Plast Surg.2009;33(5):687-694
21. Shiffman MA, Di Guseppe A. Liposuction Principles and Practice. Berlin, Germany: Springer-Verlag; 2006.
22. Flynn TC. Powered liposuction: an evaluation of currently available instrumentation. Dermatol Surg. 2002;28(5): 376-82.
23. Taufig AZ. Hydro-jet-liposuction: a new method for liposuction. Presented at Vereinigung der Deutschen Plastischen Chirurgen meeting, Cologne, Germany, September, 2000.

CHAPTER 8

Preoperative Analysis and Protocol

INTRODUCTION

After the consultation and initial clinical evaluation, the next step is thorough preoperative analysis and establishing the safety protocol for a successful outcome.

For a successful body-contouring surgery it is important to follow a standard protocol. This helps to ensure nothing is missed out and it gives uniformity to the system. The protocol can be customized to fit your practice; it can be improved with time, and it becomes a common language for the entire unit.

Most surgical procedures are performed in one of three settings[1]: hospitals, free standing ambulatory surgery centers, or office-based surgery facilities. The office-based surgery setting, in particular, has many advantages including greater control over the schedule, greater privacy for the patient, convenience, and more economical to both surgeons and patients.

But there is little scientific evidence available on patient's safety issues and even less than that specifically addresses liposuction performed in the office-based surgery setting. The published materials available focus more on the techniques and complications rather than on the provision of safe care.

We should have a strategy to manage our patients safely and provide the best outcome possible. Protocol list that I follow in my organization includes the following:
1. Patient medical history.
2. Preoperative instructions.
3. Preoperative worksheet and planning.
4. American Society of Anesthesiologists (ASA) risk assessment.
5. Thromboembolic prevention protocol.
6. Postoperative instructions.
7. Consent forms.

DOCUMENTATION

Patient Medical History (Form 8.1)

Sometimes patients forget to narrate all the medical history or may not find it necessary to narrate it to the surgeon during the first consultation. Some patients deny about the medical history, For example, I had a patient who on

---

Form 8.1: Past Medical History (PMH)

Patient Name: _____ Date of Birth: _____ File No. _____

Your appointment for surgery will be canceled if this form has not been completed and returned 3 weeks prior to the date of procedure.

Aesthetic surgery has risks and complications like any other surgery. In order to minimize these, it is important to give accurate and full information about your medical history and status of health.

1. Describe your past medical history. _____
   _____
2. Have you undergone any surgical procedures?　　　　Yes ☐　　No ☐
   If yes, please specify and give dates: _____
3. Have you undergone any cosmetic surgical procedures?　　Yes ☐　　No ☐
   If yes, please specify and give dates: _____
   _____
4. Have you had General Anesthesia?　　Yes ☐　　No ☐

Contd...

Contd...

5. Have you had Local Anesthesia? Yes ☐ No ☐

6. Did you have any problems with the Anesthesia, Surgery or Recovery period? Yes ☐ No ☐
   Adverse effect to any anesthetic or surgery (If so, please specify)_____

   ____Angina

   ____Blood Clots in Legs

   ____Heart Attack

   ____Pacemaker (cardiac)

   ____Pulmonary Embolism

   ____Stroke

   ____Congestive Heart Failure

   ____Cancer

   ____Asthma

   ____Frequent Pneumonia

   ____Diabetes

   ____Hepatitis

   ____Jaundice (skins turns yellow)

   ____High Blood Pressure

   ____Bronchitis

   ____Easy Bruising Tendency

   ____Prolonged Bleeding

   ____Recurrent Infections

   ____Poor Wound Healing

   ____Keloids

   ____Heart Rhythm Disturbances

   ____Blood Disorder

7. Are you allergic to any medication? Yes ☐ No ☐
   If Yes, Please mention the name/s of medication: _____
   Please check any medications (s) which you are allergic to:

   ____Aspirin

   ____Codeine

   ____Demerol

   ____Erythromycin

   ____Ketamine

   ____Lidocaine

   ____Morphine

   ____Neosporin ointment

   ____Penicillin

   ____Sulfa

   ____Marcaine

   ____Tetracycline

   ____Tylenol

   ____Valium

   Other medication (specify) _____
   Are you allergic to?
   _____Adhesive tape _____Iodine

8. Have you ever suffered from?
   Heart condition Yes ☐ No ☐
   Kidney condition Yes ☐ No ☐
   Liver condition Yes ☐ No ☐
   Eye condition Yes ☐ No ☐
   Dryness ☐ Discharge ☐ Glaucoma ☐
   Any other eye complains? _____

9. Have you ever been diagnosed as having Hepatitis A, B, or C? Yes ☐ No ☐
   If yes, describe when you were diagnosed, where, and by whom _____

10. Have you been tested for HIV virus? Yes ☐ No ☐
    If yes, what was the result of the test? _____
    Current Health Status

1. Mention all the medications and pills you are taking with dosage and duration:

2. Do you have any ongoing chronic conditions?
   ☐ Diabetes ☐ Hypertension ☐ Asthma ☐ Others

3. Are you undergoing any emotional stress? Yes ☐ No ☐
   If yes, please describe: _____

4. Briefly state why you are seeking a plastic surgery consultation: _____
   Please state why you would like to have your particular disorder corrected: _____
   Do you have any specific concerns about any contemplated operation? _____
   Please mention current weight: _____ height: _____

5. Has your weight increased or decreased a lot in the last year? Yes ☐ No ☐

6. How do you rate your tolerance to pain/discomfort?
   Please encircle:
   Very low Low Fair High Very High

Contd...

Contd...

7.	Do you have any bleeding or other blood disorders? Yes ☐ No ☐
	If yes, name the disorder and describe any treatment you have undergone: _____
8.	Do you smoke? Yes ☐ No ☐
	If yes, since when? _____
	How often _____
	Sticks per day _____
9.	Do you consume alcoholic beverages? Yes ☐ No ☐
	If yes, state how may units of alcohol you drink per day (One unit = half a glass of beer, one single shot of spirits, or one glass of wine): _____
	Only for Females
	When was your last menstrual period? _____
	Are you on any oral contraceptives? Yes ☐ No ☐
	Are you pregnant? Yes ☐ No ☐
	If you feel there is anything else of relevance to your medical history that we should know please use this sheet to tell us about it.
	Please give us the date and month you prefer to have the procedure _____
	Signed _____ **Date** _____
	Please fax this document to _____, Hand over to the staff of the clinic or email it to _____

asking about his health, said "I am very healthy Doc!" On leading questions he said, "Oh, I am just taking this pill to reduce my blood pressure and sometimes I take a tablet to reduce my blood sugar." He went on and said, "I take aspirin because the doctor said it is good for my heart after I had angioplasty last year." So, it was now obvious that he is hypertensive, diabetic with a previous cardiac history.

A medical history form consists of detailed leading questions that patients should fill out. They will come forward if they do not understand any part of it. An example of such a form is attached and it can be modified to suit your practice. This also serves as a legal document if the patient does not reveal any medical history that may comprise the surgical outcome.

Preoperative Instructions (Form 8.2)

Once the surgery is planned, provide a detail written instruction to the patients so that they are aware of do's and don'ts.

A successful surgery requires proper planning and necessary precautions. A clear written instructions well in advance psychologically prepares, the patient for the surgery. It also means that it is a significant event that requires commitment by the patient. This may avoid patients who deny the seriousness of the procedure and think of it as insignificant.

There are often many questions in patient's mind, sometime they are reluctant to call the surgeon or office.

In many occasions patient forget oral instructions and some important advice such as "Nil by Mouth" may be overlooked.

The preparation starts 3 weeks in advance particularly in smokers who need to stop smoking prior to the surgery. This is also the time they need to schedule there days off from work and make necessary arrangements for their after-care.

Two weeks prior to the surgery, they need to stop medications that can cause blood thinning or interfere with intraoperative medications. This will minimize excessive bleeding, bruising and other side effects due to drug interactions. It is preferred that patient buys all their prescription well in advance to avoid last minute running around particularity the first postoperative day, if they are discharged on the same day. There are incidences of patient having vaso-vagal attacks standing in a pharmacy waiting for their prescription in the postoperative period. A preoperative visit is planned within two weeks to review, the surgical plan and recent changes in their medical history. This is the time when all medical records, photography, documentation and informed consent are prepared.

One week prior to the surgery ensure the patient has properly fitting pressure garment. They are advised that they may need an additional garment of smaller size as the swelling subsides.

It is preferable to have few options to get the correct fitting. The day prior to surgery they need to be reminded about fasting and antiseptic preparation.

Form 8.2: Presurgery Instructions: Abdominal Contouring by Liposuction

Patient Name: _____Date: _____

Surgical Facility: _____Surgery Date: _____

Arrival Time: _____

A successful surgery requires proper planning and necessary precautions. Please go through the details to understand how to prepare for your procedure.

Three Weeks or More before Surgery

There may be several weeks between your decision to have surgery and your actual surgical date. During that time, there are several important considerations:

Practice proper fitness. Stretching exercises and low-weight strength training now can help to enhance your posture and your strength in the weeks following surgery.

Good nutrition. Eat well during the weeks prior to surgery. Crash dieting, overeating or high alcohol intake can greatly affect your overall health and well-being. Also, begin taking the following supplements daily_____.

Stop smoking. Smoking can greatly impair your ability to heal. You must be nicotine and smoke free for at least 4 weeks prior to surgery. You must also be free of any nicotine patch or nicotine-based products for a minimum of 4 weeks prior to surgery.

Lead a healthy lifestyle. A lingering cold, virus or other illness can result in your surgery being rescheduled. Make certain to address any illness immediately, and advise our office of any serious illness or change in your health.

Prepare and plan. Schedule any time off of work, and any support you will need at home in the days following surgery. Make certain a responsible adult is enlisted and confirmed to drive you to and from surgery, and that one is confirmed available to stay with you around the clock for 24 hours, at least, following surgery.

Preoperative testing. Make certain to schedule all of the preoperative testing and clearance you have been given. Make certain all test results are received by the doctor.

Two to Three Weeks before Surgery

This is an important planning and preparation time. Follow all of the good health habits you have begun in addition to the following:

Prepare and plan. Put your schedule together for the day before, day of and first few days following the surgery. Share this with all of your key support people

Fill your prescriptions. Some pain medication prescriptions may need to be filled on the day these prescriptions are written. Our office will advise you accordingly. Your prescriptions include:

Antibiotic:

Pain medication:

Muscle Relaxant:

Other:

Supplements:

STOP taking the following for the duration before your surgery. Taking any of the following can increase your risk of bleeding and other complications:

☐ Aspirin and medications containing aspirin ☐ Garlic supplements

☐ Ibuprofen and anti-inflammatory agents ☐ Green tea or green tea extracts

☐ Vitamin E ☐ Estrogen supplements

☐ St. John's Wort ☐ All other medications indicated

Preoperative clearance and information. If they have not been completed and results filed with our office make certain to undergo all preoperative testing. Make certain that all test results are received by the doctor.

Vital information. A preoperative visit or call is essential to review your health, your goals, and any vital information including allergies and health considerations.

Your preoperative (visit)(call) is scheduled for:_____

Fitness. Do not overdo it. Avoid anything strenuous or that could potentially cause injury.

Good nutrition. Continue taking your supplements as directed.

Contd...

Contd...

NO SMOKING. Stay away from second-hand smoke, too. Your healing and health depend heavily on this.

Lead a healthy lifestyle. Practice good hand washing and avoid risk catching a virus or cold.

Avoid sun exposure. Sun damaged skin can more readily produce irregular scars or cause pigmentation irregularities following surgery.

One Week before Surgery

Confirm your day of surgery plans. This includes your transportation and after-care (a responsible adult for the first 24 hours, around the clock).

Review your prescription orders and instructions.

Purchase ointment as recommended.

Purchase any compression garments required. You may wish to purchase more than one garment for laundering purposes.

Confirm all lab results and paperwork have been received by the doctor.

Continue to practice healthy habits, nutrition and fitness. No strenuous exercise. No saunas, hot tubs, steam baths or mud wraps. No smoking or alcohol.

Find your comfort zone. Locate the most comfortable place where you can gently recline and recover. You do not want to be testing locations or pillows the day of surgery. Shop for magazines, books and other things to keep you busy and entertained in the day or two following surgery.

Wax or shave your bikini area and legs. It may be uncomfortable to do so in the days immediately after surgery.

One Day before Surgery

Pack your bag for the day of surgery. This should include:

- ☐ All paperwork
- ☐ Your identification
- ☐ All prescription medications
- ☐ Reading glasses
- ☐ Warm, clean cotton socks
- ☐ Saltines or other crackers in case of nausea during your ride home

Expect a pre-anesthesia call to review your state of health and anesthesia for surgery.

Confirm your route to and from surgery or the recovery center, with the responsible adult who will drive you. Also confirm plans with your 24-hour support person and make certain he or she has all of your postoperative instructions.

Shower as directed. Use an antibacterial, fragrance-free soap. Shampoo your hair. Do not use any hair gel or other styling products, scented skin creams or moisturizers. Do not use any deodorant, hair spray, perfume or cosmetics. Remove all finger nail and toe nail polish.

Do not eat or drink anything 8 hours prior to time of surgery. No candy, gum or mints. Anything more than a small amount of water as needed for brushing teeth or swallowing medication may result in the need to cancel surgery.

RELAX! Get plenty of rest and avoid unnecessary stress.

The Day of Surgery

NOTHING by mouth. Anything more than a small amount of water as needed for brushing teeth or swallowing medication may result in the need to cancel surgery. This includes candy, gum, mints.

Dress appropriately.

Do not wear cosmetics, jewelry of any kind, contact lenses, hair clips, body piercing. If there is something you cannot remove, let the admitting nurse know right away.

Wear comfortable, clean, loose-fitting clothing. Do not wear jeans or any tight-fitting bottom. You may wear a robe. Wear slip on, flat shoes with a slip-proof sole; no heels. Wear clean cotton socks, as the operating room can feel cool. For your comfort, wear a zip or button front top. No turtlenecks.

I have read and understand all of the above instructions. I understand that following these instructions is solely my responsibility. I understand that it is also my responsibility to ask my doctor and his or her staff any questions. I have related to these instructions or about my procedure, health and healing.

Patient Signature _____   Date _____

Printed Name of the Patient _____

Signature of the Practice
Representative and the Witness

Preoperative Worksheet and Planning (Form 8.3)

A systematic examination is carried out to understand the distribution of fat, skin elasticity, and musculoskeletal structure of the torso in a manner that covers all the aesthetic zones of the abdomen. The details are documented as in the form provided. This ensures that we do not miss out irregularities or asymmetries that may or may not be corrected.

Repeated examination in a systematic pattern as shown in Form 8.3 allows to train our mind to examine the patient before and after the surgery. Junior colleagues are encouraged to practice this protocol. This has significant importance in postoperative period to assess the outcome and understand the behavior of the skin in different regions of the abdomen.

ASA Risk Assessment (Table 8.1)

The ASA's classification is a rating system of physical status based on systemic disease. It is useful to follow this system in each and every patient undergoing surgery. This will improve the outcome, increase patient safety, and ensures medicolegal medicolegal safety for the surgeon.

ASA I is a fit patient with no underlying systemic disease and not taking any medications. ASA II is a patient with a mild systemic disease, i.e. slightly limiting organic heart disease, mild diabetes, essential hypertension or anemia, obesity, chronic bronchitis, or any healthy individual under 1 year or over 70 years age. Chronic smokers and alcoholics come under this category.

ASA III is a patient with a systemic disease or multiple significant mild systemic diseases, organic heart diseases,

---

Form 8.3: Presurgery Worksheet: Abdominal Liposuction

Patient Name: _____ Date: _____

Surgical Facility: _____ Surgery Date: _____ OR (Operating room) Booked: _____ Hours: _____ Time: _____

    Overnight Stay: _____ ☐ Yes ☐ No   Confirmed: _____

_____ Anesthesia   ☐ Consent Signed (date)   ☐ Ordered

_____ Allergies

_____ Health Alert

_____ Smoker   ☐ Yes   ☐ No

_____ HIV   ☐ Consent   ☐ Yes   ☐ No

_____ Photos   ☐ Consent   ☐ Yes   ☐ No

_____ Imaging   ☐ Consent   ☐ Yes   ☐ No

_____ Payment   ☐ Received   Date: _____   ☐ Not yet received

_____ Insurance   ☐ Yes   ☐ No   ☐ Pre-cert authorized

_____ Informed Consent   ☐ Signed   Date: _____

_____ Medical Clearance   ☐ Ordered   ☐ Received (date)

_____ Labs

☐ HCG	☐ PT/PTT	☐ EKG
☐ CBC (with differential)	☐ Platelet function analysis	☐ Chest X-ray
☐ CMG	☐ Liver functions (SGOT, SGPT, Alk Phos)	☐ Medical clearance
☐ HIV (consent of file)	☐ Thyroid	
☐ Chem panel	☐ HCG-qualitative	
☐ Electrolytes	☐ Urine analysis	
☐ SMA-7	☐ Stress test	

_____ **Prescriptions**

Antibiotic _____   _____ mg   _____ × per day

Pain medication _____   _____ mg   _____ × per day

Muscle relaxant _____   _____ mg   _____ × per day

Other _____   _____

Supplements _____   _____

Mark the concerned areas:

Contd...

Contd...

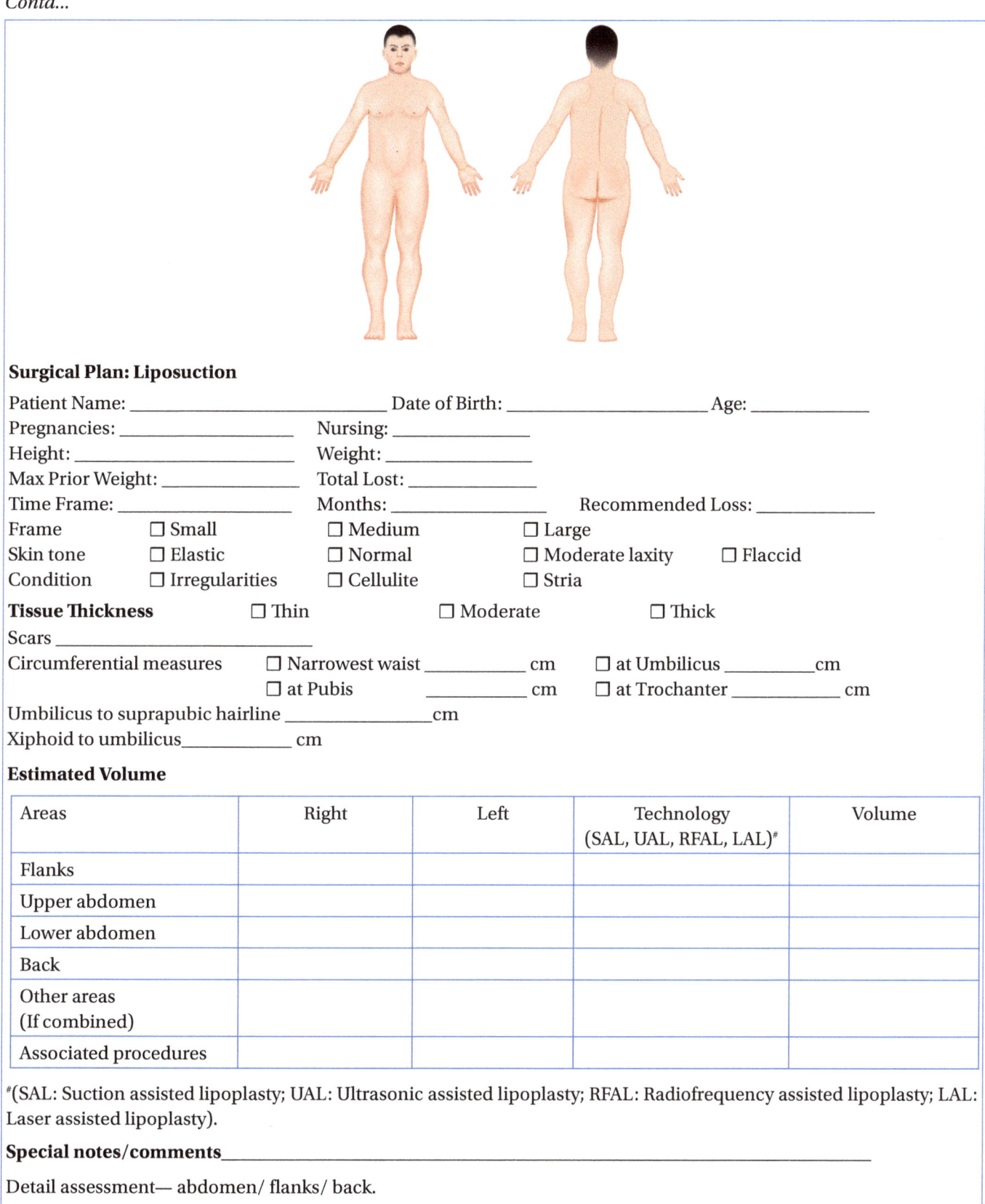

Surgical Plan: Liposuction

Patient Name: _____ Date of Birth: _____ Age: _____

Pregnancies: _____   Nursing: _____

Height: _____   Weight: _____

Max Prior Weight: _____   Total Lost: _____

Time Frame: _____   Months: _____   Recommended Loss: _____

Frame   ☐ Small   ☐ Medium   ☐ Large

Skin tone   ☐ Elastic   ☐ Normal   ☐ Moderate laxity   ☐ Flaccid

Condition   ☐ Irregularities   ☐ Cellulite   ☐ Stria

Tissue Thickness   ☐ Thin   ☐ Moderate   ☐ Thick

Scars _____

Circumferential measures   ☐ Narrowest waist _____ cm   ☐ at Umbilicus _____cm

                             ☐ at Pubis   _____ cm   ☐ at Trochanter _____ cm

Umbilicus to suprapubic hairline _____cm

Xiphoid to umbilicus_____ cm

Estimated Volume

Areas	Right	Left	Technology (SAL, UAL, RFAL, LAL)#	Volume
Flanks				
Upper abdomen				
Lower abdomen				
Back				
Other areas (If combined)				
Associated procedures				

#(SAL: Suction assisted lipoplasty; UAL: Ultrasonic assisted lipoplasty; RFAL: Radiofrequency assisted lipoplasty; LAL: Laser assisted lipoplasty).

Special notes/comments_____

Detail assessment— abdomen/ flanks/ back.

Contd...

Contd...

Assessment standing position	Findings	Patient concern	Remark
Frontal: Skin			
Tone			
Creases			
Scars/stretch marks/pigmentation			
Umbilicus			
Fat deposits			
Upper abdomen			
Lower abdomen			
Lumpiness/cellulite			
Musculoskeletal			
Muscle tone			
Hernia			
Rib cage/pelvis			
Lateral: Skin			
Creases/folds			
Scars/stretch marks/ pigmentation			
Fat deposits			
Waist line			
Flanks			
Bra roll			
Lumpiness/cellulite			
Musculoskeletal			
Oblique muscles			
Lumbar area			
Hernia			
Posterior area: Skin			
Creases/folds/pigmentations			
Fat deposits			
Paravertebral			
Lumbar area			
Sacral			

Table 8.1: American Society of Anesthesiologists' classification.*

I	Healthy patient, no medical problems
II	Mild systemic disease
III	Severe systemic disease, but not incapacitating
IV	Severe systemic disease that is a constant threat to life
V	Moribund, not expected to live 24 hours irrespective of operation
VI	Donor patient for organ harvesting

*ASA description (ASA: American Society of Anesthesiologist).

severe diabetes with vascular complications, moderate-to-severe degrees of pulmonary insufficiency, angina pectoris, or healed myocardial infarction.

ASA IV is a patient with organic heart disease showing marked signs of cardiac insufficiency, persistent anginal syndrome, active myocarditis, advanced degrees of pulmonary, hepatic, renal, or endocrine insufficiency.

Patients with ASA I and II are candidates for ambulatory and office-based surgical procedures; type III patients are candidates for an office-based procedures with local anesthesia (with or without sedation); and type IV patients are only candidates for office-based operations with local anesthesia and without sedation.[2]

Thromboembolic Risk Assessment Protocol (Form 8.4)

The term venous thromboembolism refers to a spectrum of disease that includes deep venous thrombosis and pulmonary embolism.[3] They are often clinically silent and therefore difficult to diagnose. An acute incidence can be very fatal. Hence it is important to prevent this problem. Certain factors are known to increase the risk of venous thromboembolism. Based on these factors, risk category is assigned to the patient. A thorough history and review of the patient's medications are essential for detecting and assigning risk. Caprini et al. along with recommendations of American College of Chest Physicians streamlined a protocol to prevent this complication.[4]

It is important to discuss these details with the patient and inform the patient of his or her risk category and prevention method that you propose.

Low-risk group consists of healthy patients having outpatient surgery. Moderate-risk group patients have up to four risk factors mentioned in the list and who require hospitalization. High-risk group have more than four risk factors. Prophylaxis depends upon the category of risks. Low-risk patients require comfortable position in the OR with knees flexed by using pillows. Moderate-risk group additionally requires intermittent pneumatic compression device starting before the induction of anesthesia and continuing until patient is ambulatory. High-risk category require the same measures as above and low-molecular-weight heparin 2 hours before surgery and daily until patient is ambulatory.[5]

Postoperative Instructions (Form 8.5)

The patients are given postoperative instruction sheet at the time of preoperative visit so they can understand what it involves and how to be prepared. Patients are not aware of what they will go through, not only immediately post-surgery but in long term. Giving them an idea of what to expect in future helps them to improve their lifestyle to maintain result for longer period of time.

Form 8.4: Thromboembolic Risk Assessment Protocol

Patient's Full Name: _____ File No:_____

Procedure: _____ Date:_____

DVT Prevention Protocol

Risk factors include:

_____Major surgery		_____Erythropoiesis	
_____Trauma		_____Paroxysmal	
_____Nocturnal hemoglobinuria			
_____Immobility of lower extremities		_____Medications	
_____Cancer (excluding skin)		_____Myeloproliferative disorders	
_____Cancer therapy (chemo/radiation)		_____Obesity	
_____Venous insufficiency		_____Central venous access	
_____Family history		_____Nephrotic syndrome	
_____Age above 40 years old		_____Inflammatory bowel disease	
_____Pregnancy		_____Acute medical illness	
_____Oral contraceptives		_____Selective estrogen receptor	
_____Hormone replacement			

Risk group:

_____Low risk. Healthy patients having outpatient surgery.

_____Moderate risk. Patients with zero to four risk factors, surgery requiring admission and recovery in the hospital.

_____High risk: Patients with more than four risk factors, having surgery requiring admission and recovery in the hospital.

Contd...

Contd...

Low risk	General or regional anesthesia procedure lasting less than 1 hour or sedation procedure less than 2 hours	Proper positioning and early ambulation ☐
	General or regional anesthesia procedure lasting more than 1 hour or sedation procedure more than 2 hours	IPC (Intermittent Pneumatic Compression Devices) ☐ VFT (Venous Foot Pumps) ☐
Moderate risk	Normal risk of bleeding and 3–4 risk factors	Enoxaparin 30 mg subcutaneousdaily. First dose given 12-hour postop ☐
	High risk of bleeding or 0–2 risk factors	IPC (Intermittent Pneumatic Compression Devices) ☐ VFT (Venous Foot Pumps) ☐
High risk	Normal risk of bleeding	Enoxaparin 40 mg subcutaneous daily. First dose given 12-hour postop ☐ IPC (Intermittent Pneumatic Compression Devices ☐ VFT (Venous Foot Pumps) ☐
	High risk of bleeding	IPC (Intermittent Pneumatic Compression Devices ☐ VFT (Venous Foot Pumps) ☐

Thromboprophylaxis Orders

Reducing the Risk While Travelling

Deep vein thrombosis can occur in passengers in any seating class of an aircraft. It can also happen to people on long rides in cars, trains, or buses.

A 2-hour flight would not be a problem, but a 12-hour flight would be "a big problem" if a person sits inactive the entire time.

It is important for passengers to keep moving their legs to help the blood flow, even when waiting in the airport terminal. Another way to help move blood to the heart is to wear compression stockings, which put gentle pressure on the leg muscles. Studies have shown that wearing compression stockings minimizes the risk of developing DVT after long flights.

Avoid regular socks with very tight elastic bands at the top and sitting with your legs crossed for long periods of time, which constricts the veins. Travelers who cannot walk around frequently are advised to exercise their legs by curling or pressing the toes down, which causes the muscles to contract and squeeze on the leg veins, helping to pump the blood along.

It is also advisable to drink plenty of fluids to prevent dehydration. Dehydration causes blood vessels to narrow and blood to thicken, increasing the risk for DVT. Reducing alcohol and coffee consumption, which both contribute to dehydration, is also recommended.

Form 8.5: Post-Surgery Instructions: Liposuction

Patient Name: _____   Date: _____

                                            Surgery Date: _____

Once your surgery is completed, you must follow all the instructions given to you in order to heal properly and have a good outcome. The following instructions are your obligation.

Typical Postoperative Symptoms

Typical symptoms of liposuction and signs to watch for after liposuction include the following:

Contd...

Contd...

Tightness and stiffness in treated areas: Bruising, swelling and redness: Tingling, burning or intermittent shooting pain skin firmness, hypersensitivity or lack of sensitivity
Shiny skin or any itchy feeling
If the skin becomes red and hot to the touch, contact our office immediately.
Asymmetry: both sides of your body heal differently.

Call the Office Immediately if you Experience any of the following

- A high fever (over 101°) severe nausea and vomiting, continued dizziness or incoherent behavior, such as hallucinations.
- Any pain that cannot be controlled by your pain medication.
- Bright red skin that is hot to the touch.
- Excessive bleeding or fluid seeping through the incisions.
- A severely misshapen region anywhere that has been treated with liposuction, or bruising that is localized to one specific point of the lower body.

To alleviate any discomfort, and to reduce swelling, you may apply cool, not cold compresses to the treated region. Crushed ice or ice packs must be wrapped in a towel before being applied to the skin. Do not apply ice or anything frozen directly to the skin. Apply cool compresses for no longer than 20-minute intervals.

Day of Surgery Instructions

Rest. While rest is important in the early stages of healing, equally important is that you are ambulatory, at regular interval.

Recline, do not sit down. This will be more comfortable for you, and can reduce swelling. Sitting for prolonged period of time causes swelling in the dependent part of the abdomen.

Good nutrition. Fluids are critical following surgery. Patients are encouraged to drink plenty of water and fruit juices. It is best to avoid carbonated and alcoholic drinks.

Take all medication, exactly as prescribed.

Change your incision dressings. Your incisions will seep fluid and some blood for a short time after surgery. Keep dressings clean and dry. Do not remove any steri-strips even if they are over stitches. Apply anti-bacterial ointment over the steri-strips.

Replace any compressions garments. Do not cover the wound with water proof dressings.

Wear your compression or elastic wraps around the clock. Follow the instructions specifically removing any compression wraps only to cleanse your incision or to shower.

Do not smoke. Smoking can greatly impair your safety prior to surgery and your ability to heal following surgery. You must not smoke.

Relax. Do not engage in any stressful activities. Do not lift, push, or pull anything.

Two to Seven Days Following Surgery

During this time you will progress as each day passes. Ease into your daily activities. You will receive clearance to begin driving or return to work at your postoperative visit, or within days:

- Continue to cleanse wounds as directed; you may shower. Take a warm, not hot shower. Do not take a bath. Limit your shower to 10 minutes. Apply a fragrance free moisturizer to the surrounding skin, however, not on your incisions.
- Take antibiotic medications and supplements as directed.
- Continue to wear your elastic wraps or compression garment around the clock.
- Do not resume any exercise other than regular walking. Walking is essential every day to prevent the formation of blood clots.
- No sun exposure.
- Maintain a healthy diet. Do not smoke. Do not consume alcohol.

Contd...

Contd...

One to Four Weeks Following Surgery

As you resume your normal daily activities, you must continue proper care and healing:
- Continue your wound care as directed.
- Refrain from weight-bearing exercise.
- Do not smoke.
- Continue to wear your elastic wrap or compression garment as directed. This is essential for your skin to conform to new contours.
- Practice good sun protection. The skin in areas treated with liposuction is highly susceptible to sunburn or the formation or irregular, darkened pigmentation.

Six Weeks Following Surgery

Healing will progress and your body settles into a more final shape and position:
- You may ease into your regular fitness routine. However, realize that your body may require some time to return to previous strength.
- Discomfort or tightness and tingling of the skin will resolve.

Your First Year
- Continue healthy nutrition, fitness, and sun protection.
- Your scars will continue to refine. If they become raised, red or thickened, or appear to widen, contact our office. Early intervention is important to achieving well-healed scars.
- A 1-year post surgery follow-up is recommended. However, you may call our office at any time with your concerns or for needed follow-up.

Your body will change with age. The appearance of your body will change too. Although the outcomes of liposuction are generally permanent, any significant weight gain or loss, pregnancy as well as the normal influences of aging can cause changes to your appearance.

I have read and understand all of the above instructions. I understand that following these instructions is solely my responsibility. I understand that it is also my responsibility to ask my doctor and his or her staff any questions I have related to these instructions or about my procedure, health, and healing.

Patient Signature _____   Date _____
Printed Name of the Patient _____

Signature of the Practice
Representative and the Witness

Typical postoperative symptoms after liposuction of abdominal region include:

1. *Pain*: Pain is aggravated on direct pressure or abdominal muscle movement. A combination of non-steroidal anti-inflammatory medications along with centrally acting pain medications will improve the pain. Comfortable pressure garment and adequate rest will imrpove the symptoms.

2. *Swelling, tightness and stiffness*: Patients feel puffy and swollen. Often their weight will increase due to fluid retention in the body. Patient feels tightness and firmness which progresses in the first 2–3 weeks. Swelling starts subsiding after 3–4 weeks and reduces regularly until 5–6 months. People with lax abdominal wall develop more swelling than patient with firm abdominal skin.

3. *Bruising and redness*: It happens depending upon individual patient types. Incidence of excessive bruising is very less due to tumescent infiltration, atraumatic liposuction and adequate postoperative drainage in first 24 hours.

4. *Excessive blood tinged fluid discharge*: Keeping the incisions open allows excessive fluid drainage in the first 24 hours. Although it can be inconvenient to the patient but prevents fluid retention, seroma and excessive bruising. Using adequate padding and providing patients with water proof sheets are comfortable for them.

5. *Dysesthesias*: Hypersensitivity or lack of sensation on the operated site is normal postoperatively. It takes 3–4 months to resolve.

6. *Excessive itching*: It can happen for various reasons such as type of garment material, increased vascularity of the operated site and dryness of the skin. They are adviced against applying hot fomentation or scratching with their nails. This can lead to skin damage and scras.

7. *Asymmetry and irregularities*: These are common in the initial postoperative period. Regular follow-up is important to manage the problem.

Patients are instructed to call the surgeon or office immediately, if they experience following signs and symptoms.

1. *High fever*: It may be sign of onset of infection.

2. *Severe nausea and vomiting*: Nausea and vomiting may be drug induced but can happen if their is inadvertent injury to the intraperitoneal structures.

3. Continued dizziness may be sign of excessive bleeding.

4. Incoherent behavior is a sign of lidocaine toxicity.

5. *Uncontrolled pain, severe redness and shiny skin*: These are signs of hematoma or early onset of infection.

6. *Excessive bleeding or fluid discharge*: Patient is called back to the office for adequate management.

Patient are also provided written instructions for the subsequent postoperative period as described in Form 8.5

A regular follow-up is arranged, so the surgeon can inspect the operated site and take necessary actions to improve the result.

REFERENCES

1. Iverson RE, Lynch DJ, American Society of Plastic Surgeons Committee on Patient Safety. Practice advisory on liposuction. Plast Reconstr Surg. 2004;113(5):1478-90.

2. Horton JB, Reece EM, Broughton G II, et al. Patient safety in the office-based setting. Plast Reconstr Surg. 2006;117 (4):61-80e.

3. Davison SP, Venturi ML, Attinger CE, et al. Prevention of venous thromboembolism in the plastic surgery patient. Plast Reconstr Surg. 2004;114(3):43-51e.

4. Caprini JA, Arcelus JI, Reyna JJ. Effective risk stratification of surgical and nonsurgical patients for venous thromboembolic disease. Semin Hematol. 2001;38(2):12-9.

5. Most D, Kozlow J, Heller J, et al. Thromboembolism in plastic surgery. Plast Reconstr Surg. 2005;115(2):20-30e.

CHAPTER 9

Three-Dimensional Liposculpturing

■ INTRODUCTION

Three-dimensional liposculpturing is a modern concept which is the process of removing fat from all around the abdomen, sides, and back encompassing all aesthetic sub-units of the abdominal region.

Upper Midline Aesthetic Unit

The upper midline unit overlies the midline of the abdomen (linea alba) extending from xiphoid sternum to the umbilicus. This unit adds a characteristic and aesthetic feature to the abdomen in men and women.

Two Upper Rectus Aesthetic Units

There are two upper rectus units overlying the rectus muscles extending from the lower costal margin to the level of umbilicus. Upper rectus units are concave in a healthy women and has visible intersections in physically fit man.

Lower Recti Aesthetic Unit

Single lower rectus unit overlying both the recti muscles below the umbilicus and extends down to the upper pubic hair line. The lower aesthetic unit has a mild bulge and it may have additional depressions in a physically fit man or woman. These depressions overlie the pyramidalis muscle.

Two Lateral Abdominal Aesthetic Units

Two lateral abdominal units on either side of the rectus units extend from the lower four costal areas superiorly and extend inferiorly over the oblique muscles to the iliac crest and inguinal regions. In women these lateral aesthetic units has curves that enhances the aesthetic appearance. A healthy men may have visible serrated anterior muscle slips.

Two Lumbar Aesthetic Units

Two lumbar units overlie the lumbar muscles extending superiorly from the posterior costal region and inferiorly to the gluteus region. In women there is an aesthetic curve that starts in the posterior part of the costal region and extends to the buttocks.

Posterior Midline Aesthetic Unit

Posterior midline unit is overlying the spinous processes of the lower thoracic and lumbar vertebras and sacral area. The upper part of posterior midline unit often has a groove and the lower part overlies the sacral area.

Pubic Area

It is overlying the pubic region.

The aim of three-dimensional liposculpturing is to create aesthetic curves of the body in frontal, oblique, and lateral views, particularly in women. In men, the aim is to enhance the muscular silhouette of the abdomen and back. In addition to curves and angles, it allows skin draping in a wider area and results in uniform skin contraction.

Superficial liposuction is a key component of three-dimensional liposculpturing.[1] At the same time, it is fraught with risks; during superficial liposuction if you damage the dermis, it could lead to visible induration and peau d' orange appearance of the skin. If the superficial fat is not removed uniformly, it can lead to visible and/or palpable lumps. Hence, there is a long learning curve but once you have mastered the art, the results are amazing.

Three-dimensional liposculpturing can be performed using suction-assisted liposuction (SAL), laser-assisted liposuction (LAL), ultrasonic-assisted liposuction (UAL), or radiofrequency-assisted liposuction (RFAL) on the basis of your expertise and availability of the technologies. But at the end, it is the manual work and artistic perception of the surgeon that give the result.

■ PREOPERATIVE MARKING

It involves marking the midline, and all the 10 aesthetic units of the abdomen, sides, and back. Patients with body mass index (BMI) > 28–30 may need extended liposuction involving the upper back/bra roll area.

In patients with good muscular built or BMI < 25, you can identify the rectus muscle borders and mark accordingly. The areas of fat bulges are marked; any creases, folds, or adhesions are marked. Ask the patient to sit on a chair to look for rolls. Further marking can be confirmed by asking the patient to lie down. The marking in the men differs from women; at the same time it also varies in different BMI groups. Men with BMI 28–30 may not look normal with six packs. In men lines, angles and triangles are desirable such as "V" shape of the back, triangular appearance of the lower abdomen. A man with excess fat loses these angles and develops curves.

On the other hand, women desire curves and contours in their body.

Markings in Men (Figs. 9.1A and B)

The aim of marking in BMI 25 and less is to enhance the muscular silhouette and give them a muscular look with "six-packs" definition. In BMI 25–30 patients, the aim is to give them a masculine and physically fit look. BMI above 30 requires liporeduction to reduce the waist size and abdominal bulge.

Begin with marking the midline and lateral border of the rectus muscles. Mark the intersections on the upper rectus muscle region if "six-packs" is desired. Then mark the lateral abdominal aesthetic unit giving emphasis on costal margin, subcostal depression, and the lower part overlying the external oblique muscles. This is followed by marking the pubic region area if it requires fat removal. Mark the maximum bulges of the flank area and then mark complete lumbar aesthetic unit starting from the lower part of latissimus dorsi to the upper part of buttocks. Finally, the posterior midline aesthetic unit with emphasis on erector muscle group and lower back triangle over the sacral region.

Markings in Women (Figs. 9.1C and D)

The aim of marking in female patients with BMI < 25 is to enhance the curves and give an athletic look. In the case of BMI 25–30, the focus is on creating curves, whereas in the BMI > 30 case it is to reduce waist and abdomen size.

Mark all the 10 aesthetic units as described earlier except the muscular intersections of the rectus muscles. Highlighting on the muscles and intersections is not desirable in most of the women as it gives them a "masculine" appearance.

Infiltration

Measure the estimated fluid volume accurately. Ensure that lidocaine and adrenaline are freshly prepared just prior to the start of the procedure. Adrenaline may lose its efficacy if it is preopened or nearing its expiry date. The fluid should be warmed to body temperature prior to its use.[1]

Both superficial and deep infiltration are performed using a predetermined volume with a ratio of 1:1–1.5:1. Ensure symmetric volume of infiltration on either side of the abdomen and back. Infiltrate the tissue uniformly in the deep and superficial layers all over the abdomen and back.

However, thorough infiltration is required in following situations:
1. If the procedure is performed under local anesthesia (LA) and intravenous (IV) sedation.
2. In the superficial region for vibration amplification of sound energy at resonance-assisted high-definition liposculpturing.
3. Tough fibrous areas such as costal and subcostal regions.
4. Secondary or redo liposuction.

Limited infiltration is performed in following situations:
1. If LAL or RFAL is performed, as the infiltration fluid hampers the heat-induced collagen contraction. In this situation, SAL can be performed first and then laser or radiofrequency device can be used for tissue tightening.
2. If simultaneous abdominoplasty procedure is planned.
3. In simultaneous body lift procedure as excessive infiltration and liposuction can damage the integrity of fascia system. Turgid tissues does not hold sutures well.

■ EMULSIFICATION AND PRETUNNELING

The author prefers to start the procedure in supine position. If UAL is used in the emulsification process, then start in the superficial plane with pulsed mode until all the skin is undermined. Then deep emulsification is performed (as described in earlier chapters).

In SAL, it is useful to do some pretunneling without suction using 3 mm and 4 mm cannulas to uniformly undermine the skin and break the adipose tissue. Spending 10–12 minutes literally emulsifies the fat to some extent.

Pretunneling is also useful to release the subdermal fibrous component that causes cellulite, deep adherence in the costal region and in the flexion creases. In the upper abdomen area pretunneling will allow easy cannula movement thus reducing the risk of inadvertent cannula injuries and over-resection of fat preventing depressions.

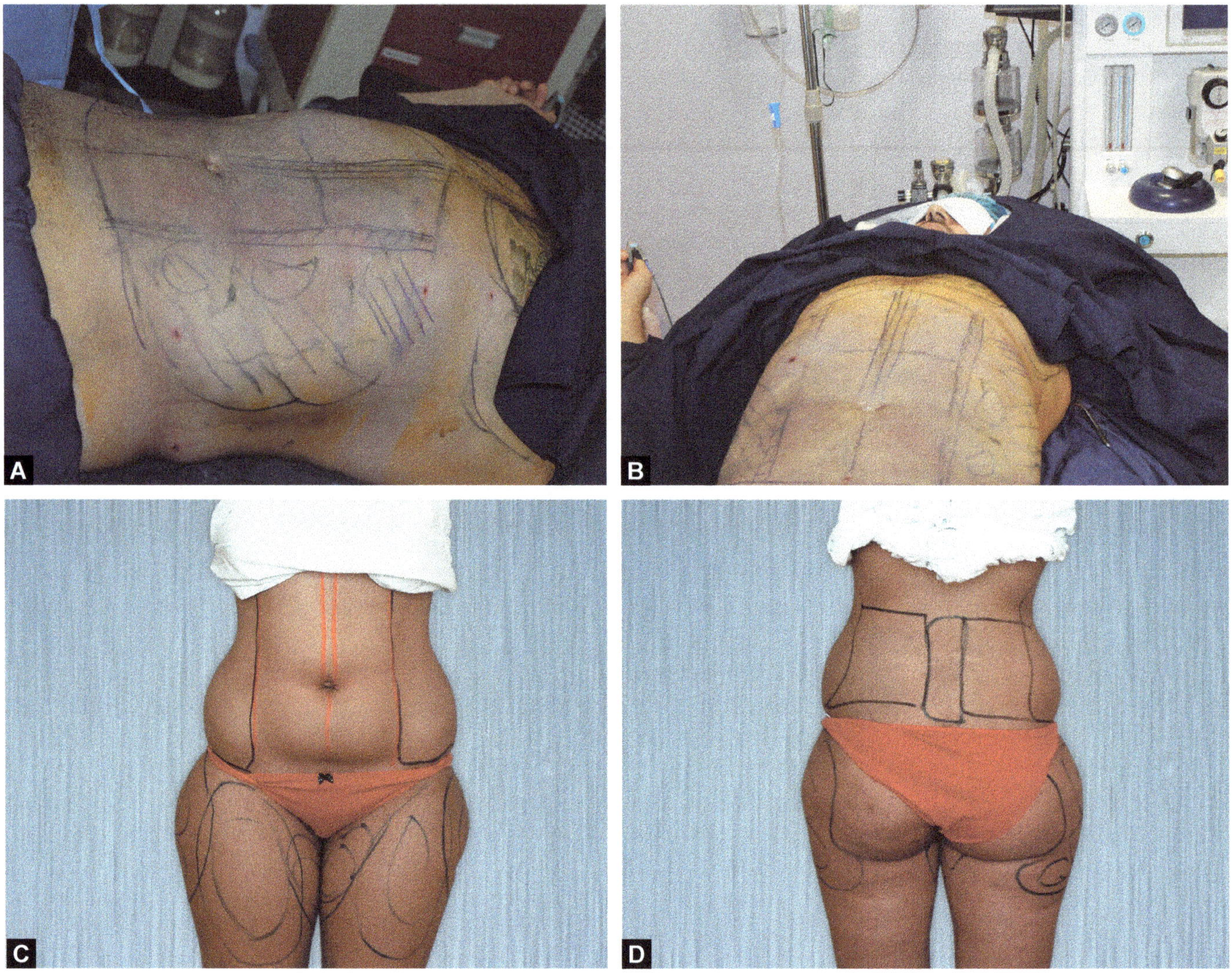

Figs. 9.1A to D: Marking of the aesthetic units: roadmap.

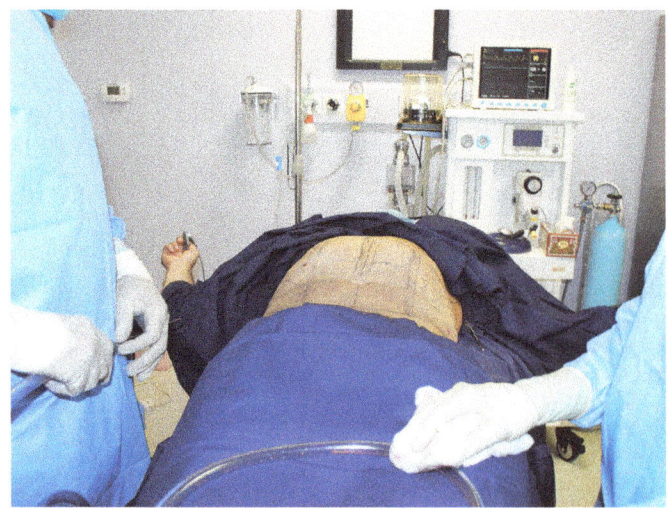

Fig. 9.2: High costochondral area: caution.

Be careful if the costal region is very prominent, particularly in men (Fig. 9.2). To avoid risks of injury to the peritoneum, diaphragm, and lungs, following maneuvers will help:
1. Flex the OR table.
2. Use incisions in the chest area so direction of the cannula is toward south.
3. If you are using umbilical incision, either use a curved cannula or use short strokes in a slow and gentle way.
4. Remember to direct the cannula away from the body by lowering your hand.

LIPOSUCTION

Procedure starts with either emulsification using ultrasonic machine or pretunneling without suction. A 3 mm cannula is used in the upper midline aesthetic unit, upper

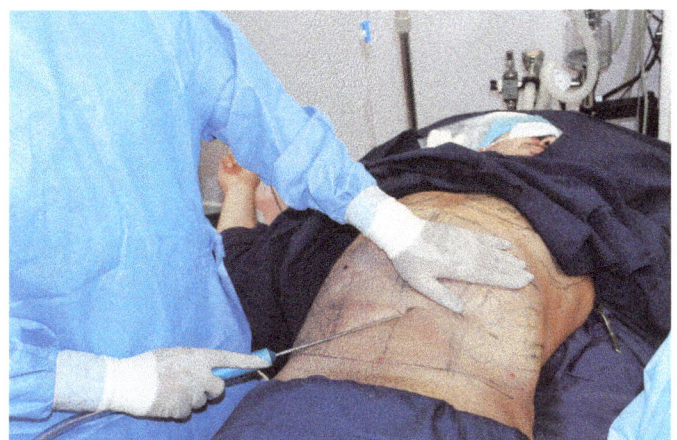

Fig. 9.3: Umbilical incisions, contouring subcostal area, lateral aesthetic units.

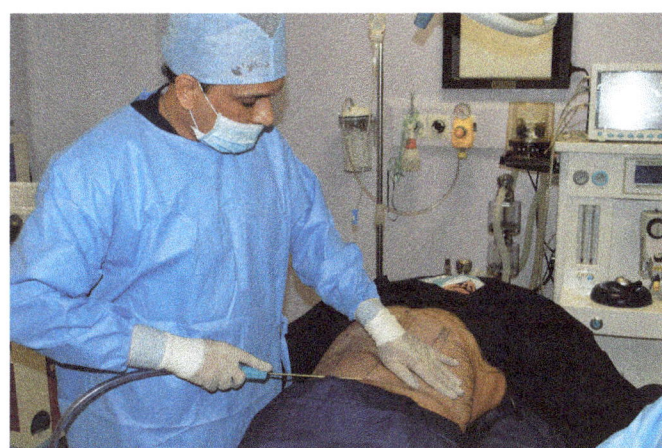

Fig. 9.4: Stabilization of skin with palm of the hand.

rectus aesthetic units, lower rectus aesthetic unit, and pubic unit. Do not use one incision port for a long time. This will prevent friction burns and over resection of an aesthetic unit. Rotating between left and right and using all incision ports sequentially ensure uniform fat removal. After medium-layer liposuction, proceed with superficial liposuction. This will allow pinching, holding, and grabbing of the skin for deeper liposuction.

Extensive deep liposuction with a 4-mm cannula is performed in subcostal region, iliac fossa region to ensure that the skin caves (Fig. 9.3). The nondominant hand is used to stabilize the skin and feel the cannula movement (Fig. 9.4).

Superficial liposuction[2] is further performed in the upper midline region, linea semilunaris/lateral border of rectus muscle, and at the tendinous intersection of the rectus sheath if a high-definition liposculpturing is desired in men. In women, the tendinous intersection is left alone. However, midline linea alba liposuction gives a youthful appearance to the abdomen in women.

LUMBAR AESTHETIC UNIT

After anterior abdominal aesthetic unit I proceed to the lumbar region in supine position.

In supine position, the fat in the lumbar unit falls away from the underlying musculoskeletal structure allowing deep liposuction. After doing a reasonable amount of liposuction the patient is turned in the lateral position. In this position the skin drapes the underlying musculoskeletal structures. In men, particular attention is paid to ensure liposuction does not create a feminine curve. On the contrary, in women a thorough liposuction is performed in

the lumbar aesthetic unit to achieve a nice curve. The fat in the lumbar region extends toward the midline parallel to the costal margin. Deep liposuction will help improve the posterior curve. Do not perform extensive superficial liposuction in this region and it is easy to cause lumpiness and tunnels that will be palpable and/or visible after the swelling subsides.

Posterior Midline and Sacral Area

Liposuction over the erector spinae muscle group and sacral triangular area will help to improve the posterior contour. There is no need for liposuction in the posterior midline over the spinous process of vertebras.

Roll the patient in an oblique position to further enhance the sides and back. This position allows us to see the skin draping over the muscles.

Extended Liposuction and Transitioning

Extended liposuction is performed if other surrounding areas are bulging with excess fat and most common area is the scapular area or "bra rolls." Other extended areas may be upper buttocks, pectoral areas in men, and lateral breast areas.

Transitioning is a part of liposuction where the interface of muscles is treated such as lateral border of rectus and external oblique, pectoralis major and serratus anterior in men. It is also performed in women for smooth transition of the curves such as in the iliac crest region, posterior buttocks, upper back, or bra roll areas. Using finer cannulas, superficial and controlled deep liposuction are performed with regular checking of the contours.

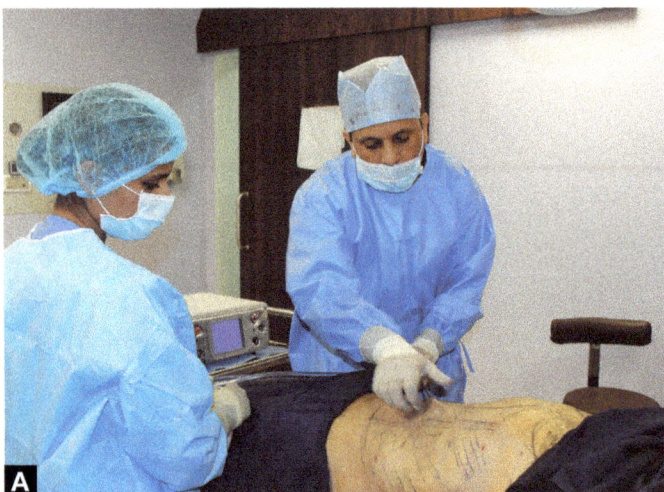 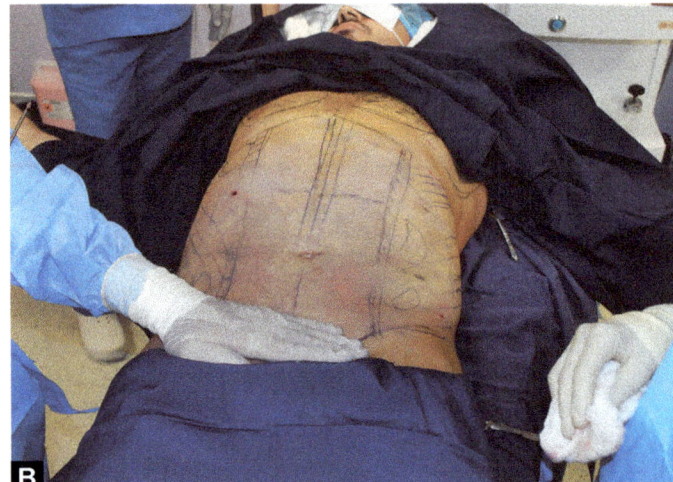

Figs. 9.5A and B: Endpoint of liposuction.

Any lumpinous, waviness, and tunnels require immediate correction using superficial and crisscross technique.

Feathering

This is liposuction of the peripheral region of the aesthetic subunits. It is performed by using a 3 mm cannula to prevent step deformities and blend the contours.

The surgical endpoint is free movement of cannula without much fat aspiration, visible endpoint of the curves and contours and uniform pinch test (minimum 1 cm pinch thickness) (Figs. 9.5A and B).

Post-tunneling and Crisscrossing

I always end the procedure using a 4 mm cannula in a crisscross manner breaking all the palpable lumps without aspiration.[3,4] After doing this method, use your eyes and hands to visualize any residual lumps of fat.

Postoperative Management

I personally do not prefer to use drains or suture the wounds. I apply padded dressing and use elastoplast with compression. If patients are allergic to adhesives than I use an abdominal binder. I encourage the patient to sleep in all positions possible. We provide the patients with Incopad and extra absorptive pads to prevent soiling their beds.

Next day morning they remove the dressing and take a quick shower. Most of the wounds stop oozing and close within 24–36 hours. Occasionally one or two wounds might seep some fluid for few days.

They use compression garment from next day onward. I use compressive foams to apply additional compressions in areas that appear swollen during postoperative visits.

All patients are advised to follow-up initially on a weekly basis for a month than monthly for 3 months finally at 6th and 12th month postoperatively.

I recommend them to start mild exercise after 1 week to 10 days. Manual massages after 10 days and if necessary put them on equipment that performs vacuum and roller massage.

I educate them about diet management and regular exercise and warn them not to gain weight to enjoy long-term results.

The results are visible in the first month and improve every month thereafter. Most of the result is noticeable in 4–6 months' time (Figs. 9.6 and 9.7).

CONCLUSION

The three-dimensional liposuction allowed us to reduce the number of abdominoplasty procedure due to the great retraction of the skin that can be obtained by near circumferential liposuction, extensive superficial liposuction, and release of fibrous adhesions.

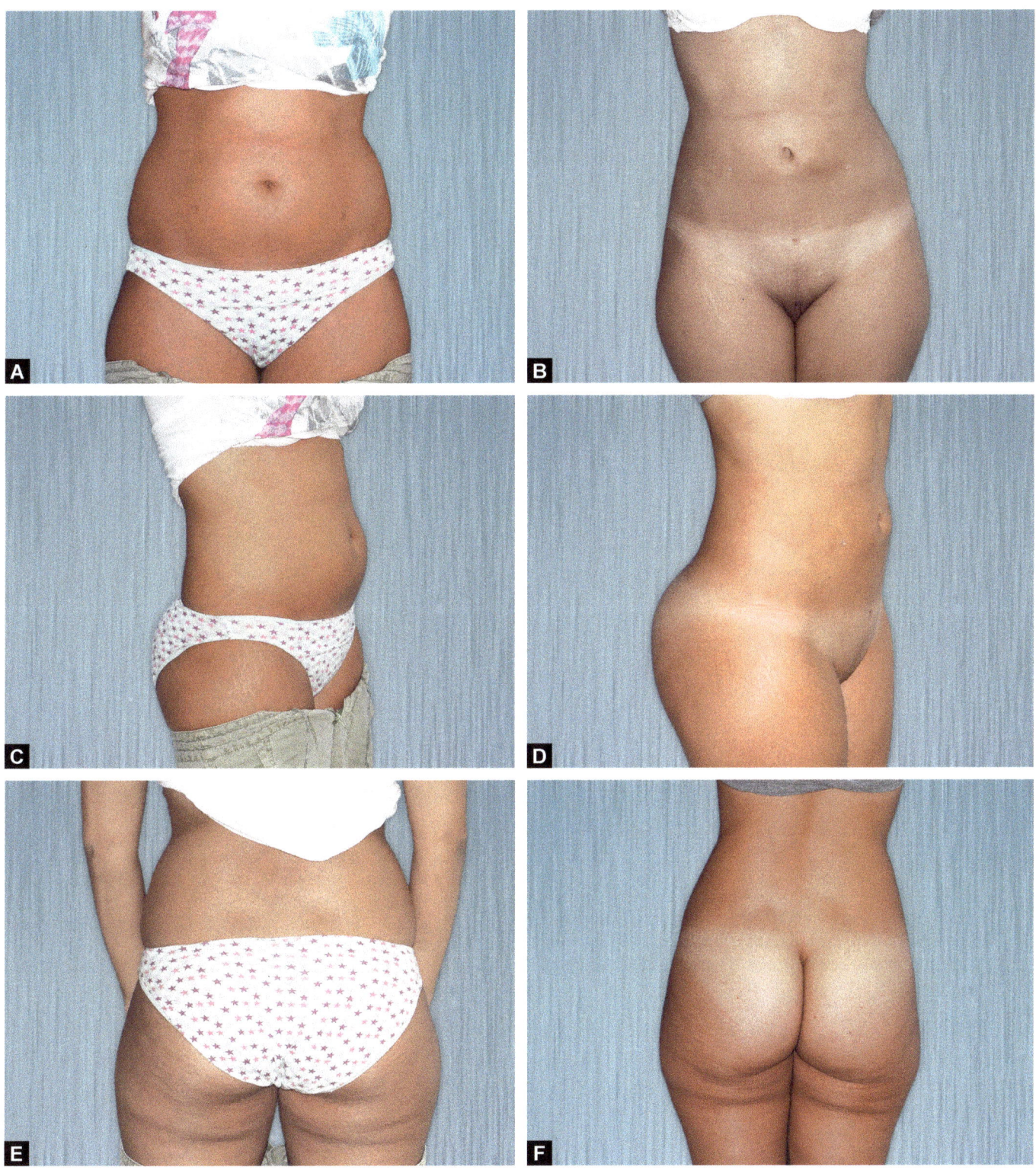

Figs. 9.6A to F: (A, C and E) Preoperative views of patient with BMI 26, (B, D and F) Postoperative views after three-dimensional liposculpturing.

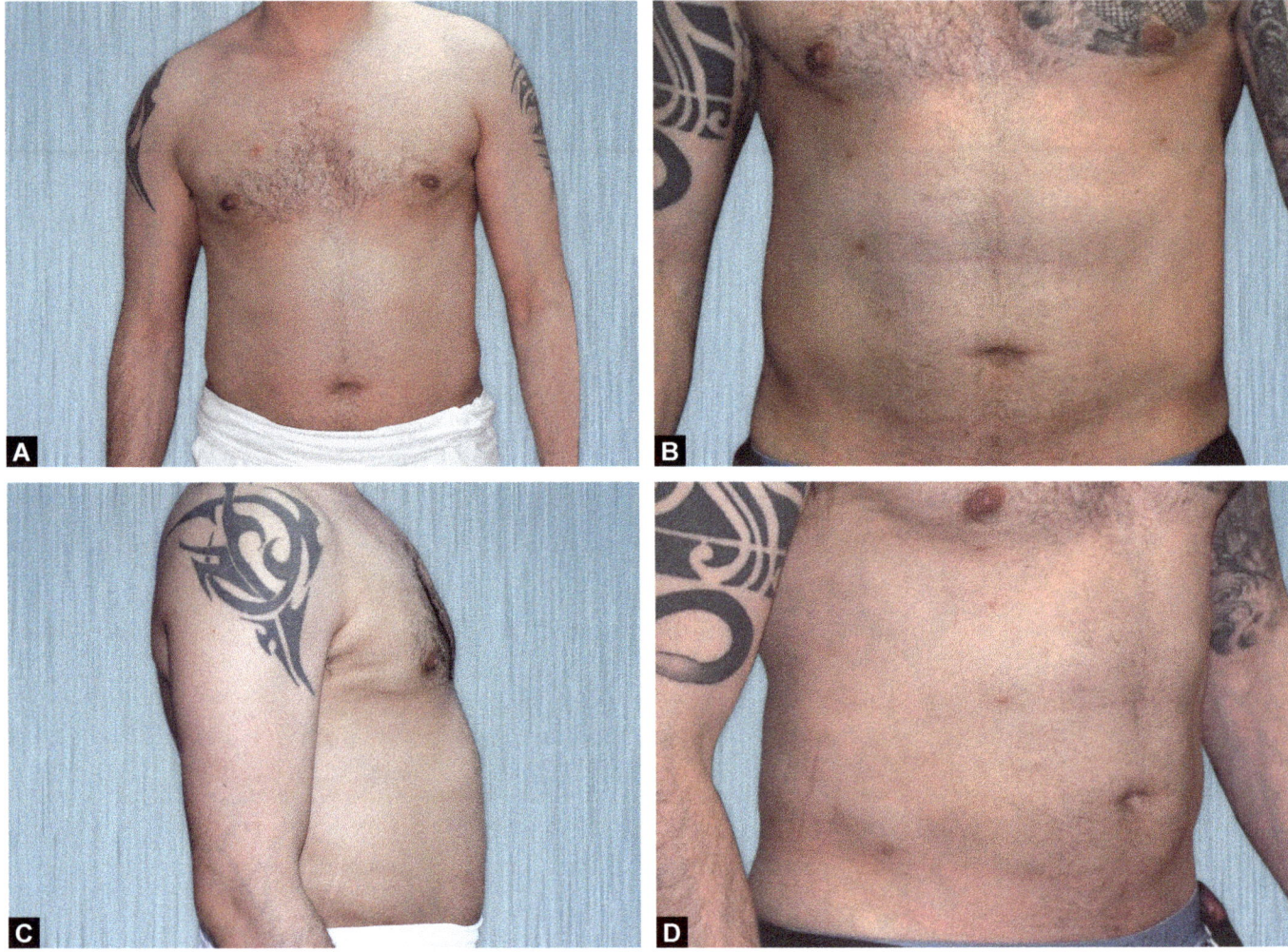

Figs. 9.7A to D: (A and C) Preoperative views of male patient with BMI 29. (B and D) Postoperative views after high-definition liposculpturing.

REFERENCES

1. Robles-Cervantes JA, Martinez-Molina R, Ca´rdenas-Camarena L. Heating infiltration solutions used in tume-scent liposuction: minimizing surgical risk. Plast Reconstr Surg. 2005;116:1077-81.

2. Gasparotti M, Lewis CM, Toledo LS. Superficial Liposculp-ture: Manual of Technique, 1st edition. New York: Springer-Verlag; 1993. pp. 1-28.

3. Mladick RA. The big six: six important tips for a better result in lipoplasty. Clin Plast Surg. 1989;16:250.

4. Chang KN. Surgical correction of postliposuction contour irregularities. Plast Reconstr Surg. 1994;94:126.

CHAPTER 10

Waist Sculpturing

▌INTRODUCTION

Waist liposculpting is usually performed as a part of three-dimensional liposculpting. But there is a rising trend for a narrow waistline in all groups of patient's normal weight to obese patient. Women desire a waistline, either a thin waistline like "Kim Kardashian" or at least a curvaceous shape of the waist area if none is existing.

By definition waist is the narrowest part of the trunk between costal margin and iliac crest. In women it follows an aesthetic curve known as "Hogarth curve." William Hogarth in his publication of "Analysis of Beauty" (1753) described S-shaped curve as line of beauty that signifies liveliness and activity and excite the attention of the viewer as contrasted with straight lines, parallel lines, or right-angled intersecting lines, which signify stasis, death, or inanimate objects (Figs. 10.1A and B).[1]

Waistline is a three-dimensional curve visible anteroposteriorly, laterally, and in oblique positions.

Two-dimensional waistline is visible only anteroposteriorly (Figs. 10.2A and B).

Accumulation of fat in the waistline causes the following:
1. Bulge called "love handle."
2. Increased waistline.
3. Makes the trunk look short.
4. Masks the underlying musculoskeletal contour.

▌ANATOMY OF WAIST

The waist comprises of two aesthetic units on each side (Figs. 10.3A and B).

Lateral Abdominal Aesthetic Units

The anterior part of the waistline is formed by the lateral abdominal aesthetic units in either side. The lateral abdominal units on either side of the rectus units extend from the lower four costal areas superiorly, to the oblique muscles, iliac crest and inguinal regions inferiorly.

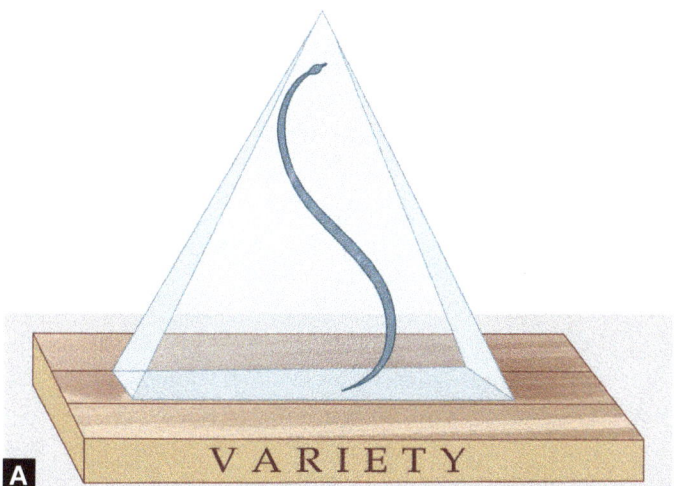

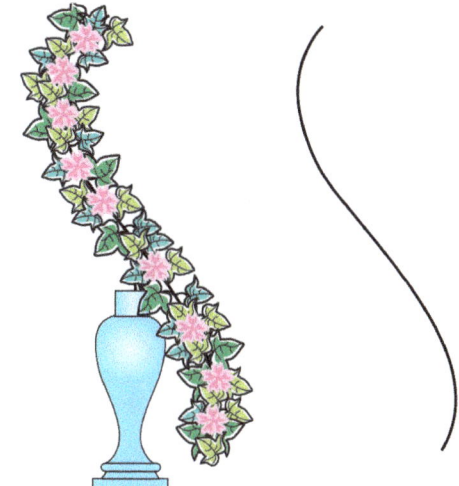

Figs. 10.1A and B: An illustration from the page of "the analysis of beauty." Anything arranged in a curve form is beautiful.

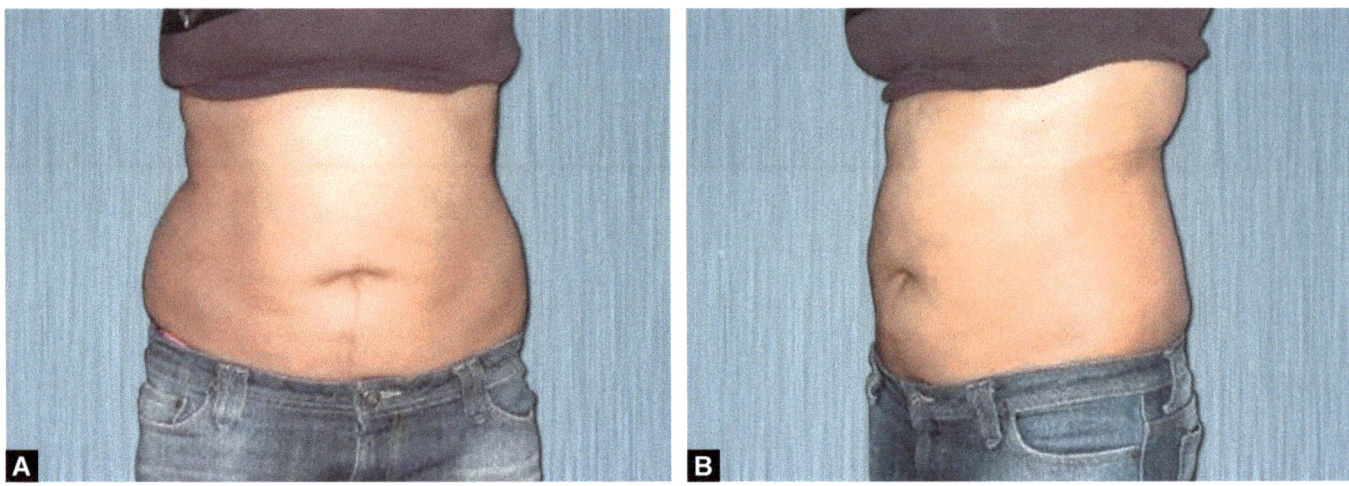

Figs. 10.2A and B: Two-dimensional waistline. (A) Waistline visible in frontal position. (B) Absence of waistline curve in profile view.

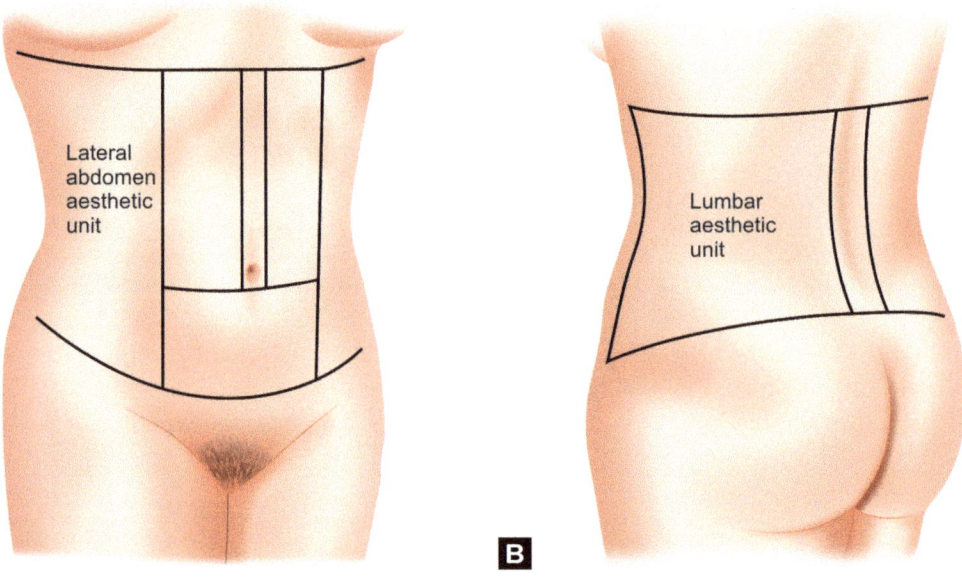

Figs. 10.3A and B: Aesthetic units of the waist. (A) Lateral abdomen aesthetic unit, and (B) Lumbar aesthetic unit.

Lumbar Aesthetic Units

The posterior part of the waistline is formed by the lumbar aesthetic units on either side of the spinous processes of the vertebrae. The lumbar units are overlying the lumbar muscles extending superiorly from posterior costal region and inferiorly to gluteal region.

Refer to the earlier chapters for detailed description of the anatomy of waistline in these aesthetic units.

The waistline gets obliterated either due to accumulation of fat in the subcutaneous region, excess skin flap, and in some patients due to musculofascial laxity because of increased intra-abdominal fat (Fig. 10.4).

The key to success lies in understanding the layers of fat in the different parts of the waist such as subcostal, lumbar and supratrochanteric areas. The fat is very compact in the central waistline zone. In the standing position sometimes fat in the bra roll areas and upper part of waistline gravitates down to obliterate the waist.

In order to understand it more clearly let us divide the waist by a line called as "waistline" going across at the narrowest part of the abdomen (Fig. 10.5).

"Suprawaist" is the area above the waistline and it overlies the ribs.

"Infrawaist" is the area below the waistline and is the true "love handles" or flank area. This is the most common

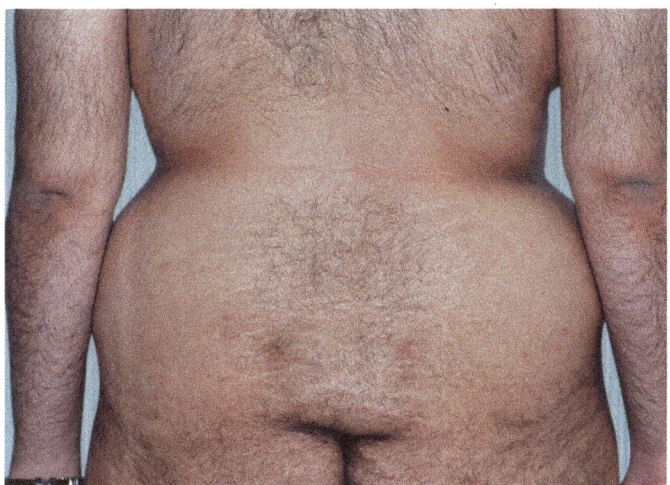

Fig. 10.4: Patient with excessive weight loss and persistent flank bulge due to musculofascial laxity.

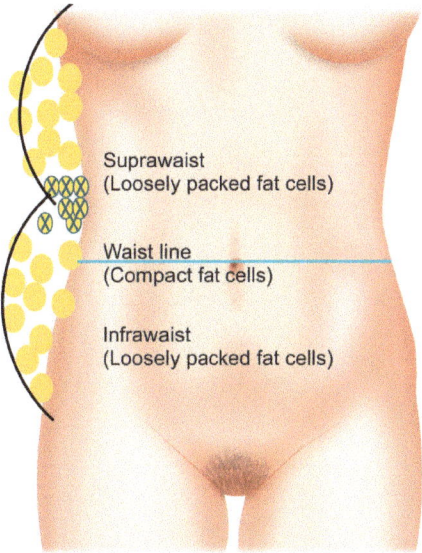

Suprawaist
(Loosely packed fat cells)

Waist line
(Compact fat cells)

Infrawaist
(Loosely packed fat cells)

Fig. 10.5: Waistline: Suprawaist area with compact fibrofatty tissue and infrawaist area with loosely packed fatty tissue.

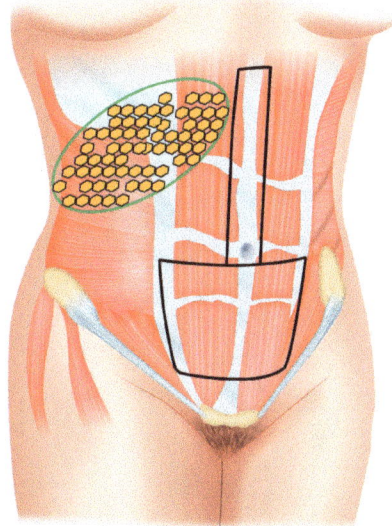

Fig. 10.6: Fibrofatty deposits in subcostal region. Removal of this fat meticulously gives an aesthetic curve to the waist.

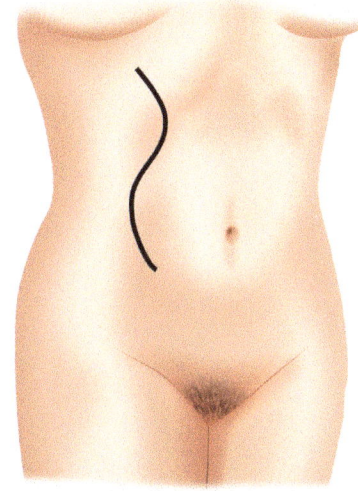

Fig. 10.7: S-shaped curve in lateral abdominal aesthetic unit.

area to collect fat even in patients with low body mass index (BMI). These are also called "muffins" as they bulge out of the tight Jeans.

The fat in the waistline area is more compact with dense fibrous tissue network. Fat accumulation in this area increases the waist size of the patient. Fat in suprawaist and infrawaist area is less compact and fibrous, and bulges in these areas form the bra roll folds and flank bulges.

In the anterolateral part of the abdomen that includes the lateral abdominal aesthetic unit there is dense fibrofatty tissue in the subcostal area with accumulation of fat over the lower costal area and subcostal recess (Fig. 10.6).

Removal of fat from this area exaggerates the silhouette and gives a lazy S-shaped curve that is desired by women (Fig. 10.7).

In the lumbar aesthetic unit the fat occupies the lumbar triangle and extends in an oblique fashion to the paraspinous region. Removing this fat carefully enhances the posterior curve of the body (Figs. 10.8A and B).

In some patients, it may be seen that the fat is only deposited in the flank areas (infrawaistline) and this can be pinched horizontally like grasping a handle. But the actual waistline is also increased due to fat accumulation as depicted in the illustration and this can be grasped vertically.

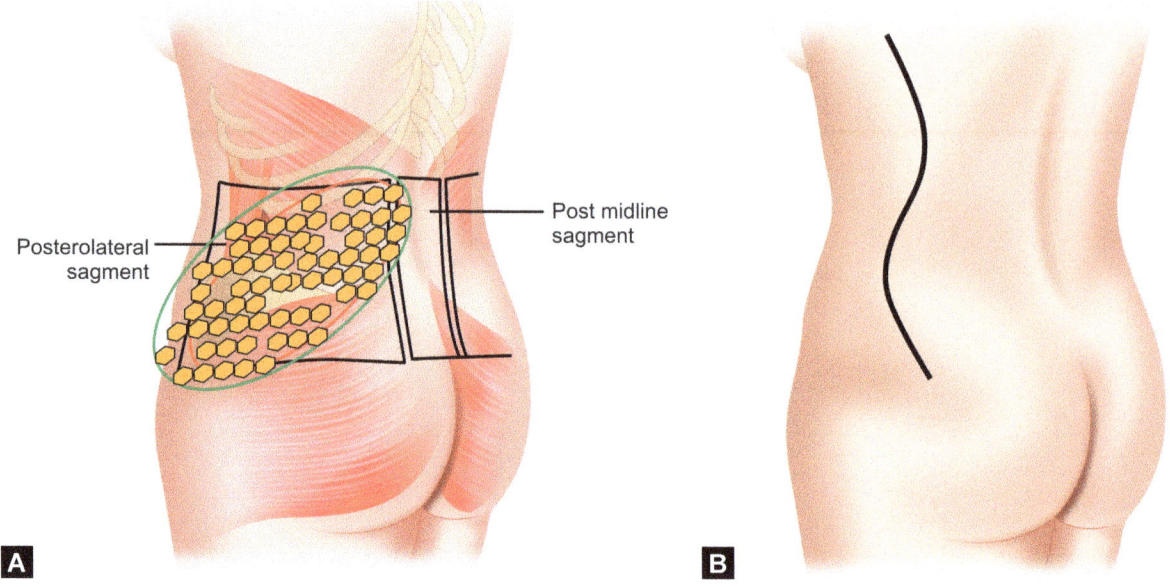

Figs. 10.8A and B: Fat accumulation in lumbar aesthetic unit and S-curve in the posterior part of the trunk.

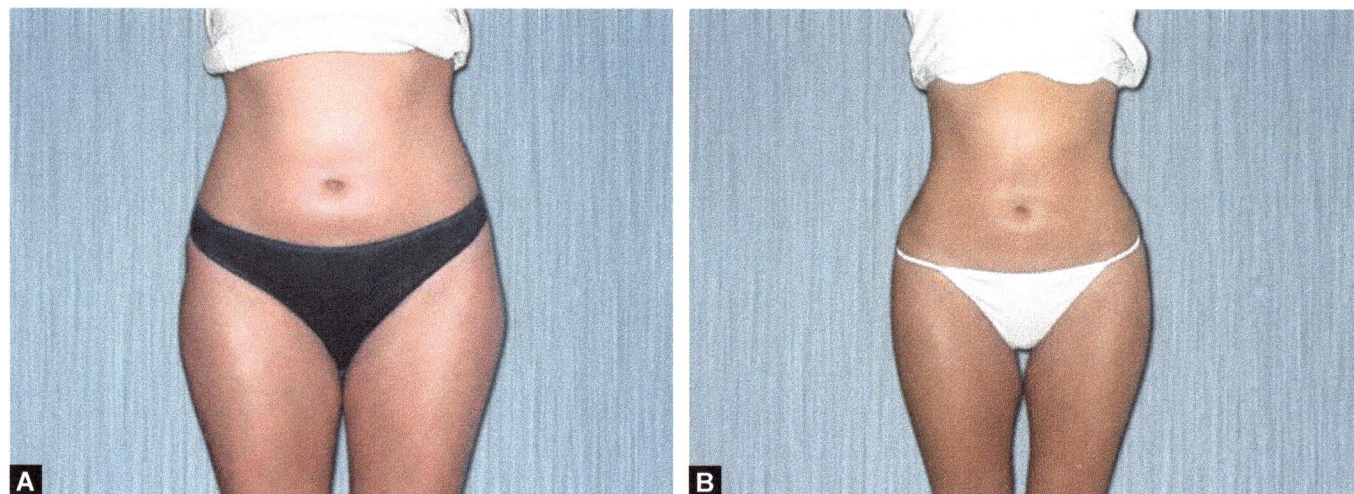

Figs. 10.9A and B: (A) Type I, patient with BMI 22 has a good waist shape but increased waistline. (B) After waist sculpting, note the curves in the lateral abdominal aesthetic unit and lumbar units. Also note the reduction in waistline.

▌ TECHNIQUE OF WAIST SCULPTING

Waist sculpting can be done in most of the BMI groups except excessively obese patients (Figs. 10.9 to 10.13). It is performed as isolated waist sculpting in patients with localized fat or excessive accumulation in patients with a past history of liposuction abdomen and lipoabdomino-plasty. It can also be done along with three-dimensional abdominal liposculpting or lipoabdominoplasty. The results of the procedure are visible very early in most patients as

the skin elasticity in this region is better than the lower abdomen region. Even an obese patient is happier if he/she sees a narrow waistline. In my opinion it has more predictable outcome than the abdominal liposculpting.

Marking (Figs. 10.14A to C)

Marking is performed in standing position and as per the aesthetic units described earlier. If there is excess fat in the surrounding areas such as bra roll, that should be marked as well.

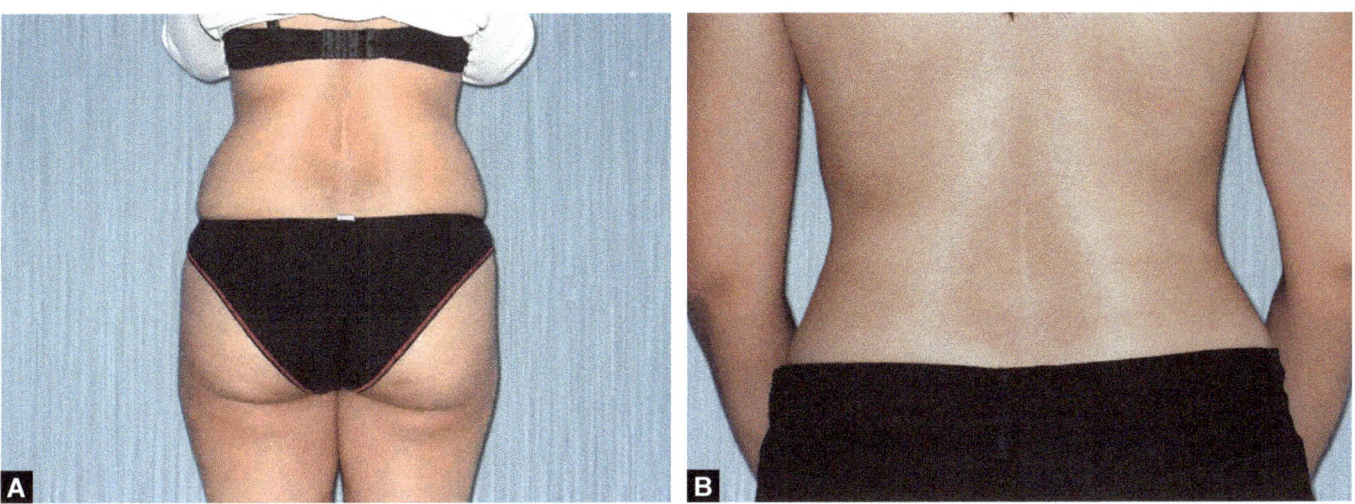

Figs. 10.10A and B: (A) Type II waistline in a female with BMI 26, increase in waistline and prominent bulge in flank region. (B) Postoperative view after waist sculpting.

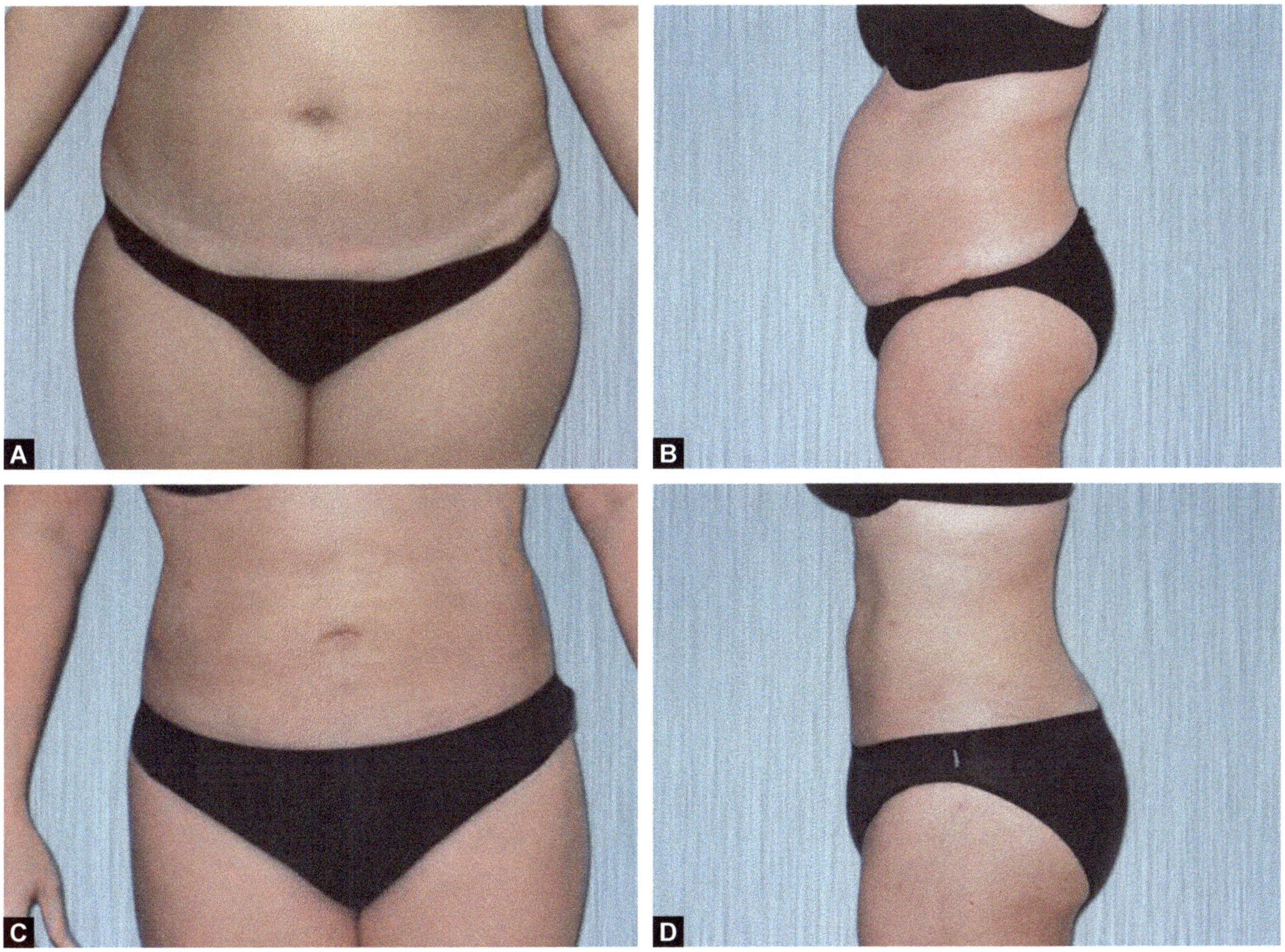

Figs. 10.11A to D: (A) Type III waistline in patient with BMI 34, frontal view. Increase in waistline and abdominal bulge. (B) Lateral view (C) Postoperative view after three-dimensional liposculpturing. (D) Postoperative profile view, note significant reduction in the waistline.

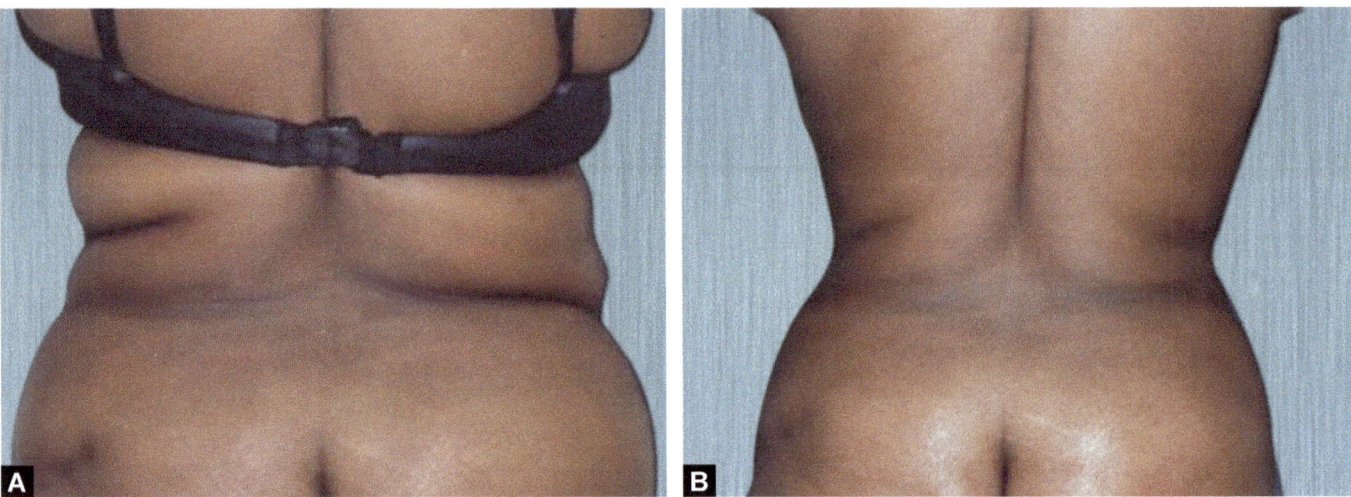

Figs. 10.12A and B: (A) Type IV waistline with supra- and infrawaist line bulges in a patient with BMI 34. Note suprawaist rolls also known as bra rolls. (B) Postoperative view after waist sculpting.

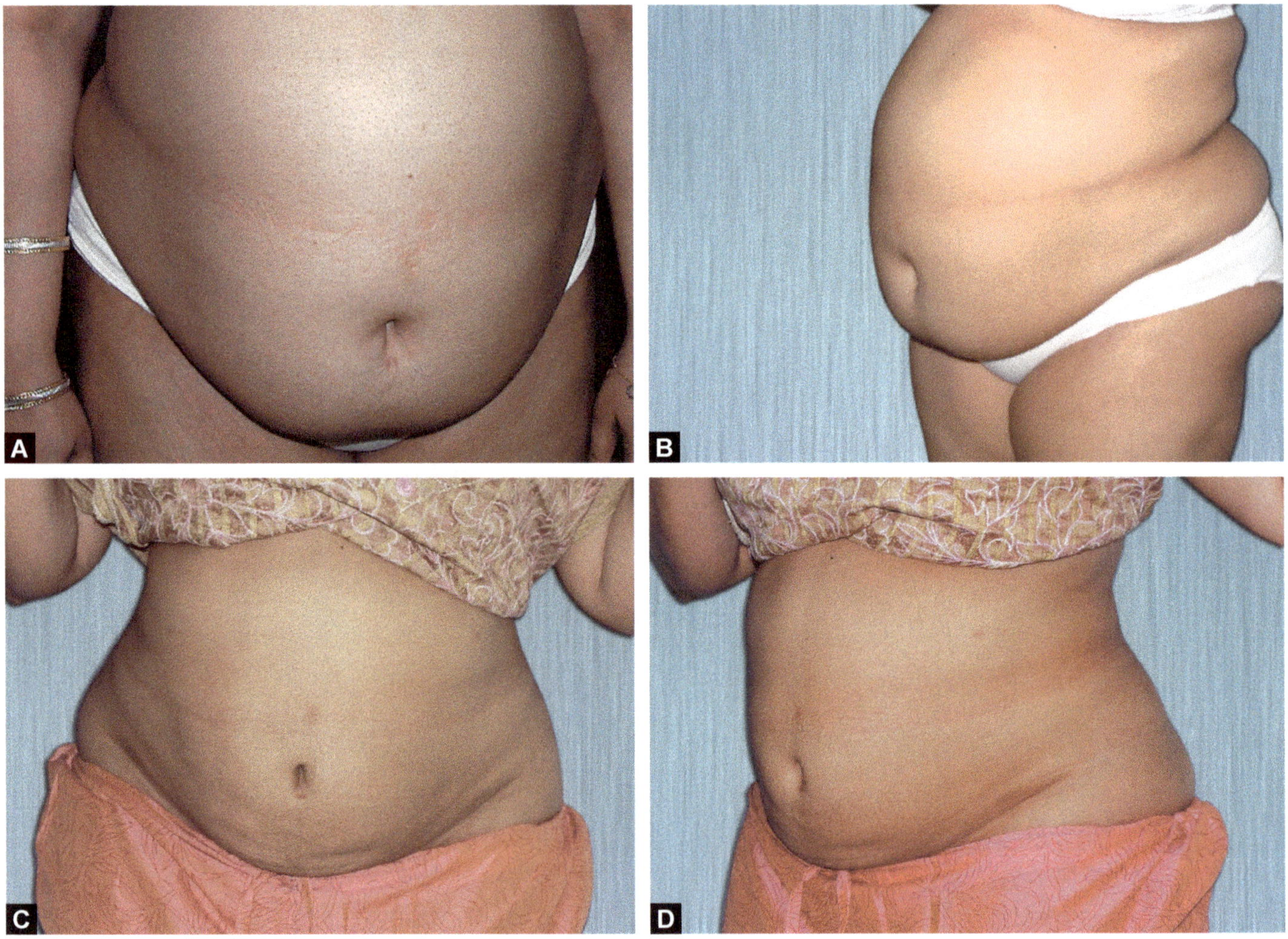

Figs. 10.13A to D: (A) Type V waistline in and obese patient with BMI 40. (B) Oblique view of the same patient. (C) Postoperative view after 1 year. (D) Postoperative result, oblique view.

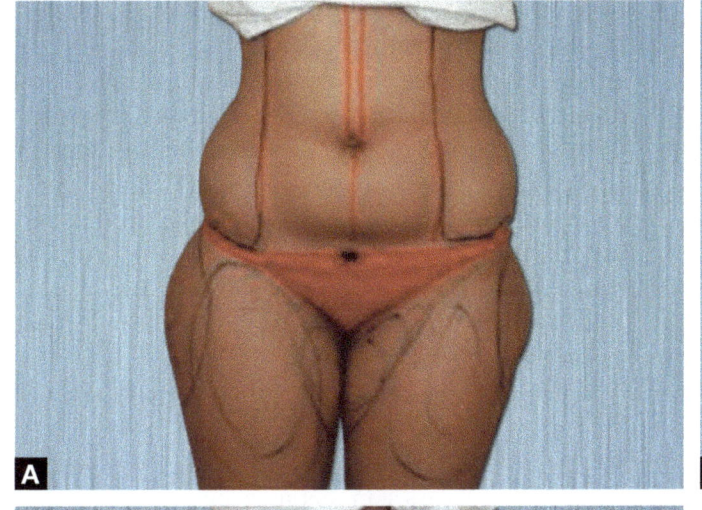
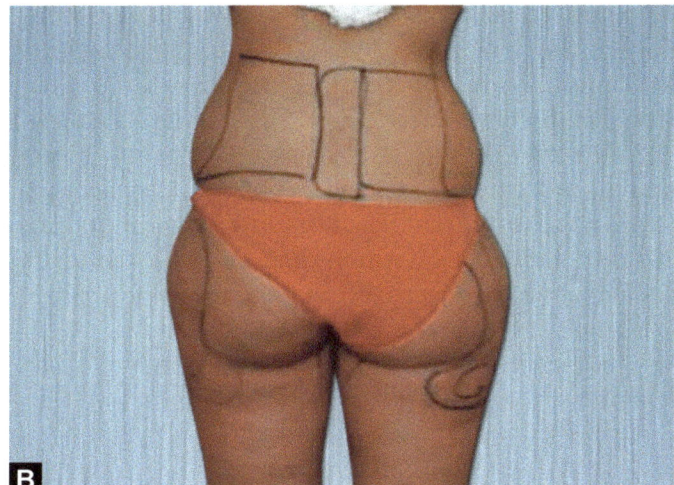
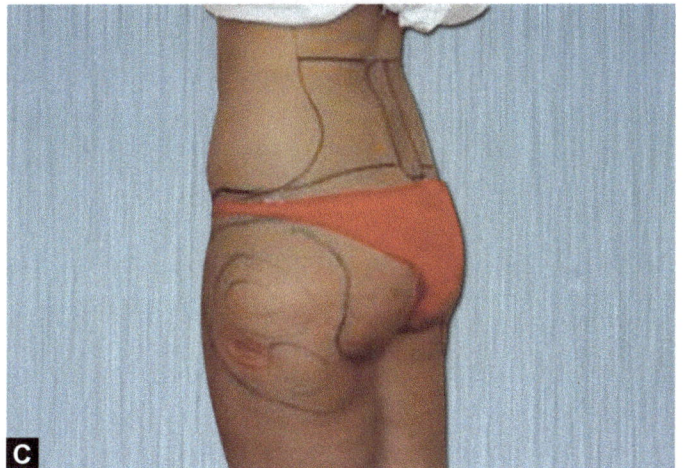

Figs. 10.14A to C: (A) Markings of the abdominal aesthetic unit and waistline, frontal view. (B) Markings, posterior view. (C) Oblique view.

Anesthesia

It can be performed under local anesthesia as an office-based procedure. Occasional patients may need deep sedation or general anesthesia. The procedure starts with local infiltration of the incision sites. Then a standard wetting solution is used on the basis of maximum dosage of lidocaine (45 mg/kg) to infiltrate the entire area extending beyond the margin of the marking to prevent pain due to cannula tip impinging the skin (this also causes bruising at the impinged site).

Emulsification and Liposuction

Procedure starts in supine position. This allows emulsification of fat in the lateral aesthetic units from the costal areas down to the lateral inguinal area. Particular attention is paid to subcostal region fat. Removal of fat over the external oblique muscles can be performed using incision in the umbilicus and/or inguinal region.

It can be performed using laser, ultrasonic, syringe-assisted or conventional technique based on the availability in your center. But as I mentioned earlier, it is the artistic use of the cannula and manual work that results in a perfect sculpted waistline. The lateral part of the waist, lumbar, and bra roll areas can also be reached in supine position. In fact, it is easier as the fat falls away from the underlying musculoskeletal system (Fig. 10.15A).

The cannula is inserted through an incision near the anterior superior iliac region. The other hand guides the cannula to prevent inadvertent deep penetration. The correct technique of liposuction in the flank region is short stroke and fanning technique. The cannula is moved along the undersurface of skin with the other hand constantly guiding the tip of the cannula. Pinch test will allow assessment of residual fat and uniformity of liposuction (Fig. 10.15B).

Curved cannula can be used to contour along the flanks and bra rolls (Figs. 10.15C and D). Then the patient is turned in lateral position for final contouring. In this position the skin and fat drapes the underlying muscular structure. So you can accurately visualize the contour (Fig. 10.15E). It also helps us to tilt the patient oblique for better definition. Cross-tunneling is important to prevent grooves and tunnels that can easily happen in patients with firm adipose tissue and skin. Plan the incision at the time of liposculpting for cross-tunneling. Incision planned in supine position may change its location when the patient is turned.

I use standard 3 mm and 4 mm Mercedes-type straight and curved cannulas for most of my liposculpturing. Endpoint of liposuction of waist is determined by pinch test and visual assessment of the contour (Figs. 10.15F and G).

Finally the patient is turned back to supine position to assess the contour in both sides and confirm symmetry.

Symmetry is very important in waist sculpting and that can be accomplished by the following:
1. Identifying pre-existing asymmetry and marking.
2. Equal infiltration in each aesthetic unit on either side.
3. If you are using an ultrasonic or laser device then the timing of energy delivery must be equally distributed.
4. Equal volume of suction unless there is pre-existing asymmetry.
5. Pinch test at specific sites equally on both sides.
6. Visual comparison in supine or standing (if only local anesthesia is used).

In supine position if the patient is awake, ask him/her to lift his/her buttocks up in the air and look for any asymmetry from the head end of the table. This is useful if the patient has excess skin that may appear as bulges in supine position.

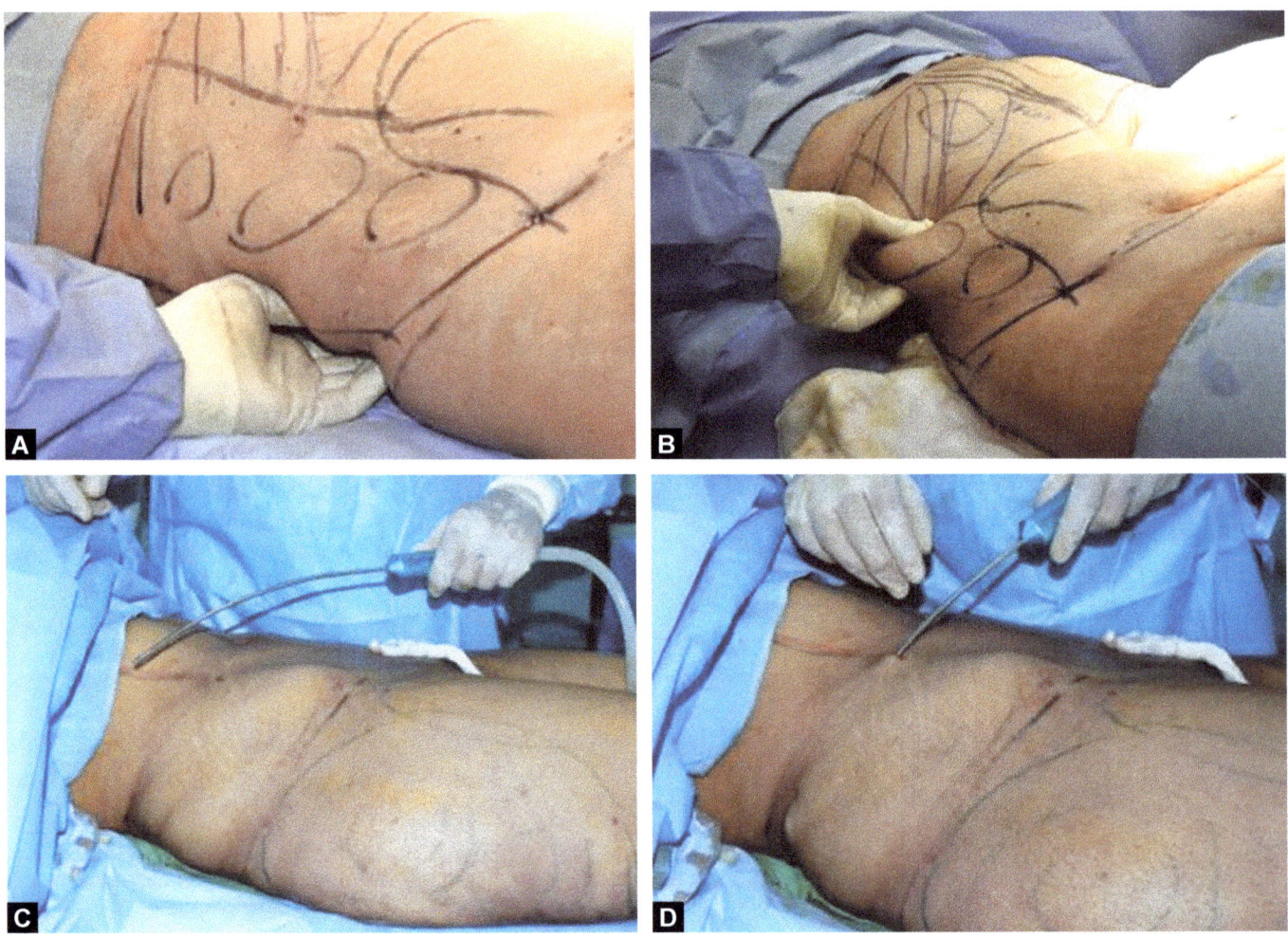

Figs. 10.15A to D

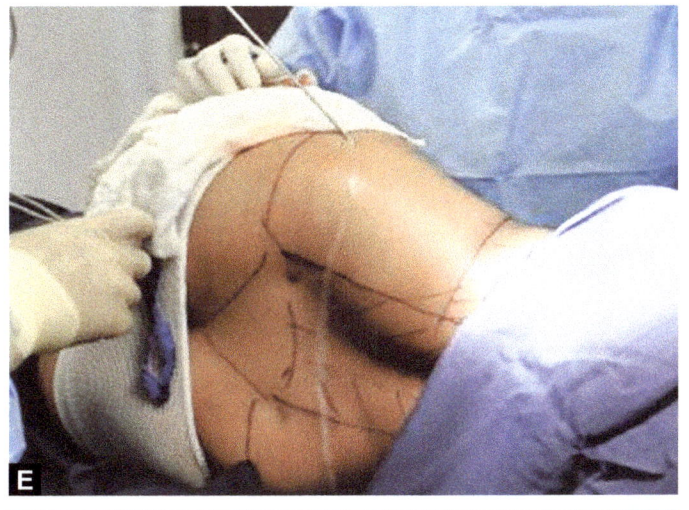

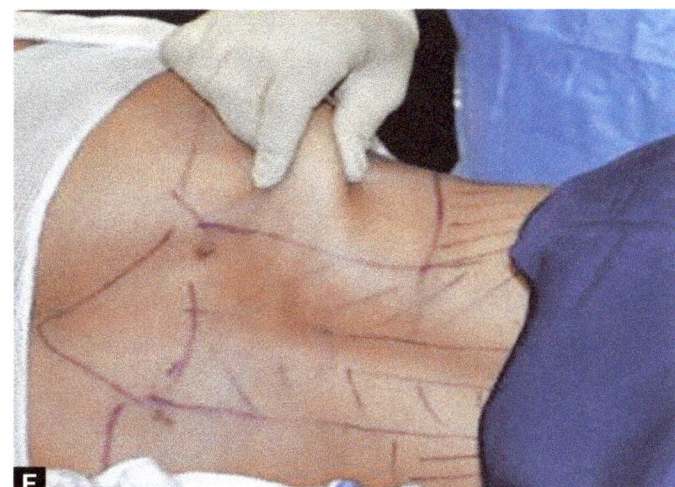

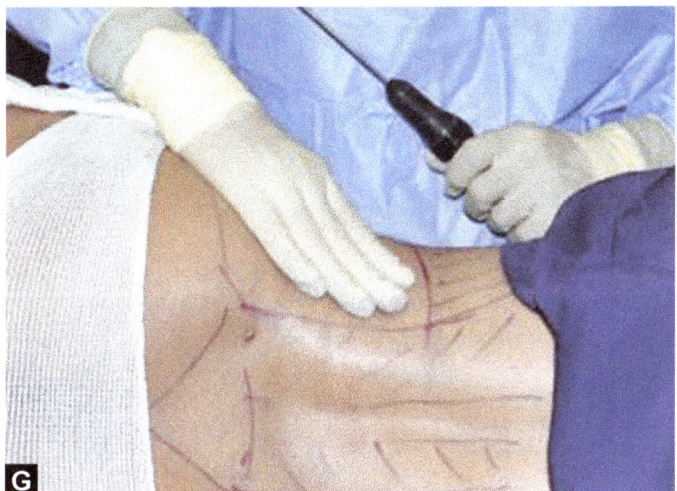

Figs. 10.15A to G: (A) Flanks and bra rolls are easily accessed in supine position. (B) Pinch test to assess adequacy of liposuction in supine position. (C) Curved cannula used to contour along the flanks. (D) Curved cannula used to contour along the flanks. (E) Lateral position to complete contouring of the waist line. (F) A pinch test to assess the endpoint of liposuction. (G) Assessing the contour of the waist.

If these maneuvers are not performed it is easy to over-resect the fat causing caves and depressions postoperatively.

POSTOPERATIVE DRESSINGS

This is similar to other area liposuction as described earlier. To improve the result, some additional points are included:

using foam under the garment, avoiding tight jeans that can lead to persistent bulge and postoperative massages either manually or with equipment.

REFERENCE

1. Hogarth W. The Analysis of Beauty, 1772 edition. London: W. Strahan; 1772.

CHAPTER 11

Nonsurgical Technologies

INTRODUCTION

Liposuction is the gold standard in fat removal technique; there are several advantages that we are aware of. Many patients do not prefer to go the route of "liposuction" for several reasons such as anesthesia, pain, recovery, and risks. They are looking for simpler ways to reduce fat. I have come across the term lipolysis and it is being used to describe various noninvasive or minimally invasive procedures for reducing subcutaneous fat volume.[1] There are several methods I have come across in the literature and in the Internet. There are medications [i.e. phosphatidylcholine (PDC) or deoxycholate] that impact the content and integrity of adipocytes that are injected subcutaneously,[1] or technologies such as ultrasound shock waves, lasers, and radiofrequency that are applied to skin with the aim of reducing fat and remodeling collagen, thereby improving the appearance of cellulite and tightening skin.[2,3] None have been studied clinically, only one US Food and Drug Administration (FDA)-approved technology that uses bipolar radiofrequency and optical energy (either laser or light) has been approved to treat the appearance of cellulite but not underlying fat.[4]

Let us go through these and see how effective they are and how can we apply them in our practice. We as plastic surgeons are often cynical about any nonsurgical methods. But let us understand and put aside the scalpel of cynicism.

FAT REDUCTION METHODS

Fat cells can be reduced by two methods:
1. Burning calories and reducing calorie intake. This is done by nutrition and exercise.
2. Destroying fat cells under the skin by nonsurgical techniques utilizing technologies.

There are different ways of targeting fat cells under the skin to reduce in size. It is important to evaluate the medical history of the patient, lifestyle, and identify the distribution pattern of fat. Only after this analysis a particular technology or combination of technology can be used to mobilize the fat cells. The equipment do not work on visceral fat.

EXTERNAL ULTRASOUND

Noninvasive ultrasonic energy may be delivered to the tissue in one of two forms: nonfocused or focused waves. Focused ultrasound can be concentrated in a defined subcutaneous focal area to produce fat cell lysis and limit damage to blood vessels, nerves, connective tissue, and muscles (Fig. 11.1).[5]

The transcutaneous focused ultrasound device (Contour I; UltraShape, Inc., Yoqneam, Israel) is composed of a transducer, a power control unit, and a tracking and guidance system. Brown et al. conducted a study to demonstrate stable cavitation on porcine skin and histologically demonstrated fat cell lysis without any epidermal or dermal changes. He further mentions that the "high"-intensity focused ultrasound (HIFU) works in the similar fashion as a lithotripsy machine shattering the fat cells. The tissue temperatures are raised very rapidly (in < 3 seconds) to an excess of 56°C causing instantaneous cell death.[6] On the contrary, "low"-power ultrasound works by raising the temperature that causes increased blood circulation and

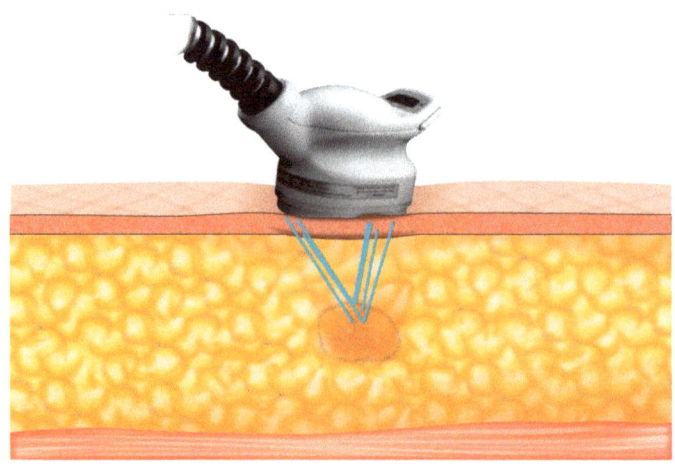

Fig. 11.1: High-intensity focused ultrasound.

has been used in gene therapy and bone healing. Histological assessments of multiple experiments using many animals consistently show discrete holes in the layers of adipocytes. They conclude by saying that the energy from this device is delivered as cavitation and not as thermal energy, which has very important clinical implications for wound healing. However, to date, there are not many randomized controlled trials regarding the effectiveness of this technology. The only multicenter trial was a nonrandomized, controlled clinical study with 164 subjects, with only 27 in the control group. A reduction in approximately 2 cm in the treatment area was achieved within 2 weeks after a single treatment, which lasted for 12 weeks.[7]

External ultrasound has been used immediately prior to liposuction procedure by many surgeons. Cook et al.[8] report that the application of ultrasonic energy to the adipose tissue liquefies the fat effectively, releasing a combination of triglycerides, normal interstitial fluid, and the infused tumescent solution. These components form an emulsion, which can be removed using vacuum suction. They further discussed that the ultrasonic waves selectively target the fat cells without affecting the intervening connective tissue and neurovascular structures. The depth of penetration is inversely proportional to the frequency used.

There have been reports that postoperative external ultrasound is a very useful modality for properly selected patients, namely those with firm or persistent induration or swelling.[9,10] In such patients, postoperative external ultrasound can speed up recovery and improve patient comfort.

Low-frequency focused ultrasound (LOFU) has also gained some popularity. It operates at low frequency (20–200 kHz) and low intensity (up to 17.5 W/cm^2 to induce cavitations through mechanical stress rupturing the adipocytes. There are few publications in the United States on the biological effects but there are still no randomized clinical trials or comparative studies. In one of the studies on 20 women with maximum fat thickness of 4 cm in skin fold test, LOFU was used for total five sessions at 2-week intervals.[11] After efficacy assessment with bioelectric impedance analysis device and various measurements, there was a significant reduction of 1.5 cm in waist circumference, 2.1 cm in abdominal circumference, and 1.9 cm in the umbilical circumference.

Adipose cells are composed of 80–90% triglycerides that are released into circulation after LOFU and follow the normal physiologic pathways after treatment.

INJECTION LIPOLYSIS

In this technique, combination of medications such as PDC is injected deeper into the fat cells that cause disruption of the fat cells. But it is currently not approved by US FDA.

In mesotherapy, medications and other substances are injected into the mesoderm (the layer of fat and connective tissue under the skin). When PDC is used for body contouring, a "recommended dosage is 100 mg per 5 × 5 cm^2 area every 2 weeks for 3–6 treatments. In a double-blind, prospective study, a single-body region was treated by mesotherapy on a weekly basis for 5 weeks, followed by monthly maintenance therapy. I reported that majority of patients observe noticeable difference in the treated area. Circumference measurements decreased in the majority of treated patients. The average decrease in circumference was 2.6 cm at the waist and 1.8 cm at the thigh; the greatest circumference decrease was 3.8 cm at the waist and 2.5 cm at the thigh.

The mechanism by which injectable PDC may result in decreased localized fat collections is not well understood. One hypothesis is that concentrated amounts of PDC injected subcutaneously would emulsify fat, allowing tissue lipases to hydrolyze fat and producing glycerol and free fatty acids. Alternatively, PDC may act to stimulate β-receptors or inhibit α-2-receptors, thus producing increased lipolysis activity.[12]

A survey was published in 2006[13] that reviewed data on 17,276 patients who were treated with a PDC-based compound by a large number of practitioners. Most of the surveys reported a maximum safe limit of 2,000–2,500 mg of PDS-based solution per treatment area. At a dilution of 25 mg/mL, 100 mL per session could be safely used. Larger doses can have side effects such as nausea, diarrhea, and dizziness. Among the reporting physicians 26.6% used additives including L-carnitine, aminophylline, and vitamin. The commonest contraindications were pregnancy, allergies to soy product, autoimmune disease, anticoagulant treatments, etc.

Recently FDA has approved a new drug, Kybella (Deoxycholic acid) for submental fat reduction.

It was based on evidence from two clinical trials on 1,022 adult patients with the appearance of moderate or severe amounts submental fat. There was significant reduction in the submental fat thickness after 12 weeks of the final treatment.

Kybella is a cytolytic drug that physically destroys the cell membrane causing lysis. This has opened a new avenue to fat reduction by injection technique.

LOW LEVEL LASER THERAPY

The biologic and physiologic effects of laser have been extensively researched since 1960. Neira et al. identified the ability of low-level laser to emulsify the fat using scanning electron microscopy and magnetic resonance imaging.[14]

The commonest wavelength used is 650 nm (635–680 nm) and it is absorbed by cytochrome-c-oxidase unit in mitochondria causing ionic (H^+ and Ca^{2+}) efflux and altering the pH inside the cell. This stimulates lipase enzyme breaking down the triglycerides into glycerol and fatty acids.[15] Glycerol and fatty acids are then released in the interstitial tissue and absorbed by lymphatics. Energy levels used are low level, around 40 mW and is referred to as cold laser.

There is very limited literature to demonstrate significant reduction in body circumference when used in isolation nor there is comparative data to compare with other nonsurgical devices.[16,17]

CRYOLIPOLYSIS

This is approved by the US FDA for the reduction of focal adiposity. Cryolipolysis is the controlled application of cold to subcutaneous tissue to reduce adipose tissue. The procedure is performed on an outpatient basis and suction is used to pull the skin into a cup-shaped hand piece, in which contact is established between the skin and subcutaneous tissue and two opposing cooling panels. Intense cooling of tissue called cooling intensity factor causes an inflammatory process culminating in necrotic cell death at temperatures between – 2°C and 7°C.[18,19]

Some studies suggest that the inflammatory response begins within 3 days after treatment and peaks within 14 days. From day 14 to day 30, macrophages and phagocytes engulf dead lipid cells. In humans, cryolipolysis for isolated fat deposits in the flank or on the back has been associated with a reduction in fat content of approximately 20–26% at the treatment site 4–6 months after treatment. Side effects include pain, bruising, erythema, and numbness. The destruction of adipocytes does not significantly affect serum lipid levels or liver function tests. Since cryolipolysis does not use heat, it does not produce skin tightening. Consequently, a skin-tightening procedure may be required after cryolipolysis.[20]

In a study by Ferraro et al.,[21] 50 patients were treated with a cryolipolysis protocol. They reported a mean reduction in fat thickness of 3.02 cm and a mean reduction in circumference of 4.45 cm after treatment. Recently, Zeltiq

(Zeltiq Aesthetics, Inc., Pleasanton, CA, USA) and Zerona (Erchonia Corp., McKinney, TX, USA) have received US FDA approval for noninvasive body contouring and fat reduction.

RADIOFREQUENCY

This is a skin-tightening technology and no radiofrequency device has been approved for body sculpting in the United States or Canada. Radiofrequency works primarily through skin tightening rather than destruction of adipose tissues.

In monopolar radiofrequency devices, energy is passed from a single electrode into the skin and subcutaneous tissues and directed to a return pad in another area of the body, whereas in multipolar radiofrequency, two or more electrodes are positioned at different points on the skin so that the waves pass between them to create heating. Radiofrequency waves travel between the two plates heating the tissues in between. This increases the risk of skin damage and is nonselective for fatty tissue. Typically, the devices require a cooling system to prevent epidermal damage and prolonged period to adequately heat the fatty tissue.[22]

In some clinical trials, 6–10 radiofrequency treatments have produced 2 to 3.5 cm reductions in waist and thigh circumferences. Radiofrequency causes skin tightening, and it also has been proposed that reductions in circumference with radiofrequency therapy are temporary and secondary to skin tightening.

Radiofrequency is a painful procedure and has risks of scars, burns, and fat atrophy. Thus, as a fat-reduction technology, it is unpredictable but it surely has skin toning and tightening effect.[23]

CARBOXYTHERAPY

Carbon dioxide (CO_2) therapy or carboxytherapy is the transcutaneous administration of CO_2 for therapeutic purposes. Brandi et al.[24] published the efficacy of CO_2 in treating localized adiposities, and showed measurable reductions in circumferences of the abdomen, thigh, and knee regions.

Carbon dioxide is infused subcutaneously into the affected areas using the carbomed programmable automatic carbon dioxide therapy apparatus (Carbossiterapia Italiana SRL, Via Zanella, MI, Italy) and 30-gauge needles. The depth of infusion is 10–13 mm. The device controls the temperature and calibrates the flow rate. Approximately 500–1,000 mL of CO_2 gas is infused in areas such as abdomen and thighs with a flow rate of 50–100 mL/min.[25]

In a histologic study, Brandi et al. reported fracturing of the adipose tissue with release of triglycerides in the intercellular spaces. He also reported microcirculatory changes after CO_2 therapy, reflected by increased perfusion as measured by laser Doppler flowmetry and increased oxygen tension as measured by transcutaneous oxygen tension. This is due the Bohr effect on the oxygen dissociation curve.

COMBINATION OF TECHNOLOGIES

Noninvasive techniques such as radiofrequency, cryolipolysis, injection lipolysis, external low-level lasers, laser ablation, nonthermal ultrasound, and HIFU may be particularly appropriate options for nonobese patients requiring modest to moderate body sculpting. Each of these treatments can be performed in a clinical setting without any downtime or significant risks. However, with the exception of HIFU, these procedures require multiple treatments to achieve meaningful results.

INDICATIONS AND CLINICAL APPLICATION

There are a wide range of technologies and nonsurgical options available for fat reduction. How does one decide the best technology and what results are to be expected? There are no straightforward answers to these questions.

In my practice, I have used many of these technologies and with my experience of over 8 years in nonsurgical fat reduction, there is no single technology that has given objective outcome.

We use a variety of combinations and the results are unpredictable. The technologies can be used as one of the armamentarium to deal with body contouring patients.

So what is the advantage of having such options for the patients? There are several benefits of nonsurgical fat reduction options for the patients:

- It is a scientific method to reduce fat and patients should be aware of this option.
- There are a large percentage of patients who do not want to go through invasive procedures. You can offer them a comprehensive nonsurgical management for weight reduction. Many of these patients decide later to opt for invasive procedures.
- Medically compromised patients who are not good candidates for invasive procedures can be benefitted with noninvasive and comprehensive weight-reduction methods.
- It will drive more patients to your practice, like the mouth of the funnel that will always stream down to ideal patients for invasive procedures. This is "funnel effect" in our practice.

Postliposuction treatment: noninvasive technologies help reduce swelling, contour the body, and stimulate skin contraction. I have found it very useful in challenging patients with lumpiness and skin irregularities, etc.

However, the cost of these technologies is the limiting factor. Other disadvantages include lack of standard protocol, quantifying the result objectively and noncompliance of the patients.

Some of the Technologies that can be Combined

External Ultrasound and Endermology Therapy

After ultrasound cavitation, a few sessions of endermology therapy help to mechanically displace the adipose tissue with the help of a roller and a vacuum cup. It can be used as lymphatic massage by a therapist. Mendes[26] published a report on 30 patients where they used external ultrasound energy on waist, hips and thighs for 15 minutes each for 24 sessions. Each session of ultrasound treatment was followed by "endermosuctioning massage" with negative suction device. They noticed a significant reduction in subcutaneous fat and reshaping of the skin.

Bipolar Radiofrequency, Infrared/Low-level Laser, and Pulsatile Suction Devices

This machine have a combination effect due to low-level laser and radiofrequency on the skin and subcutaneous tissue. The suction device sucks a fold of skin to stabilize the skin and fatty tissue, and it discharges laser energy and radiofrequency energy simultaneously targeting the subcutaneous fat and dermal collagen.[26,27]

In our office, we combine HIFU with low-level laser, radiofrequency, and suction device. Addition of carboxytherapy in some patients has given us objectively visible results. Some of the clinical results with objective evidence of contouring of the abdominal region (Figs. 11.2 to 11.7).

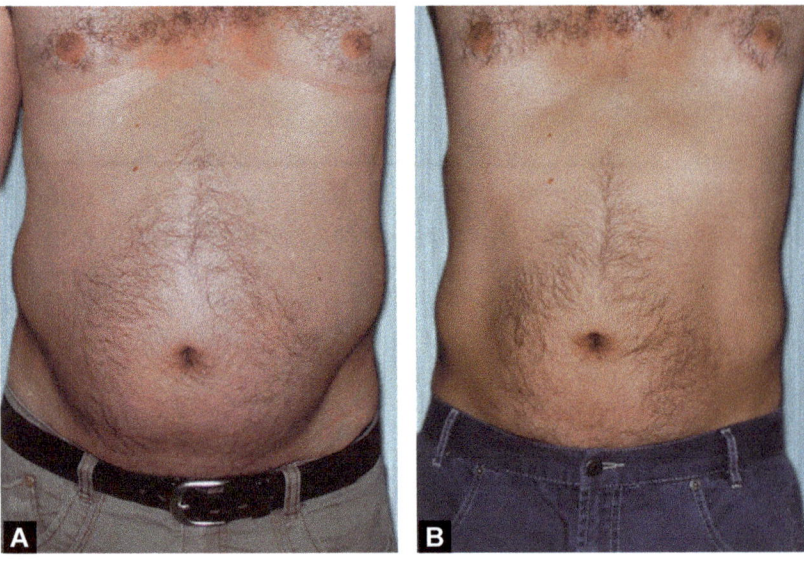

Figs. 11.2A and B: Case study 1 (A) Patient with BMI 24, requested nonsurgical reduction of abdomen. (B) Combination cavitation, PowerShape, carboxytherapy used in weekly sessions for eight weeks.

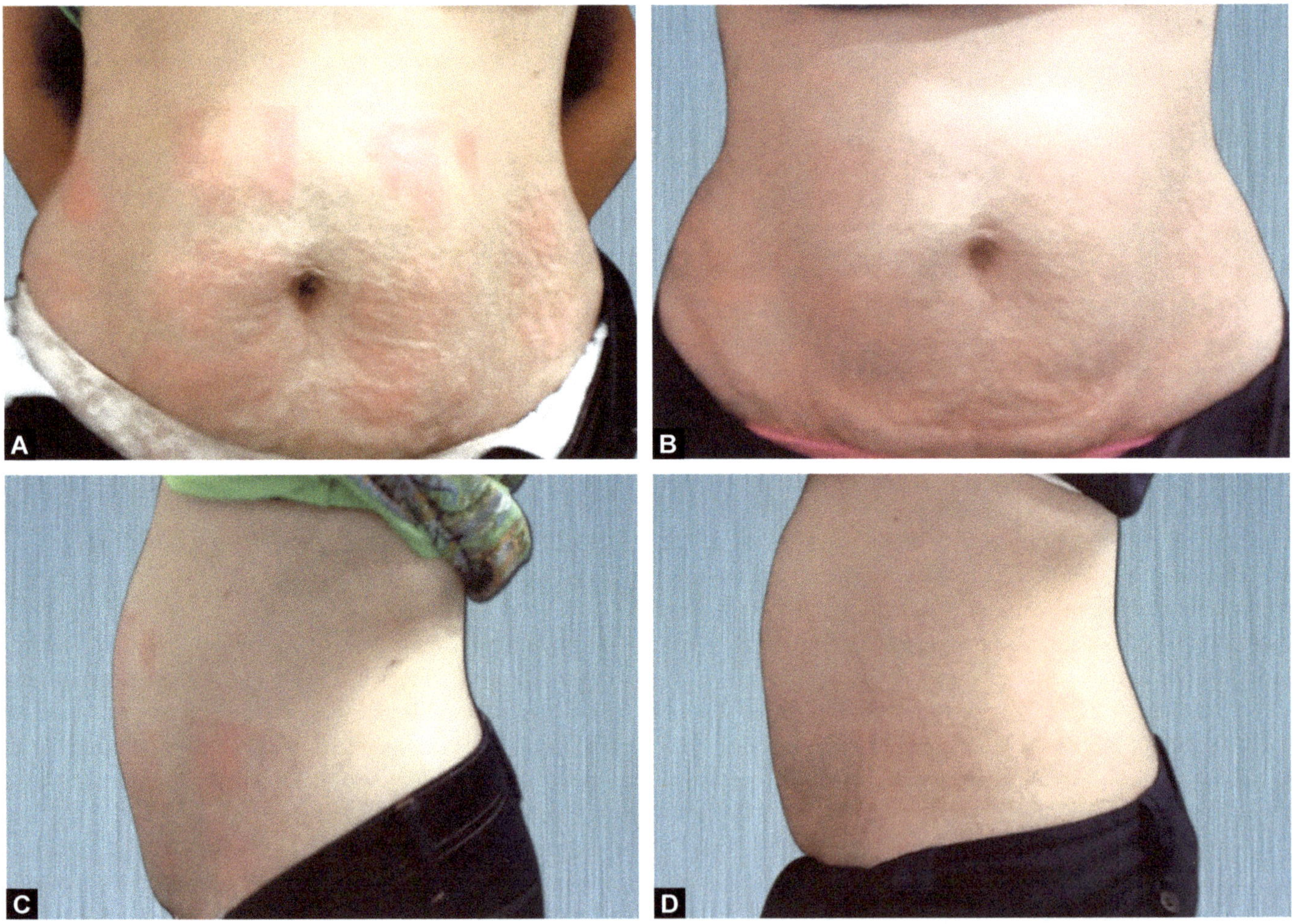

Figs. 11.3A to D: Case study 2. (A and C) A 38-year-old patient with BMI 28, history of multiple pregnancies refusing to undergo invasive procedure. A combination treatment using radiofrequency, PowerShape, carboxytherapy used as weekly session for 10 weeks. (B and D) Results after ten sessions with improvement in the tone of the skin and stretch marks.

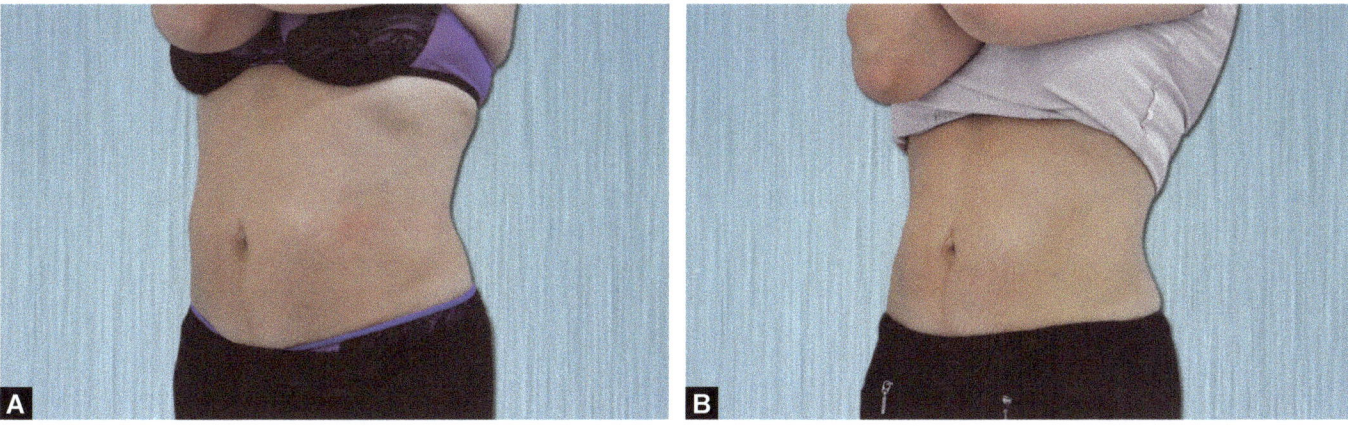

Figs. 11.4A and B: (A) A 32-year-old patient with BMI 24, mild abdominal wall laxity and moderate amount of subcutaneous fat. Combination of PowerShape, cavitation and radiofrequency used once a week for six weeks. (B) Reduction in abdomen by 2.8 cm at the level of the umbilicus and improvement in quality of the skin.

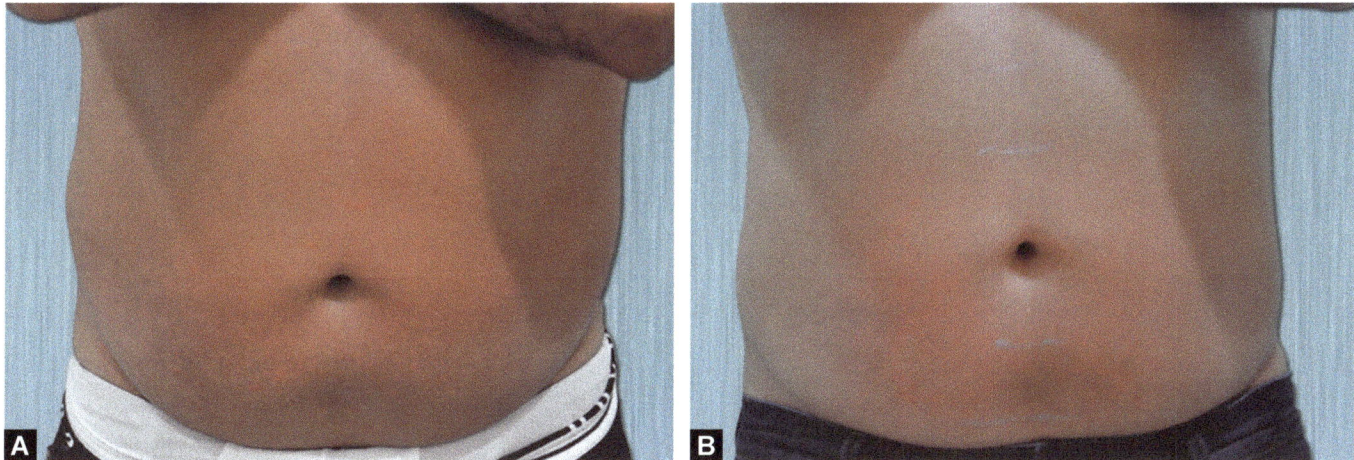

Figs. 11.5A and B: (A) A 32-year-old male patient with BMI 28. (B) Combination of cavitation, carboxytherapy and PowerShape for six weeks. (B) Reduction of waist circumference by 3.2 cm with visible improvement in the contour of the abdomen and flanks.

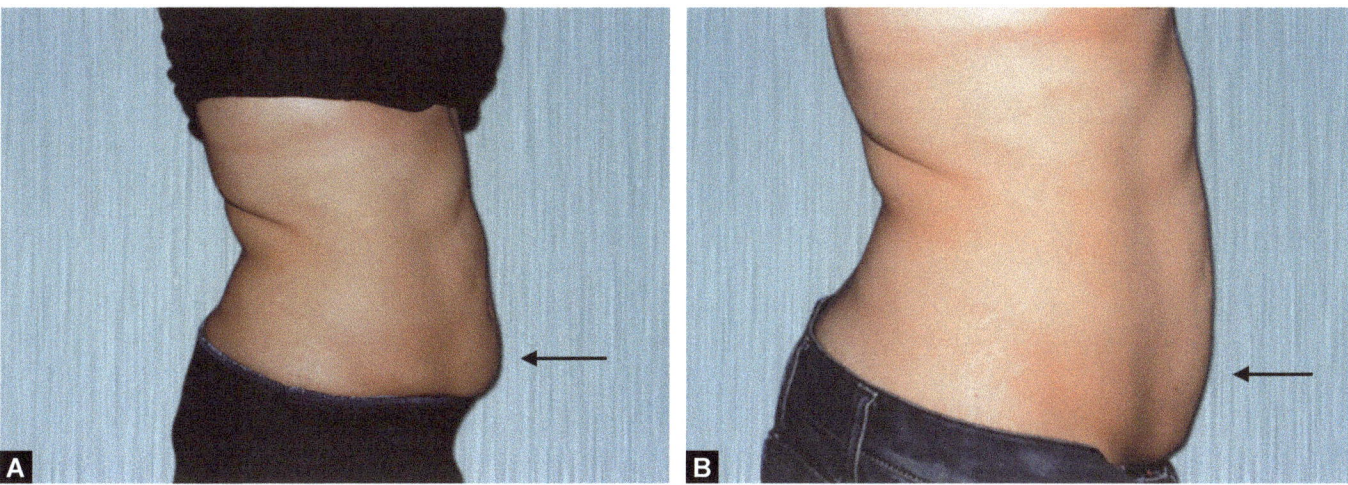

Figs. 11.6A and B

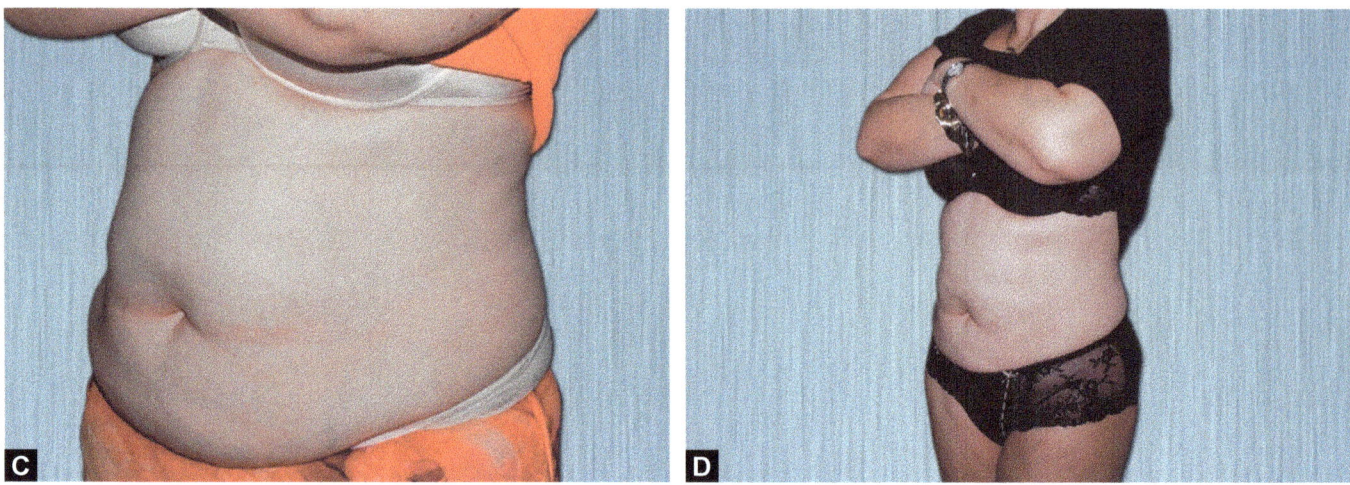

Figs. 11.6A to D: (A and C) A 42-year-old patient with 2 normal deliveries. (B and D) Combination therapy for eight weeks improved the circumference from 88 cm at the umbilicus to 82 cm. Also note the improvement in the panniculus in the lower abdomen.

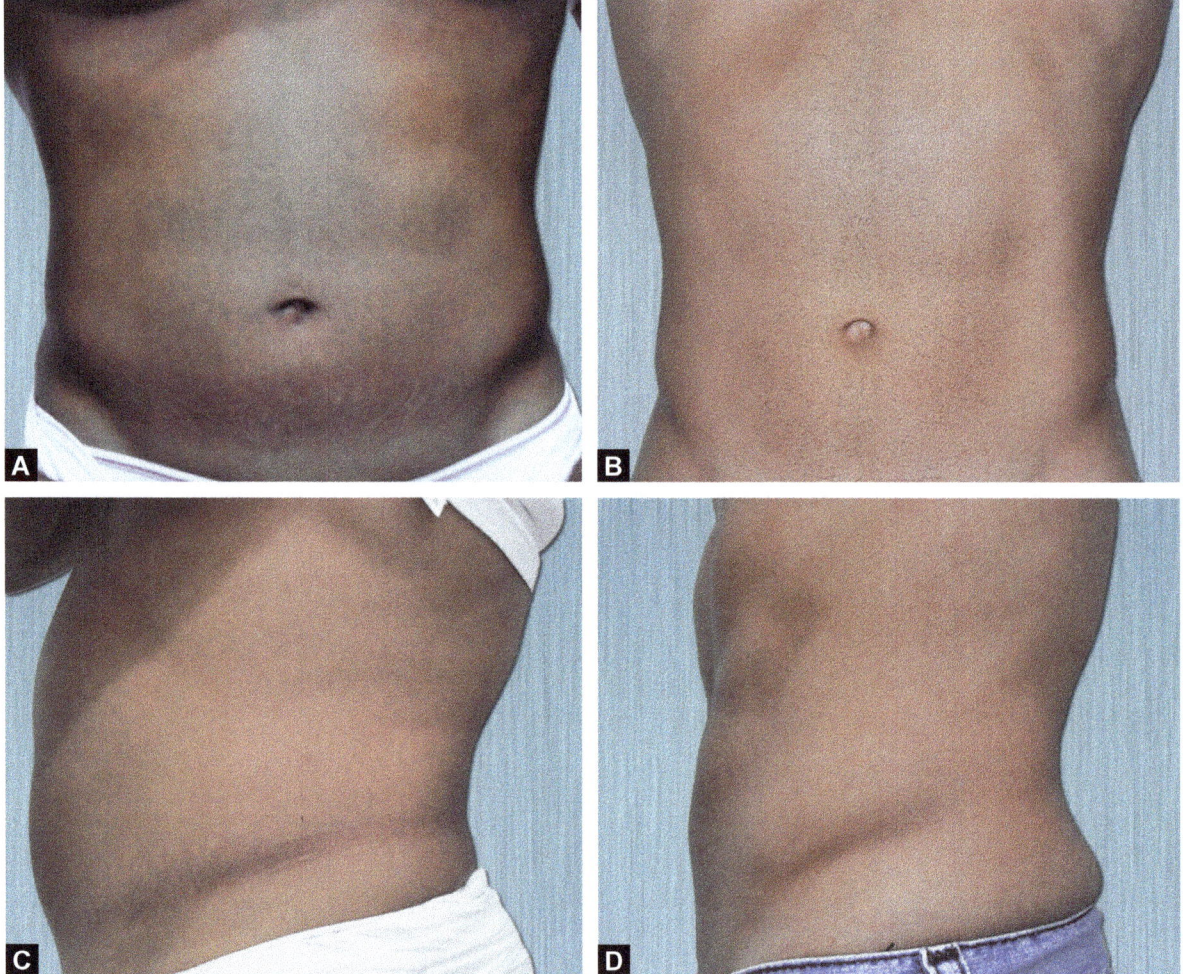

Figs. 11.7A to D: (A and C) A young male regularly visiting the gym was unable to reduce the subcutaneous fat. (B and D) After six sessions of combination therapy the pinch thickness in lower abdomen reduced from 7 cm to 3 cm. Also note the enhancement of the muscular contour of the abdomen.

▍ REFERENCES

1. Toledo LS. Emerging techniques in aesthetic plastic surgery. Clin Plast Surg. 2009;36:177-80, v.
2. Paul M, Blugerman G, Kreindel M, et al. Three dimensional radiofrequency tissue tightening: a proposed mechanism and applications for body contouring. Aesthetic Plast Surg. 2011;35:87-95.
3. Wong L, Vasconez HC. Patient satisfaction after Nd:YAG laser-assisted lipolysis. Ann Plast Surg. 2011;66:561-3.
4. Sadick N, Magro C. A study evaluating the safety and efficacy of the VelaSmooth system in the treatment of cellulite. J Cosmet Laser Ther. 2007;9:15-20.
5. Brown SA, Greenbaum L, Shtukmaster S. Characterization of nonthermal focused ultrasound for noninvasive selective fat cell disruption (Lysis): technical and preclinical assessment. Plast Reconstr Surg. 2009;124(1):92-101.
6. Ferraro GA, De Francesco F, Nicoletti G, et al. Histologic effects of external ultrasound-assisted lipectomy on adipose tissue. Aesthetic Plast Surg. 2008;32:111-5.
7. Teiselbaum SA, Burns JL, Kubora J, et al. Noninvasive body contouring by focused ultrasound: safety and efficacy of the contour I device in a multicenter, controlled, clinical study. Plast Reconstr Surg. 2007;120:779-89, discussion 790.
8. Cook WR Jr. Utilizing external ultrasonic energy to improve the results of tumescent liposculpture. Dermatol Surg. 1997; 23:1207-11.
9. Butterwick KJ, Tse Y, Goldman MP. Effect of external ultrasound post liposuction: a side-to-side comparison study. Dermatol Surg. 2000;26:433-5.
10. Bernstein G. Ultrasound therapy for postoperative liposuction care. Dermatol Surg. 1997;23:211.
11. Tonucci LV, Mourao DM. Noninvasive body contouring: biological and aesthetic effects of lowfrequency, low intensity ultrasound device. Aesthetic Plast Surg. 2014;38:959-67.
12. Matarasso A, Pfeifer TM. Mesotherapy for body contouring. Plast Reconstr Surg. 2005;115(5):1420-4.
13. Duncan DI, Chubaty R. Clinical safety data and standards of practice for injection lipolysis: a retrospective study. Aesthetic Surg J. 2006;26(5):575-85.
14. Neira R, Arroyave J, Ramirez H, et al. Fat liquefaction: effect of low level laser energy on adipose tissue. Plast Reconstr Surg. 2002;110 (3):912-22.
15. Karu T, Kolyakov SF. Exact action spectra for cellular responses relevant to phototherapy. Photomed Laser Surg. 2005; 23(4):355-61.
16. Caruso-Davis MK, Guillot TS, Podichetty VK, et al. Efficacy of low-level laser therapy for body contouring and spot fat reduction. Obes Surg. 2011;21(6):722-9.
17. Jackson RF, Dedo DD, Roche GC, et al. Low-level laser therapy as a non-invasive approach for body contouring: a randomized, controlled study. Lasers Surg Med 2009; 41 (10):799-809.
18. Avram MM, Harry RS. Cryolipolysis for subcutaneous fat layer reduction. Lasers Surg Med. 2009;41:703-8.
19. Klein KB, Zelickson B, Riopelle JG, et al. Noninvasive cryolipolysis for subcutaneous fat reduction does not affect serum lipid levels or liver function tests. Lasers Surg Med. 2009;41: 785-90.
20. Zelickson B, Egbert BM, Preciado J, et al. Noninvasive cooling of fat cells to induce lipolysis for noninvasive adipocyte cell death: initial results from a pig model (poster 25). In: ASDS 2008—American Society of Dermatologic Surgeons, Orlando; November, 6–9, 2008.
21. Ferraro GA, De Francesco F, Cataldo C, et al. Synergistic effects of cryolipolysis and shock waves for noninvasive body contouring. Aesthetic Plast Surg. 2012;36:666-79.
22. Goldberg DJ, Fazeli A, Berlin AL. Clinical, laboratory, and MRI analysis of cellulite treatment with a unipolar radiofrequency device. Dermatol Surg. 2008;34:204-9, discussion 209.
23. Manuskiatti W, Wachirakaphan C, Lektrakul N, et al. Circumference reduction and cellulite treatment with a TriPollar radiofrequency device: a pilot study. J Eur Acad Dermatol Venereol 2009;23:820-7.
24. Brandi C, D'Aniello C, Grimaldi L, et al. Carbon dioxide therapy in the treatment of localized adiposities: clinical study and histopathological correlations. Aesthetic Plast Surg. 2001; 25:170-4.
25. Lee GS. Carbon dioxide therapy in the treatment of cellulite: an audit of clinical practice. Aesthetic Plast Surg. 2010; 34:239-43.
26. Mendes FH. Noninvasive liposculpture: an association of external ultrasound delivery with endermosuctioning massage. Plast Reconstr Surg. 1999;104(4):1206-7.
27. Wanitphakdeedecha R, Manuskiatti W. Treatment of cellulite with a bipolar radiofrequency, infrared heat, and pulsatile suction device: a pilot study. J Cosmet Dermatol. 2006;5: 284-8.

CHAPTER 12

Postoperative Management

■ INTRODUCTION

"It cannot be too often emphasized, however, that the postoperative treatment is as essential as the operation, and the surgeon is as much responsible for the postoperative treatment as for the operation."   —*Roscoe C Giles*

Our aim is to achieve the best possible outcome with minimal complications and a pleasant experience for patients. Often a patient who suffers postoperatively with excessive pain, bruising, and swelling is not encouraged to talk about your practice and will not participate in word of mouth referral. On the contrary, a patient who recovers with minimum discomfort is motivated to talk positively about it helping you increase your practice.

Postoperative management is based on pre-emptive precaution to avoid potential problems and complications that is covered in detail in the Chapter 13.

■ DISCHARGE CRITERIA

After the procedure is over and the patient is recovered from sedation and anesthesia, he or she is assessed by a qualified person to ensure that the patient is safe to discharge. We follow a strict protocol (Chart 12.1) to ensure that all criteria are met before they leave the premise.

The patient is then handed over the discharge instruction sheet that clearly explains the "do's and don'ts." The details of what to expect and care required at home are also printed for the patient and caregiver (Chart 12.2).

The commonest events that may occur on the day of the procedure, whether in the hospital or at home, are as follows:
1. Dizziness/Postural hypotension
2. Excessive oozing and discharge
3. Pain

The caregivers and nurses need to be educated that after a few hours of surgery when they are ambulated, there is a sudden drop in blood pressure causing fainting attack and panic. This could be due to excessive bleeding

Chart 12.1: Discharge criteria.

- Every patient is seen following the surgery by the anesthetists and surgeons involved in each case.
- Assessment of when the patient is ready for discharge is performed by nursing staff.
- The discharge criteria should consider social factors as well as medical assessment of sufficient recovery for discharge.
- In general, the essential discharge criteria must be met before the patient leaves the facility. These include:
  ° Stable vital signs for at least 1 hour.
  ° The patient is conscious and oriented as to time, place, and person.
  ° The patient is pain free and comfortable and has supply of oral analgesia.
  ° The patient is able to dress and walk where appropriate.
  ° There is no or minimal nausea, vomiting, or dizziness.
  ° The patient has taken oral fluids.
  ° There is no or minimal bleeding or wound drainage.
  ° The patient has passed urine (if appropriate).
  ° The patient has a responsible adult to take him/her home.
  ° The patient has agreed to have caregiver at home for the next 24 hours.
  ° The patient has written and given verbal instruction about postoperative care.
  ° The patient knows when to come back for follow-up.
  ° The patient has the emergency contact number supplied.

Patient's Name: ....
Mobile No: ....
Surgeon: ....
Mobile No: ....
Date: ....

Chart 12.2: Postoperative instructions.

The patient is advised verbally and in writing that, in the first hours postoperatively, he/she must not do the following:

1. Drive or operate machinery
2. Cook
3. Work or make important decision
4. Drink alcohol
5. Take any medication except that approved by the Daycare center

The specific information given to the patient and caregiver:

1. Medication instruction regarding analgesia, antiemetic, or antibiotics.
   ....
   ....
   ....
   ....

2. Wound care and when the patient may bath or shower.
   ....
   ....
   ....
   ....

3. Arrangements for dressing renewal and suture removal.
   ....
   ....
   ....
   ....

4. Resuming normal activities; return to work, exercise, etc.
   ....
   ....
   ....
   ....

5. What "normal" postoperative symptoms' may be expected and their situation?
   ....
   ....
   ....
   ....

6. What would be abnormal postoperative symptoms and what to do if they occur?
   ....
   ....
   ....
   ....

Contd...

Contd...

7. Arrangement for follow-up.
   ....
   ....
   ....
   ....

8. In case of emergency, contact the doctor and ambulance service on _____. Hospital for emergency _____. Doctor on call _____.
   Patient's Name: ....
   Mobile No: ....
   Surgeon: ....
   Mobile No: ....
   Date: ....

or lidocaine toxicity or vasovagal attack due to the site of blood tinged discharge.

To prevent bleeding, necessary preoperative and intraoperative precautions must be in place and postoperatively, a firm compressive dressing is applied.

Prior to ambulation, the patient is advised to sit up, take deep breaths, and slowly hang the legs on the side of the bed. If there is a mild dizziness, he/she is advised to lie flat; or if they feel well then they can stand up. The patient may have to do this for a few times before they are able to walk without severe dizziness.

The patients, nurses, and caregivers should be taught on how to deal with fainting attacks, so they are aware and do not cause panic situation, particularly, among the relatives and caregivers.

I prefer to hand over a sheet "how to deal with dizziness?" to patients before they leave the hospital (Chart 12.3).

PROTOCOL FOR POSTOPERATIVE VISIT

The patients are handed over the postoperative instruction sheet well before the surgery (*see* Chapter 8), so they are aware of the course of events. This needs to be reminded at every postoperative visit.

Protocol helps us to coordinate activities between primary surgeons, assistants, trainees, nurses, patient relatives, and patients, thus completing the "circle of patient care."

We follow a system to call back the patient at regular intervals. This is recorded in a chart and helps in preventing problems, providing high-quality postoperative care, statistics, and photographic documentation, and so on and so forth (Table 12.1).

Chart 12.3: How to deal with dizziness?

It is important to read this document for the patient and family/ friend attending the patient.

Dizziness after any procedure (*usually same night or next morning*) can happen in following circumstances:
1. Not eating and drinking adequately (lack of sugar, hypoglycemia).
2. Fall in blood pressure because of standing up suddenly from lying down position or standing for long time (postural hypotension).
3. Keeping your legs dangling for long-time.
4. Sudden release of tight garment.
5. Sight of blood, discharge (fainting attack, vasovagal).
6. Abnormal sensation during showering.
7. Sight of bruising and swelling.
8. Eating medications empty stomach.

To prevent dizziness do the following:
1. Eat and drink well; keep juices and water besides your bed.
2. Do slow movements when getting up.
3. Do not stand or sit for a long period of time.
4. Cover the soaked dressing with cotton, do not look at the operative site when you are standing under the shower.
5. Remove all dressings and garments in the bed, before you walk to bathroom for showering.
6. Have a quick shower with warm water (neither too hot, nor too cold).
7. Avoid alcohol and smoking.

If you have dizziness/fainting attack, *friends and relatives, please do not be panic!!*
1. Support the patient ensure that he/she does not fall.
2. Lie down flat wherever you are or the patient is.
3. Ask the patient to take deep breath.
4. Raise the leg of the patient, bend the knees, and gently press those against the tummy.
5. Give the patient juice and water.
6. If not improving, call your surgeon_____ and ambulance 999.

Table 12.1: Postoperative follow-up protocol.		
Duration	*Potential problems*	*Parameters and management*
First postoperative day—first 24 hours	Nausea, vomiting, pain, dizziness, fainting attacks, breathlessness, bleeding	TPR, BP, general condition, pain control, physical movement, treatment
Second postoperative day	Pain, discomfort, physical limitations, wound drains, plaster irritation, dressing spillage	Pain control physical movement wound check for irritation, allergy, blood collection, skin vascularity, sensibility
Fifth postoperative day	Pain, physical limitation, wound problems	Pain control, physical movement wound care
Seventh postoperative day	Discomfort, physical limitation, allergies, swelling	Suture removal, dressing advice, garment advice, traveling advice, work related advice, scar management
Overseas patient		Written instructions, email/telephone follow-up, arrangement to see local medical center, if necessary
1 month	Swelling, scar itching, tenderness	Scar examination, swelling, assess skin redraping
3 months	Swelling, scar, lumpiness	Result assessment
6 months	Optional	
1 year	Residual issues	Result
3 years onward		Long-term result

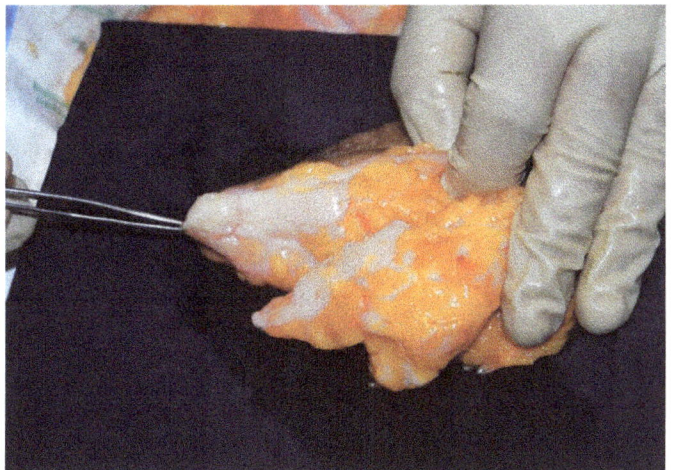

Fig.12.1: White colored internal fibrous tissue removed during abdominoplasty in a patient with previous liposuction.

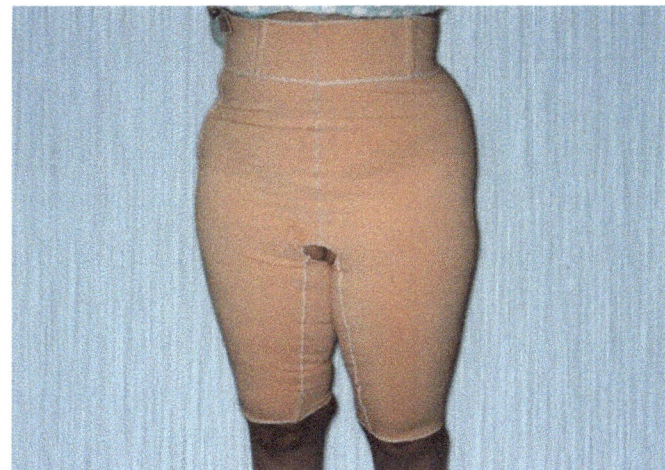

Fig.12.2: Improper garment.

DRAINAGE

Postoperative swelling, bruising, seroma, and pain occur due to the accumulation of fluid and blood. The proportion of infiltration and aspiration is important to understand the need for postoperative drainage. The following are the methods of drainage:

1. *Leaving incision ports open*: This works very good for us. I often use 8–10 small incisions particularly more in a dependent position. A good compressive dressing with elastoplast and leaving the port open allows adequate drainage in first 24 hours.

2. *Silicone or Penrose drains*: Some surgeons prefer to use an open drain in the dependent sites such as pubic and sacral incisions. These are removed after 2–3 days. If you use these drains, patients need to be monitored on daily basis as it requires dressing changes and can sometimes retrieve inside the wound if not secured properly.

3. *Closed suction drains*: This is another option many surgeons are using. In my opinion, often it fails in many occasions as it can get blocked, loose vacuum, and removal can be very painful.

It is an independent decision based on experience and acceptance by the surgeons and the patients.

COMPRESSION GARMENT

This is the most important part of postoperative management. An improper fitting garment can cause following problems:

1. Discomfort
2. Blistering
3. Pressure necrosis
4. Distal edema
5. Abnormal creases on the skin
6. Inadequate compression

After lipoaspiration if the skin is not elastic enough, the space gets filled with fluid. Depending upon the elasticity of the skin and quality of the garment, the edema may reduce over time and skin will drape over the muscles. If not, there is internal scar formation that compromises the result (Fig. 12.1).

Choosing right material and fitting is very important for a successful outcome. I prefer to use spandex or lycra material than cotton fabric as it is thinner and more breathable. Some of the modern garments are comfortable even in hot weather. Some of the garments are made of cotton but they are too thick and do not conform to the body well (Fig. 12.2).

Additional foam support under the garment is a very useful way to get an appropriate compression and splint the skin, preventing wrinkling and creasing. There are some commercially available foam such as Epifoam and Topifoam available online.

How Long to Wear the Garment?

This is the one question that has not been answered very well. The duration has ranged from 1 month to 6 months by different surgeons. Majority of publications mention 6 weeks of postoperative compression.[1]

If we look at the literature and understand the edema process, we will be able to justify the duration of compression garment.

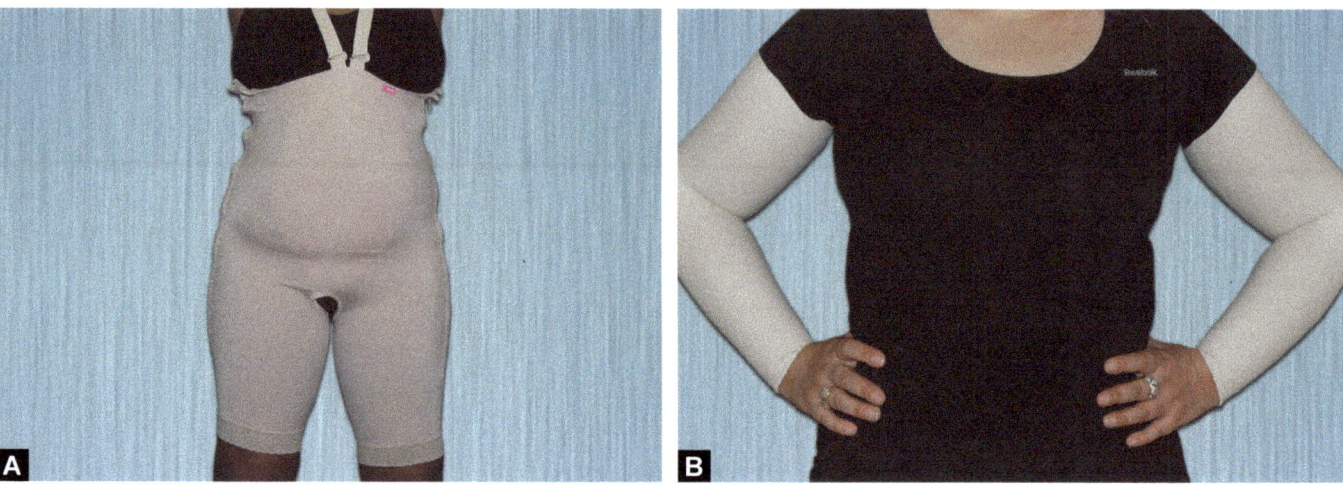

Figs. 12.3A and B: (A) Pressure garment first stage, (B) Second stage pressure garment.

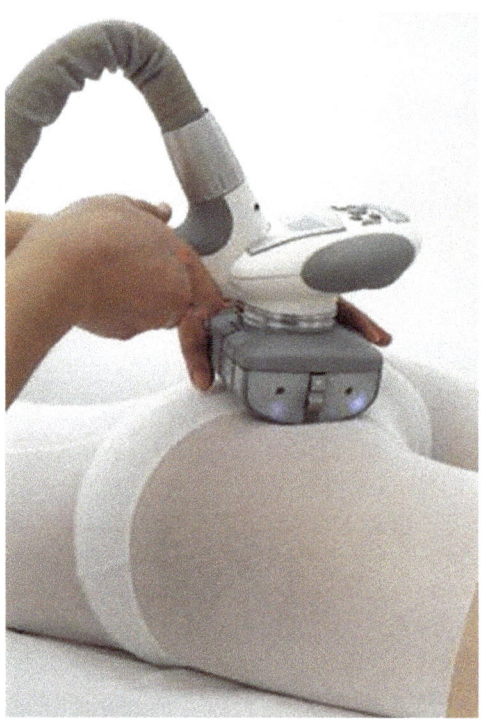

Fig.12.4: Endermologie.

Swanson addressed the issue of postoperative edema in a presentation at the 2011 American Society of Plastic Surgeons Annual Meeting in Denver, Colorado, USA.[2] He performed magnetic resonance imaging studies on three women who underwent ultrasonic liposuction of the lower body (i.e. abdomen, flanks, buttocks, thighs, and knees) using a superwet technique. He demonstrated that 66% of the swelling associated with the procedure resolved after 1 month and 87% of the swelling resolved after 3.3 months.

I usually recommend two-stage garments, first stage of surgical pressure garment for 4–6 weeks depending upon the skin elasticity and amount of swelling, followed by second-stage garment (4–6 weeks) with standard normal firm fitting garments available at stores (Figs. 12.3A and B).

MANUAL MASSAGE

Manual massage performed by patients or manual lymphatic massage performed by experts assists in enhanced healing. The strokes of massage done in certain direction help to improve blood circulation and lymphatic flow, reduce induration and fibrosis, and comfort the patient.

There are many publications emphasizing the benefit of manual lymphatic drainage (MLD) to improve microcirculation, reduce pain, swelling, and ecchymosis.[3] The patient can receive MLD every 2–3 days for 2 weeks. This can be followed by traditional massages at home.

EQUIPMENT-BASED THERAPIES

There are many devices available in the market to non-invasively improve body contour, drape the skin uniformly, and reduce cellulite formation.

Endermologie is vacuum-based equipment that has rollers that can be used on top a special garment worn by the patient during treatment. Equipped with rollers the treatment heads gently grasp the skin tissue and roll on the body using only mechanical stimulation (Fig. 12.4).

It can be started after 5–6 days when the patient is more comfortable to undergo pressure and manipulation. It is performed with low vacuum in a gentle manner and it can be repeated as a weekly session for 4–6 weeks.

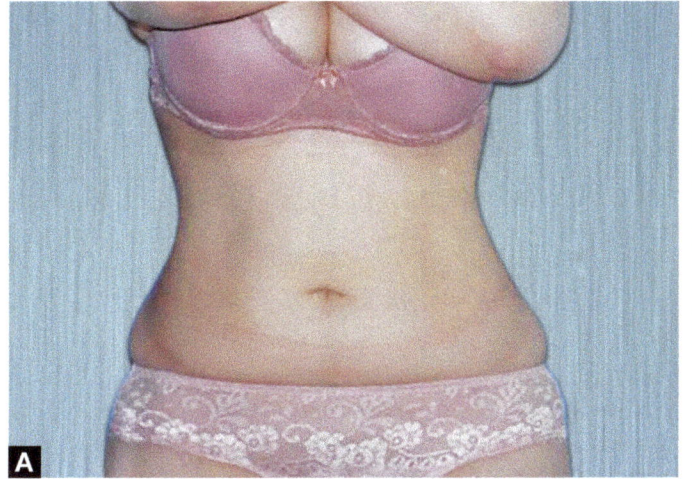

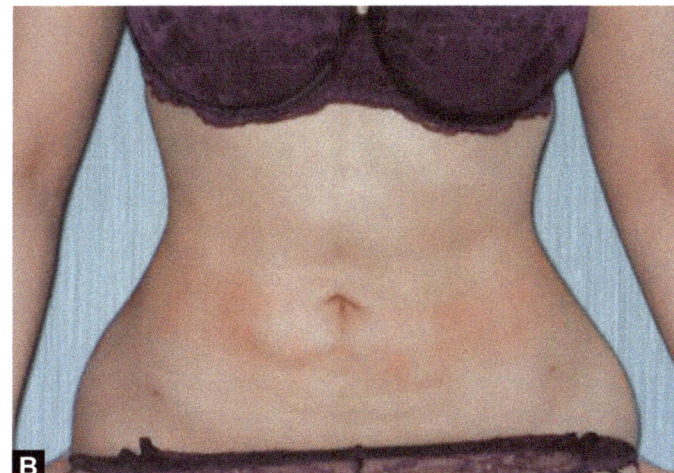

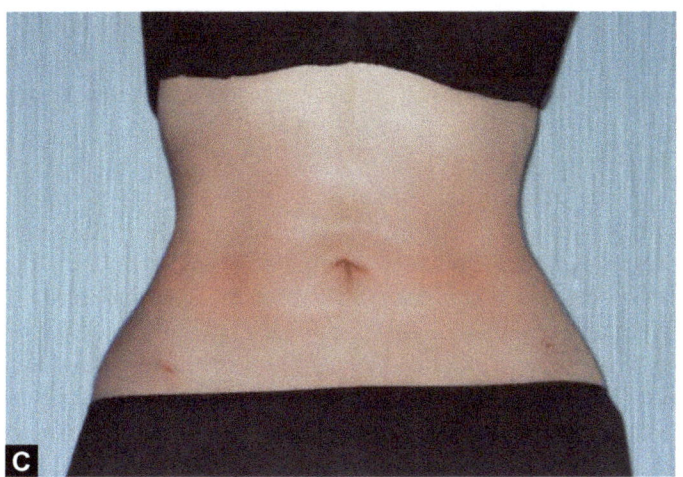

Figs.12.5A to C: (A) The patient with weight loss came for liposculpting. (B) She underwent suction-assisted liposuction and developed irregularity and lumpiness after 1 month. (C) She underwent a combination therapy using PowerShape device for four sessions, which results after 2 months of surgery.

Combination of Vacuum, Low-Level Laser and Radiofrequency

There are equipments that have the above combinations and it has combined benefit of massage, low-level laser therapy (LLT) for improved healing and radiofrequency (RF) for skin tightening.

External Ultrasound

Nonfocused ultrasound like the one used for physiotherapy and sports medicine can also be used on the treated areas. Low-frequency ultrasound penetrates deeper and works in dissipating the fluid trapped in the tissue. It works well if it is combined with mechanical displacement of fluid using MLD or endermologie.

The above treatments also help patients with early complications such as lumpiness, skin irregularity, and skin laxity. At least 4–6 sessions may be required for adequate outcome (Figs. 12.5A to C).

Warnings

Do not allow the patient to use the following:
1. Hot water bags, because of altered sensation it may cause deep burns.
2. Unsupervised external pressure like binders as this can cause pressure necrosis of the skin.
3. Herbal or any packs on the treated area as this may cause severe allergic reactions.

▌ REFERENCES

1. Iverson RE, Pao VS. MOC-PS(SM) CME article: liposuction. Plast Reconstr Surg. 2008;121(4):1-11.
2. Swanson E. Assessment of reduction in subcutaneous fat thickness after liposuction using magnetic resonance imaging. J Plast Reconstr Aesthet Surg. 2012;65:128-30.
3. Hutzschenreuter P, Brummer H, Ebberfield K. Experimental and clinical studies of mechanisms of effect of manual lymphatic drainage therapy. Z Lymphol. 1989;13(1):62-4.

CHAPTER 13

Complications of Liposuction

Anything that you explain to the patient prior to the surgery is science; any explanation postsurgery is an excuse. It is easier to stay out of trouble than to get out of it. There are many such aphorisms that convey in a sentence or two what has been learned and experienced for many years. I personally like to read the complications first, and then subsequent part to find out how to avoid them.

INTRODUCTION

Liposuction may appear easy to perform for the beginners, but if it is not understood well, learnt well, planned well, and performed well, complications can be very high. Abdominal contouring is nothing but technical artistry, aesthetic perception, and manual labor, and unfortunately it is not inborn. It is a talent that needs to be acquired. Avoiding complications plays a big role in improving your standard of care. Regular postoperative follow-up is essential to identify early signs of complications. If treated early major complications can be avoided (Chart 13.1).

Let us go through in depth what are the potential complications and how to avoid them. We will restrict our discussion to complications arising after liposuction in the abdominal region.

BLEEDING

Preoperative analysis and instruction are important to prevent bleeding episodes. Blood tests like coagulation profile, platelet counts, and hematocrit are mandatory prior to the surgery. Patients need to stop all the medications and food that can cause blood thinning at least 7 days prior to the surgery. Alcohol can cause vasodilation and increase chances of bleeding.

Intraoperatively adequate tumescene and waiting period will ensure good hemostasis. The infiltration should be diffused in all the layers, and more generous infiltration is done in areas that are more fibrous and vascular such as subcostal and periumbilical areas. Gentle emulsification and low-powered suction ensure bloodless aspirate.

Any sign of fresh bleeding indicates the change of site and further infiltration. It is common to have some bleeding at the end of the surgery. But that is indicative of surgical end point.

Use of excessive manual thrust and sharp curetting cannula can cause more avulsion injury and risk of bleeding. At the end of surgery, observe the incision ports for any fresh bleeding. If visible, identify the area and treat immediately.

Adequate postoperative compression dressing is important to prevent bleeding. Occasionally, bleeding may start after 6–8 hours when the adrenaline effect wears off. The risk is higher in large-volume liposuction (>5 L) and massive weight loss patients. Obese patients have distended and hypertrophied vessels and despite massive weight loss the vessels remain enlarged. The vessels can get damaged easily during liposuction. Because of excessive skin laxity, there is loose areolar space that can easily collect blood and get unnoticed. In suspected patients, postoperative hemoglobin will be indicative of the amount of bleeding.

If blood loss is not >15% of the blood volume, it can be treated with intravenous (IV) fluid resuscitation, dextran or albumin.[1] If the hemoglobin is < 8 gm, then patients need to remain hospitalized and managed accordingly. On discharge these patients should be on oral medications to improve the hemoglobin.

Only bruising is a sign of minimal blood accumulation that does not require active intervention, but if it is associated with tense swelling and hemodynamic changes it requires evacuation. It is less known in the liposuction procedure but can happen if it is combined with abdominoplasty.

SEROMA

It can happen due to following reasons:
1. Excessive tumescene and inadequate aspiration.
2. Closure of incision ports.
3. Excessive traumatic liposuction creating a large cavity.
4. Overenthusiastic ultrasonic emulsification.

Chart 13.1: Postoperative protocol.*

Patient's Name: _____   File Number: _____

Procedure Done: _____ Date of Surgery: _____

Post Op visits	Date called	Date attended	Photographs	Wound/Scar	Skin/Tissue	Result	Satisfaction
Post Op (day 1)							
Post Op (day 2)							
Post Op (day 5)							
Post Op (day 7)							
2 weeks							
4 weeks							
6 weeks							
2 months							
3 months							
6 months							
1 year							
2 years							
3 years							
Others							

*Follow-up examination: vital signs, assess pain/discomfort, scar or wound assessment, measurements, local sensitivity, overlying skin and tissue, contour, overall result, patient satisfaction, photographs.

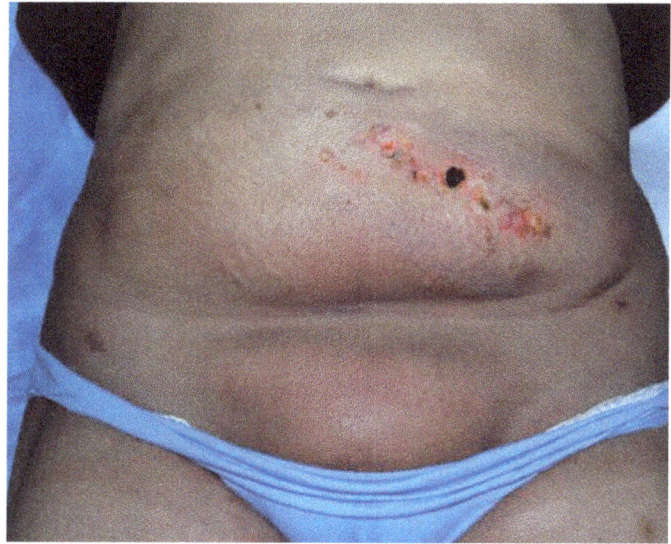

Fig. 13.1: Post vaser lipo after 1 month. Extensive seroma and skin necrosis.

5. Residual hematoma.
6. Damage to lymphatic system in the inguinal region.

On occasions, I have seen patients with seroma in spite of the use of suction device. In one patient particularly, she had seroma and pressure necrosis despite suction that was kept for a week. The cause was obviously tissue and lymphatic damage due to overenthusiastic cannula movement or prolonged ultrasonic energy delivery (Fig. 13.1).

The key points to prevent seroma are as follows:

1. Limiting infiltration to 1:1 or 1.5:1. After lipoaspiration ensure that all the fluid is drained out by turning the position of the patient and manually massaging the treated areas.
2. Plan incision port at dependent sites in inguinal and sacral areas and do not close the port. I personally do not use the plastic ports in the incision sites as they require larger incision and suturing. However, burns can be prevented on the port site by avoiding torque and leverage of the probe against the skin. Alternatively, you can use two incisions for plastic ports that can be closed and rest smaller incision for only liposuction leaving it open.
3. Do not use closed dressings (water-proof, nonabsorbent) on the incision sites, an absorbent dressing will allow free drainage.
4. The recommended ultrasonic usage is 1 minute for 200 mL aspirate recommended by the Vaser Company;

however, it does not cause adequate emulsification. I prefer to use it for 1 minute per 100 mL aspirate safely.[2] Excessive use of ultrasonic energy may damage the lymphatics and can cause seroma.

5. Avoid using traumatic cannulas with sharp edges and follow a systematic pattern of movement of cannulas to prevent extensive tissue avulsion. Large cannulas (5 mm and above) tend to create more cavities as compared to 3 mm and 4 mm Mercedes cannulas.

6. Regular follow-up as per the protocol to carefully examine the patient and detect complications early.

If seroma is present, then it requires repeated aspiration and compression until it resolves. A chronic seroma that persists for > 4 weeks requires aspiration and injection of sclerosants, surgical drainage, or surgical curettage by opening the area.

▌INFECTION

Although infection is very rare after abdominal liposculpturing, it can lead to severe morbidity and mortality.

List of infections that we need to prevent includes the following:

1. Incision site infections
2. Cellulitis
3. Fulminant bacterial infection
4. Atypical mycobacterial infection
5. Fungal infection
6. Necrotizing fasciitis
7. Toxic shock syndrome

▌PREOPERATIVE PROTOCOL

Thorough preoperative checkup to identify risk factors such as HIV, hepatitis infection, diabetes, systemic steroids, smokers, and focus of infection in the body such as respiratory tract infection, urinary tract infection, and skin infection, are mandatory. Stopping smoking, controlling blood sugar, treating infections are some of the ways to reduce postoperative infections.

Preoperative Betadine Scrub and Shower

Generally to prepare patients in the operating room, surgeons scrubbed the operative and adjacent areas with antiseptic soap and solutions. In liposuction, this method of preparation is challenging because of frequent change in patient's position during the surgery. There are different methods adopted by plastic surgeons that are inconvenient,

time consuming, and potentially embarrassing to the patients. We routinely provide povidone-iodine (Betadine scrub soap) to the patients to take home and use during bathing. They are told to begin preparation 2 days prior to surgery including the day of the surgery. Special attention must be paid to the axillae, perineal area, and feet as they have high concentration of commensals.

▌INFECTION CONTROL POLICY

Each center should have an infection control policy with a stringent protocol for highest level of cleanliness, sterilization, and sterile techniques. The cannulas are the potential source of infection, particularly, if they are not cleaned immediately after surgery. Some of the reported atypical mycobacterium and viral infections are due to contaminated instruments, operating room, and or postoperative recovery areas.[3,4]

Cannula sterilization is very challenging and the cannulas can harbor life-threatening pathogens.[5] At the end of the procedure, cannulas should be decontaminated as soon as possible. Two-piece instruments should be taken apart to facilitate cleaning. The cannulas should be soaked in water and in an enzymatic solution that aids in the breakdown of proteins. Then they should be washed either by hand with a brush and detergent or with a mechanical washer such as an ultrasonic cleaner.[6] Ultrasonic cleaning assists in the removal of small debris and particles from the cannulas. Then they are rinsed, dried, and inspected for any debris prior to autoclaving or any other standard method of sterilization.

▌POSTOPERATIVE FOLLOW-UP

Regular follow-up will ensure that infection can be detected early. Any persistent swelling, induration, redness, tenderness, free fluid needs to be managed accordingly. A course of perioperative antibiotics that starts one day prior to the surgery with oral cephalosporins, followed by IV antibiotic prior to induction of anesthesia and postoperative dose is an adequate cover. If there is any doubt, further oral antibiotics may be recommended.

If the infection appears from 10 days to 6 weeks after surgery and is in the form of a mass with overlying erythema, mycobacterium should be considered. There is no other way to diagnose mycobacterial infection. Vigorous prolonged treatment may be necessary. Rifampin, 600 mg,

2–3 times weekly combined with isoniazide, pyrazinamide, ethambutol, and/or streptomycin should be used for up to 6 months.[1]

NECROSIS

This may occur due to extensive superficial liposuction devascularing the overlying skin, chronic smoking, excessive pressure due to tight-fitting garment, overuse of foam compression, etc. Chronic seroma and hematoma with external pressure can also lead to skin necrosis. It is common in the lower abdomen with large panniculus, particularly, if extensive liposuction is followed by uncontrolled compression postoperatively (*see* Fig. 13.1). Interestingly, necrosis can happen in upper abdomen particularly in chronic smokers.

Excessive edema after liposuction also increases the risk of skin necrosis. If the patient is sitting for long hours in the early postoperative period, the edema of the lower abdomen can increase reducing the microcirculation of the skin. The patient should be advised to prevent continuous sitting for long hours, wearing tight-fitting jeans over the garment, and advise him/her to release the garment every 4–5 hours for 10 minutes. This is applicable to large-volume liposuction patients, chronic smokers, and early signs of blistering, etc. I recommends frusemide tablet 20–40 mg once a day for 2–3 days to reduce water retention and swelling if there are no medical contraindications.

Necrotizing fasciitis and toxic shock syndrome[7-9] are some lethal complications that have been reported in the literature. Necrotizing fasciitis (hemolytic streptococcal gangrene, suppurative fasciitis, or synergistic necrotizing cellulitis) is a rapidly progressive infection of the deeper layer subcutaneous tissues, easily spreading across the superficial fascial plane, with subsequent death of the overlying skin and severe systemic toxicity. In majority of cases, multiple aerobic and anaerobic organisms cause a synergistic infection of mixed aerobic-anaerobic microflora, or it may be caused by a single isolated microbe: *Streptococcus pyogenes*.

Mostly, it becomes clinically evident within the first 24 hours after surgery, which should serve as a reminder to re-examine all liposuction patients within this time period. Erythema, prominent edema, and induration accompanied by intense or intolerable pain are the warning signs. Immediate and complete surgical debridement with combined antibiotic therapy is necessary to control the progression.

THROMBOEMBOLISM

The risk of venous thromboembolism in aesthetic surgery is real, and complications may range from minor to life threatening. The basis of venous thromboembolism chemoprophylaxis is to prevent the untoward complications associated with thrombus and embolus formation and to minimize bleeding complications.

There were several venous thromboembolism risk-assessment tools reported in the literature, the 2005 Caprini scale was selected by the Task Force as the reference point because it was formally validated to stratify plastic surgery patients based on their individual risk factors. Incorporating a standard protocol in your practice ensures safety and prevents medicolegal litigations.[10] Observe the patient for calf swelling, tenderness and Homan's sign (pain in dorsiflexion of the foot).

Pulmonary embolus (PE) can happen as a consequence of deep vein thrombosis. The patient presents with dyspnea, tachypnea, chest discomfort, and tachycardia. Immediate hospitalization in intensive care unit with IV heparin is the primary management of PE.

FAT EMBOLISM

Liposuction can cause mechanical damage to the adipocytes and blood vessels, through which ultimately some lipid globules might escape into the venous circulation. In a study conducted by El Ali et al, in a rat model to determine whether intravascular fat mobilization occurs during mechanical liposuction and whether fat embolism is a real risk, they reported that on histological examination, lipid deposits and fat emboli were seen in the lungs (intravascular) of all the study group animals. On the other hand, there was no evidence of lipid deposits or fat emboli on histological examination of the brain tissues. It seems that the risk of systemic fat mobilization and fat embolism after liposuction is much more significant than we really appreciate clinically, and it may be subclinical in most individuals.[11,12] After reviewing this study, I realized that they used plain normal saline for infiltration without adrenaline. So, we still do not know what is the true incidence of fat emboli in our patients.

There are two theories as to the origin of fat emboli, one mechanical and another biochemical.[13] In liposuction, a mechanical blockage can occur when vessel rupture and adipocyte damage allow globules of triglycerides to enter into venous circulation. The fat globules are too large to pass through the pulmonary capillaries, where they get trapped. Fat embolism syndrome occurs later and is an inflammatory response to circulating free fatty acids in the pulmonary system that damage endothelial cells and pneumocytes. The three classic symptoms of fat embolism syndrome are respiratory distress, cerebral dysfunction, and petechial rash, which usually occur within 24–48 hours after surgery.[14]

Treatment includes pulmonary support, evaluation of hemodynamics, monitoring of fluid status, and, in some cases, the use of high-dose corticosteroids.[13]

PULMONARY EMBOLISM

It accounts for approximately one of every four liposuction-associated fatalities in different reports. In most cases, it occurred after an extensive procedure performed under general anesthesia, operation time over 4 hours and or large volume of liposuction.[15]

It occurs because of three mechanisms: venous stasis, activation of blood coagulation, and injury to the vascular endothelium. So the patient should be assessed for genetic and acquired conditions that predispose him or her to coagulation disorders (e.g. the factor V Leiden mutation, use of oral contraceptives, or hormone replacement therapy).[16] Once the patient's relative risk is determined, appropriate prophylaxis can be implemented, including preoperative and intraoperative interventions such as graduated compression stockings, intermittent pneumatic compression devices, and prophylactic anticoagulation therapy.

SCARS

The incision ports can leave scars and pigmented marks. They could form hypertrophic scars or keloids. The incisions should be small enough and placed in hidden areas such as umbilicus, under the breasts, bikini line, or pubic areas. The incision should be along the Langers' line and staggered in the abdomen to prevent give-away signs of surgery.

Friction burns at the incision sites can be avoided by infiltrating the port site with saline, avoiding long-time use of single port. If the wound needs suturing, nonstrangulating sutures should be used that is removed within 5 days.

Scars can also occur if the dermis is injured while doing superficial liposuction or using a sharp cannula such as basket cannula or if there is a burn due to ultrasound or laser.

CONTOUR DEFORMITIES

Contour deformities such as lumpiness, waviness, depressions, and skin wrinkling can occur due to improper technique, improper cannula size, and improper assessment of the skin.

To prevent such complications, I recommend starting liposuction with small cannulas followed by bigger cannulas and complete with small cannulas to break any left-over lumps of fat. Proper fanning technique, regular assessment of the contour as described earlier, and post-liposuction tunneling with cannulas only can prevent unevenness.

Postoperative uniform compression is also a key step to prevent unevenness. If unevenness is noted while performing the liposuction, autologous fat can be injected at that time. Liposhifting is a technique recommended by Saylan where large cannulas are used in a crisscross manner without suction to distribute the fat and it is molded by rolling the cannulas.[17]

LIDOCAINE TOXICITY

The recommend dose of lidocaine for infiltration is between 35 and 55 mg/kg. Lidocaine toxicity can occur if the concentration exceeds the recommended dose, injected rapidly in vascular areas such as face or the tumescent fluid is retained inside the body after liposuction.

The systemic toxicity of local anesthetic has been directly related to the serum concentration.

Signs of Toxicity (Versus Serum Levels of Lidocaine)

1. Circumoral numbness, lightheadedness, and tinnitus: 3–4 µg/mL for lidocaine
2. Tachycardia, tachypnea, confusion, muscular twitching, and cardiac depression: 8 µg/mL
3. Unconsciousness, seizures, and cardiorespiratory arrest: 10–20 µg/mL

However, the toxicity of lidocaine may not always correlate with the plasma level of lidocaine, because of the variable extent of protein binding in each patient and the presence of active metabolites and other factors, including the age, ethnicity, health, and body habitus of the patient, and additional medications.[18-20]

If the patient develops seizure following infiltration, proper airway management and maintaining oxygenation are critical. Seizure can be treated with IV diazepam (10–20 mg) or midazolam (5–10 mg).

Internal Scar Tissue

Like external scars, the body can form internal scars. Scars form due to fibrotic reaction to inflammatory stimulus that

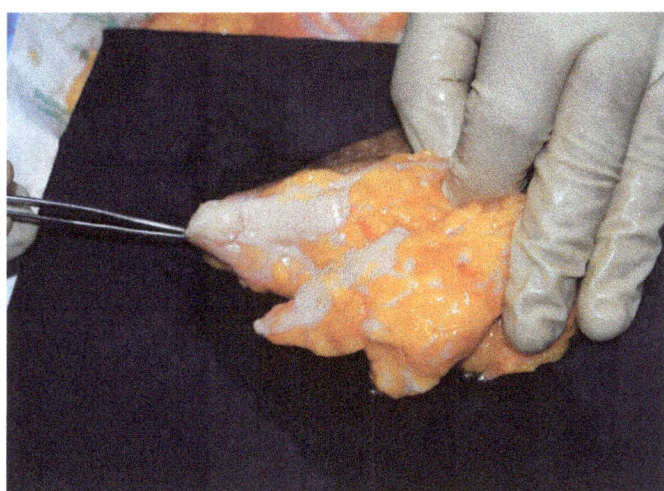

Fig. 13.2: Internal scar.

can be due to friction burns, excessive heat, infection, and traumatic avulsion of tissue. Fibrous tissue also replaces chronic hematoma and seroma.

Interestingly, if the skin does not "snap" back after liposuction or garment is not firm enough, the dead space is filled with edema fluid; part of this edema may retain and form scar tissue. This is evident if you have an opportunity to operate on this patient and get a specimen as shown in Figure 13.2. Internal scars remain as bulges and lumps. To prevent internal scars, a proper fitting garment, use of foam, and noninvasive body contouring devices are some of the known methods. The scars can be resolved with intralesional steroid injection with very diluted and careful deep injections otherwise it can cause depression and hypopigmentation.

Shiffman in his textbook describes evaluation and treatment of fibrosis. He uses 1mL, 5-fluorouracil (50 mg), 0.5 mL triamcinolone (40 mg/mL), and 1 mL lidocaine (0.5%) with epinephrine.

Postinflammatory Hyperpigmentation

There is a significant risk of hyperpigmentation after liposuction, particularly in colored skin. Inflammation due to tissue avulsion, extensive bruising, and immediate post-operation sun exposure are all the causes of hyperpigmentation. A turgid and distended skin appears pallor; once the fat is removed, the skin is contracted and it appears darker for unknown reasons. Prevention is the key as in any other complication. Ensure that there is minimal tissue avulsion, avoid using curetting cannula, prevent excessive bruising,

and avoid sun exposure during the recovery period. Hyperpigmented skin can be treated with hydroquinone 4%, moisturizing cream, and sun protection cream.

Perforation

Perforation of abdominal wall, diaphragm, and pleura is all potential life-threatening complications that one needs to be aware of. The causes are as follows:
1. Hernia
2. Abdominal wall scar
3. Sharp cannula
4. Uncontrolled movement of cannula
5. Improper direction of cannula movement
6. Devices such as vibration amplification of sound energy at resonance (VASER), laser, power assisted in inexperienced hands
7. Improper position of patients

I always advise my trainees to constantly think of what lies beneath your cannula while performing liposuction. It is the skill set that needs to be acquired to prevent inadvertent cannula movement; every movement of cannula must be in control of the surgeon. Using your wrist to cantilever the cannula, directing the cannula away from the deeper cavities, constantly feeling, or visualizing the tip of the cannula, and most importantly using the cannula smoothly (like playing violin) are some of the ways of preventing deeper injuries. Identifying the injury early and immediately implementing the action plan will prevent significant morbidity and mortality.

Patient Dissatisfaction

This is an important consideration as the procedure is meant to satisfy the patients and solve their concerns about abdominal bulges. Remember a happy patient is our greatest word of mouth referral source.

There are many reasons a patient may be unhappy of the outcome:
1. Painful procedure and painful recovery
2. Bad experience in any of the chain of event starting from arranging consultation appointment, preoperative workup, intraoperative period, postoperative recovery to the follow-up
3. Extensive bruising and swelling
4. Complications
5. Undesirable result
6. Early recurrence of fat

▌REFERENCES

1. Shiffman MA, Guseppe A. Prevention and treatment of complications. In: Liposuction Principles and Practice. Gabriele Schroder, Editor. Berlin, Germany. Springer-Verlag. 2006: 333-42.
2. de Souza Pinto EB, de Souza Pinto PC, Maciel CM. Liposuction and vaser, Clin Plastic Surg. 33;2006:107-15.
3. Meyers H, Brown-Elliott BA, Moore D, et al. An outbreak of Mycobacterium chelonae infection following liposuction. Clin InfectDis. 2002;34:1500-7.
4. Ferenczy A, Bergeron C, Richart RM. Human papillomavirus DNA in fomites on objects used for the management of patients with genital human papillomavirus infections. Obstet Gynecol. 1989;74(6):950-4.
5. Weber PJ, Wulc AE, Jaworski C, et al. Warning: traditional liposuction cannulas may be dangerous to your patient's health. J Dermatol Surg Oncol. 1988;14:1136-8.
6. Association for the Advancement of Medical Instruments. Steam Sterilization and Sterility Assurance in Healthcare Facilities. American National Standard: Arlington, VA; 2002.
7. Heitmann C, Czermak C, Germann G. Rapidly fatal necrotizing fasciitis after aesthetic liposuction. Aesthetic Plast Surg. 2000;24(5):344-7.
8. Rhee CA, Smith RJ, Jackson IT. Toxic shock syndrome associated with suction-assisted lipectomy. Aesthetic Plast Surg. 1994;18:161-3.
9. Heitmann C, Czermak C, Germann G. Rapidly fatal necrotizing fasciitis after aesthetic liposuction. Aesthetic Plast Surg. 2000;24:344-7.
10. Venturi ML, Davison SP, Caprini JA. Prevention of venous thromboembolism in the plastic surgery patient: Current guidelines and recommendations. Aesthet Surg J. 2009;29: 421-8.
11. El-Ali KM, Gourlay T. Assessment of the risk of systemic fat mobilization and fat embolism as a consequence of liposuction: ex vivo study Plast Reconstr Surg. 2006;117(7): 2269-76.
12. Ross RM, Johnson GW. Fat embolism after liposuction. Chest. 1988;93:1294-5.
13. Gingrass MK. Lipoplasty complications and their prevention. Clin Plast Surg. 1999;26:341-54.
14. Wang HD, Zheng JH, Deng C, et al. Fat embolism syndromes following liposuction. Aesthetic Plast Surg. 2008;32:731-6.
15. Haeck PC, Swanson JA, Gutowski KA, et al. The ASPS Patient Safety Committee. Evidence-based patient safety advisory: liposuction. Plast Reconstr Surg. 2009;124(4S):28-44S.
16. Wu O, Robertson L, Langhorne P, et al. Oral contraceptives, hormone replacement therapy, thrombophilias and risk of venous thromboembolism: a systematic review. The Thrombosis: Risk and Economic Assessment of Thrombophilia Screening (TREATS) Study. Thromb Haemost. 2005;94: 17-25.
17. Saylan Z. Liposhifting: treatment of post liposuction irregularities. Int J Cosm Surg. 1999;7(1):71-3.
18. Klein JA. Tumescent technique for regional anesthesia permits lidocaine doses 35 mg/kg for liposuction: peak plasma levels are diminished and delayed 12 hours. J Dermatol Surg Oncol. 1990;16:248-63.
19. Ostad A, Kageyama N, Moy RL. Tumescent anesthesia with a lidocaine dose of 55 mg/kg is safe for liposuction. Dermatol Surg. 1996;22:921-7.
20. Yukioka H, Hayashi M, Fugimori M. Lidocaine intoxication during general anesthesia (Letter). Anesth Analg. 1990;71 (2):207-8.

CHAPTER 14

Abdominoplasty

HISTORY

Abdominoplasty is performed for >100 years. There has been much significant advancement in this field. It is no longer about just removing skin and fat. It is about contouring, reshaping, body habitus, patient desires, correct indications, etc.

In 1890, Demars and Marx reported the first dermolipectomy in France. Kelly, a gynecologic surgeon, was the first to report this procedure in the United States in 1899 at John Hopkins.[1,2] He called it "transverse abdominal lipectomy." It was part of hernia repair; he was the first to note "cosmetic benefit" from this procedure. But the umbilicus was sacrificed.

In 1905, Gaudet and Morestin performed a similar procedure for umbilical hernia and preserved the umbilicus. In 1931, Passot described undermining with resection.[3] The excision design also changed a lot. Weinhold (Germany) in 1909 described cloverleaf incision that is combination of horizontal and vertical excision. Desjardin in 1911 and Amedee Morestin in the same year described vertical and horizontal excision, respectively, whereas in 1911, Jolly described low transverse incision. Pitanguy described an incision that was like an inverted arc; lateral end of the incision was turned down. Regnault modified the incision into the "W" incision. In 1973, Grazer considered the dressing pattern and suggested the "bikini line" incision that is commonly followed now.

Babcock (1916), Thorek (1924), Pick (1949), Barsky (1950), Galtier (1955), Vernon (1957), and Dufourmental (1959) did various modifications to the excision to improve the outcome. The first major aesthetic accomplishment in contour surgery is credited to Thorek, who performed the first umbilicus-preserving abdominoplasty in 1924.[4] Vernon, in the 1950s, pioneered the conventional abdominoplasty when he combined extensive undermining with the novel concept of umbilical transposition and relocation that is the basis of all our abdominoplasty procedures today.[5]

In 1967, Baroudi published his experience in abdominoplasty with particular attention to the aesthetic appearance of umbilicus. The use of quilting sutures was championed by Baroudi to minimize seromas. Grazer was the first to describe rectus plication and was published in 1973.

Of course with Illouz (1977), the whole concept of body contouring changed. Illouz encouraged abdominoplasty with adipoaspiration for further refinements. In 1977, Rebello described the reverse abdominoplasty for selected patients with laxity above the umbilicus. This added another option in our armamentarium of abdominoplasties. Klein's tumescence was further expanded by Converse, Illouz, and Hetter. This resulted in significant reduction of blood loss and thus was used concurrently with majority of abdominoplasty procedures.[6]

Then, the focus was on waistline improvement; Toranto in 1988 expanded Pitanguys and Grazer's concept of rectus plication by bringing together not only medial but also lateral borders of the rectus muscle sheath. The scar was a challenge; so Lockwood in 1991 emphasized on superficial fascial system (SFS). Wound closure by maximum tension at the level of SFS allowed skin closure with minimal tension. Thus, the quality of scar improved.

Hunstad presented advanced abdominoplasty concepts in 1999 where he combined many of the above concepts in one such as high lateral tension, SFS closure, wide rectus plication, subscarpal fat resection, and thorough concurrent liposuction to achieve more predictable results.

There will be continuous improvements and innovations to refine the practice of body contouring surgery. What also need to be addressed are safety, morbidity, longevity of the results and psychological satisfaction.

Body contouring surgery is a rapidly evolving field of plastic surgery and this is a new challenge to us. This is the result of exponential growth of successful bariatric surgery cases. The issue of obesity and weight fluctuation has deleterious effect on skin, often leaving pendulous and saggy skin folds in multiple directions and all around the torso. Somalo and Gonzalez-Ulloa extended the transverse abdominal incision circumferentially and introduced the belt lipectomy.[7,8] This started the trend of body lifting procedures.

Matarasso in 1988 expanded the use of abdominal contour surgery on the basis of variations in patients' anatomy.

TYPES OF ABDOMINOPLASTY

Why Do We Need to have this Classification?

It is important to have a thorough knowledge of various modifications of the surgery to fit each individual. The physical condition varies in each patient; the expectations are different; tissue behavior varies; and the outcome is individual specific.

Various types of abdominoplasty procedures are in fact modifications that are suited to individual patient needs.

What are these Modifications?

1. Conventional lipoabdominoplasty.
2. Miniabdominoplasty (short scar).
3. Extended abdominoplasty.
4. Circumferential abdominoplasty.
5. Reverse abdominoplasty.
6. Fleur-de-lis abdominoplasty.
7. Horseshoe abdominoplasty.

CONVENTIONAL LIPOABDOMINOPLASTY

1. With muscle plication (full/complete abdominoplasty).
2. Without muscle plication.

Introduction

The full/complete abdominoplasty is the most commonly performed method of abdominoplasty, as this procedure addresses most of the problems of excess skin, excess adiposity, diastasis recti, and abdominal striae (Figs. 14.1A to I).

In this procedure, after performing judicial liposuction, the incision extends from one anterior superior iliac spine to the other. Umbilicus is transcribed, and flap is elevated till the xiphoid process. The rectus sheath is plicated in the midline. The excess skin flap is removed and umbilicus is fixated in a new location.

Advantages

1. *Significant skin tightening supra and infraumbilical areas*: The procedure addresses the vertical excess skin and removes folds that are formed above or below the umbilicus.
2. *Umbilical position and shape are improved*: If the umbilicus is displaced inferiorly and if the shape is altered, this procedure helps reposition of the umbilicus. If it is well fixated to the rectus sheath, the shape appears youthful and aesthetic.
3. *Muscle is corrected*: The vertical bulge that is because of the diverification is corrected with plication. With modified technique as described by Toranto, the waistline can also be improved. Even if there is no diversification, the rectus plication improves the muscle strength.
4. *Myofascial component can be strengthened*: If there is lateral musculofascial laxity, it is important to plicate that as well. Otherwise, the rectus plication displaces the intra-abdominal volume laterally and obscures the contour laterally.
5. *Concurrent liposuction improves waistline, abdominal contour*: In the past, because of residual fat in the upper abdomen there was a problem of upper abdominal fullness. It was exaggerated in long-term, if the patient gains weight. Judicious liposuction of the upper abdomen prevents this problem. Similarly, liposuction improves the waistline and prevents dog ears.
6. *Thus result can last longer*: A complete abdominoplasty can have a longer-lasting result as moderate weight gain does not alter the shape of the abdomen and waistline.

Disadvantages

1. Recovery and downtime.
2. Risks of surgery.
3. *Scars*: Length of scars, risk of hypertrophy/discoloration/displacement of scars.
4. If there is limited upper abdominal skin, there may be additional or unfavorably located scars of umbilical opening.
5. If there is a large intra-abdominal volume, the bulge may remain.
6. Recurrence of fat in the upper abdomen if inadequate liposuction is performed.

MINIABDOMINOPLASTY (SHORT SCAR)

Introduction

Miniabdominoplasty is a modified abdominoplasty where some of the steps are eliminated. It is more appealing to

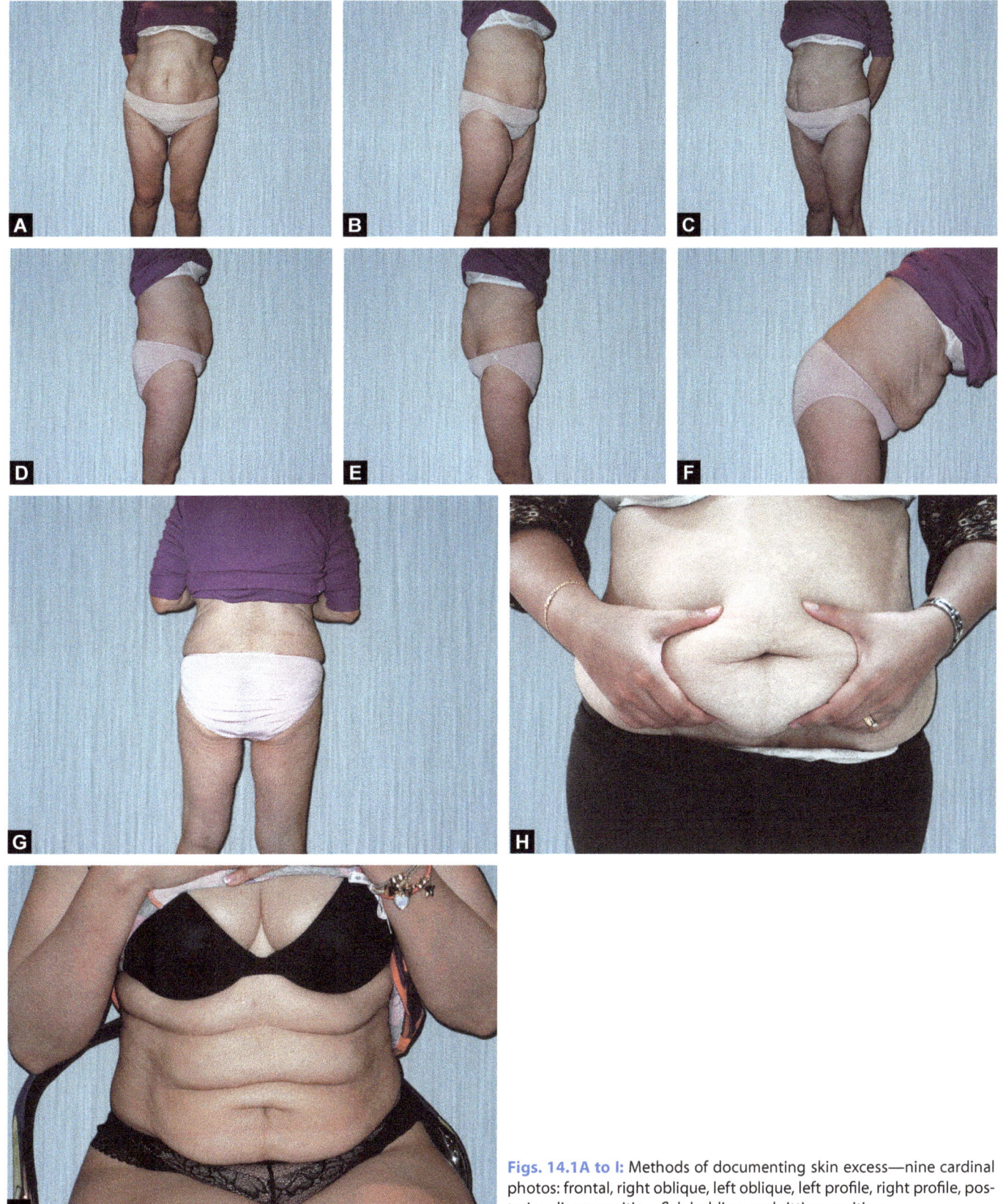

Figs. 14.1A to I: Methods of documenting skin excess—nine cardinal photos: frontal, right oblique, left oblique, left profile, right profile, posterior, divers position, flab holding, and sitting position.

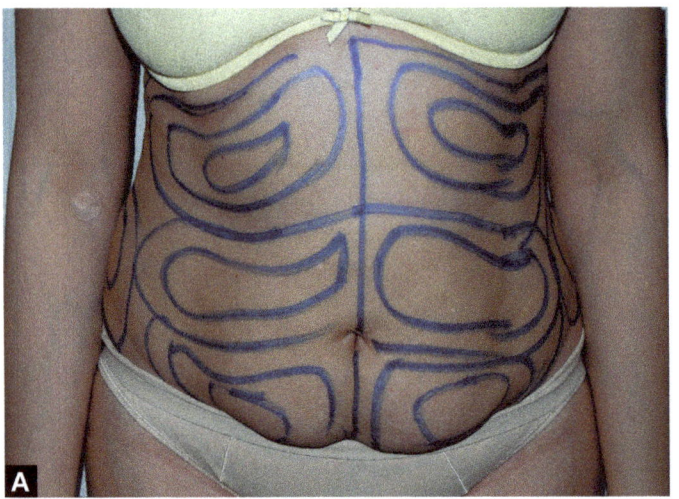 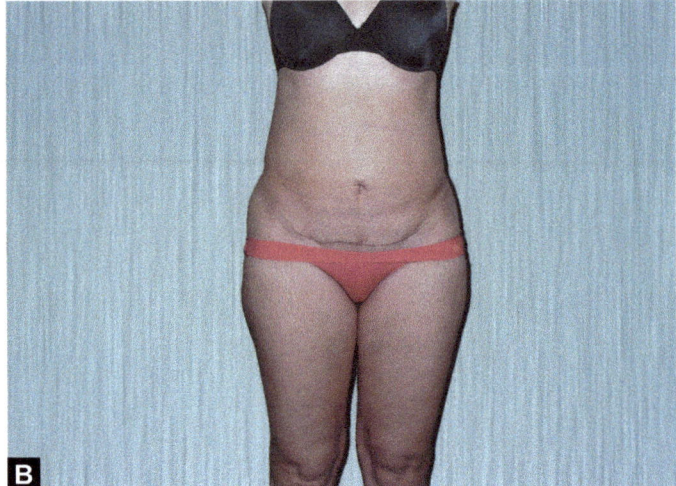

Figs. 14.2A and B: (A) Patient with excess fat in the abdominal region and moderated infraumbilical skin excess. Note the quality of supraumbilical skin is good. (B) Postoperative view after liposuction and short scar abdominoplasty.

prospective younger patients as it indicates smaller scars, less extensive procedure, and less morbid recovery. This procedure eliminates umbilical translocation. From a surgeon's perspective this is more appealing as we now understand the true potential of thorough liposuction that helps excellent skin firming and contouring.

We can subclassify this surgery according to individual needs:

1. Short scar.
2. Endoscopic-assisted miniabdominoplasty.
3. Dermolipectomy with umbilical relocation (floating umbilicus).

Short Scar Abdominoplasty

In this procedure, essentially only dermolipectomy is performed in the lower abdomen without changing the position of umbilicus. The scar length is kept as short as possible (Figs. 14.2A and B).

It can be combined with liposuction for better contouring.

Indications

1. Patient refuses to undergo conventional lipoabdominoplasty.
2. Only for lower abdominal skin excess, with no or minimal upper abdominal skin laxity.
3. Umbilicus is not or minimally altered/displaced.
4. Rectus muscle is intact.
5. No intra-abdominal bulge.

6. Usually suitable for patients with body mass index (BMI) < 30.

Advantages

1. Recovery and downtime is short.
2. Scar is short.
3. No umbilical scars.
4. Option of conventional abdominoplasty is still there in future.

Disadvantages

1. Does not address supraumbilical muscle diversification.
2. Does not address supraumbilical skin excess.
3. Patient satisfaction is limited.
4. Risk of disproportion if the patient gains weight in future.
5. Does not address circumferential/horizontal skin excess.

Technique

Mini abdominoplasty without muscle repair can be performed under local anesthesia with IV sedation. However, a nervous patient may require general anesthesia. General anesthesia with laryngeal mask is very convenient and has a smooth postoperative recovery.

Procedure begins with wet infiltration and thorough liposuction in all the aesthetic units of abdomen as indicated. Length of incision depends upon the predicted amount of elliptical skin excision. If there is a hanging panniculus, the incision extends till the end of the panniculus. Any shorter incision may leave dog ears at the end.

The flap dissection continues above the scarps fascia and the extent is till the umbilicus. Excess skin is than pulled inferiorly to mark the limit of excision. Average 8–10 cm skin should be left behind from the center of the umbilicus. Excess skin removal will either retract the scar superiorly or cause tight lower abdomen.

There is often significant disparity between the length of upper and lower incision. After addressing the "dog ears" at the end of the incision the wound is closed in two layers by stealing the extra length of the upper incision. Subcutaneous sutures are placed deep in the tissue to prevent future "suture spitting". A small penrose drain is enough to prevent hematoma provided the hemostasis at the end of procedure is achieved well.

Endoscopic-assisted Miniabdominoplasty

In this procedure, a short scar is used in the lower abdomen with an additional scar in supraumbilical crease if necessary for muscle repair above the umbilicus. It is indicated in patients with excess subcutaneous fat and rectus diversification without any skin excess.

Indications

1. Average or low BMI.
2. Only rectus diastasis.
3. Minimum to moderate subcutaneous fat in anterior abdomen and waistline.
4. Good skin tone without excessive stretch marks.

Advantages

1. Minimal scarring.
2. Early recovery.

Disadvantages

1. Technically demanding.
2. Very limited indication.
3. Improper counseling can lead to patient dissatisfaction.
4. Skin bunching in the upper abdomen.
5. There are no standard guidelines to evaluate and select the patients; it is individual judgment of the surgeon and patient.

Technique

This procedure requires general anesthesia as the dissection is cumbersome. After usual infiltration and liposuction an incision is made at the lower end of the abdomen and flap is elevated at the subscarpal level. Careful dissection is performed around the umbilicus. The perforators around the umbilicus is carefully ligated. A semilunar incision is made above the umbilicus, big enough to accommodate an endoscopic retractor.

The dissection continues above the umbilicus to expose the diastasis recti. Three retractors are positioned to accomplish this dissection and muscle repair. One lighted or endoscopic retractor through umbilical incision and two broad retractors from the lower abdominal incision. The dissection is combination of blunt and sharp. A good infiltration and liposuction helps the dissection. It is important to ensure the dissection is continuous on both sides of the umbilicus for muscle repair. A double loop ethilon number 0 is used to repair the muscle. The umbilicus is bypassed and the plication continues in the lower abdomen. If there is any bunching of the skin in the central abdomen, it is dissected using combination of blunt and sharp dissection.

The excess skin is removed similar to mini abdominoplasty technique and wound is repaired (Figs. 14.3 A to D).

Dermolipectomy with Umbilical Relocation (Floating Umbilicus)

In this procedure, lower abdominal excess skin is removed and umbilicus is disinserted and lowered to address upper abdominal skin laxity and repair of diversification of recti.

Indications

1. Younger patients with a history of pregnancy.
2. Nonpregnant patients who have lost a lot of weight.
3. Patients with moderate to excess fat deposits, mild to moderate skin excess and moderate diastasis.

Advantages

1. Relatively shorter scar.
2. No umbilical scars.
3. Relatively early recovery.

Disadvantages

1. Redo surgery requiring umbilical translocation is not possible.
2. Risk of umbilicus going to low.

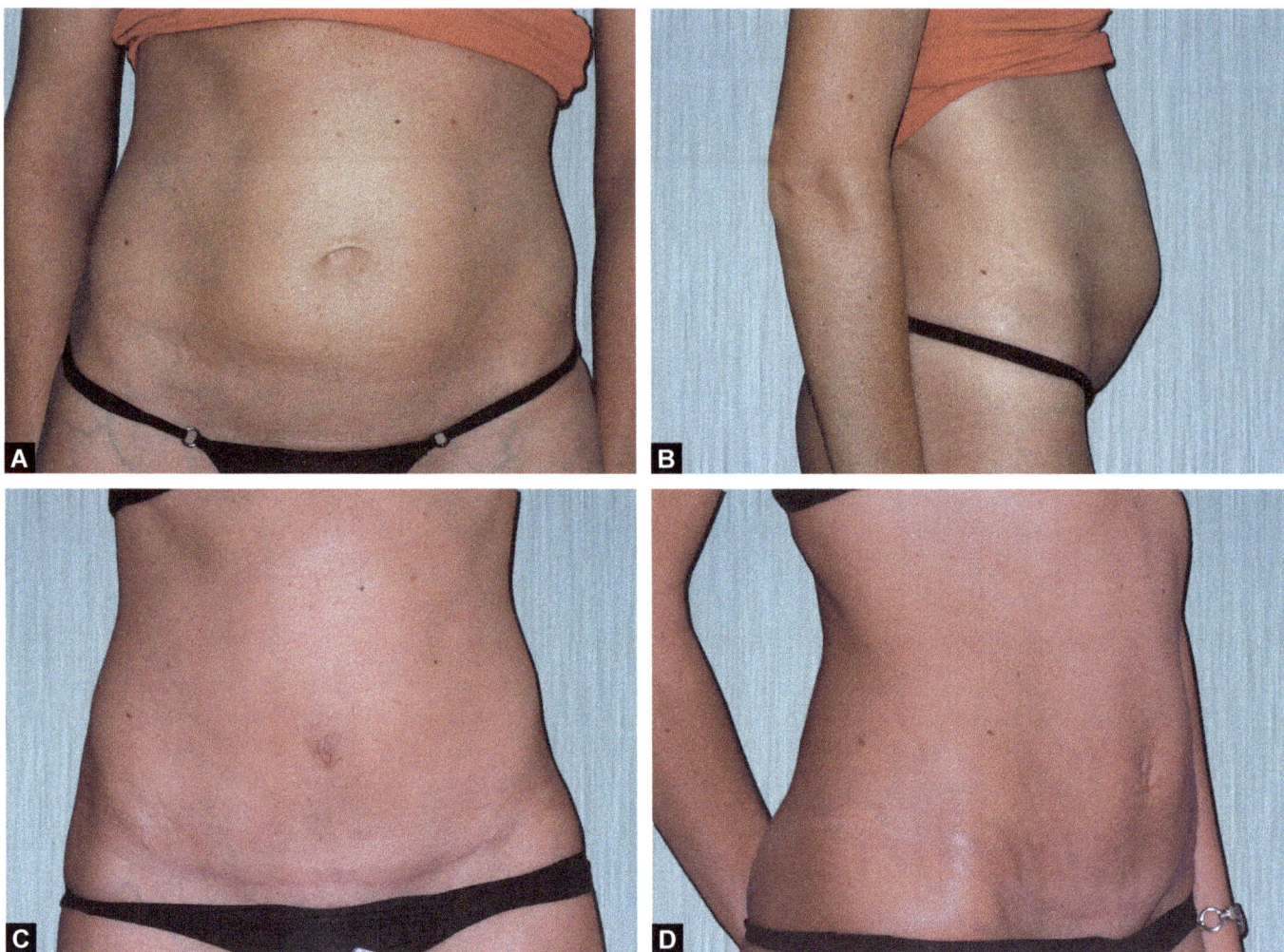

Figs. 14.3A to D: (A and B) Preoperative views of patient with bulging abdominal muscles, diversification of recti and minimal excess skin and fat. (C and D) Postoperative view after short scar abdominoplasty with endoscopic assisted repair of rectus sheath.

3. Not indicated in short stature patients.
4. Not indicated in patients with low umbilicus.

Technique

Mini abdominoplasty with umbilical relocation is performed under general anesthesia particularly if rectus sheath needs repair. The procedure starts with infiltration of solution and thorough liposuction of all the aesthetic units of abdomen.

The incision length depends upon the amount of excess skin removal. The flap is dissected above or below the scarps fascia depending upon the need to strengthen the musculofascial system. Skin hooks are applied at 12 and 6 o'clock position and it is lifted up. Ensure absence of any herniation in and around the umbilicus. A hemostasis clip is applied at the base of umbilicus flush to the rectus sheath. With an 11 number scalpel umbilicus is transected. The rectus sheath defect is closed with 2-0 vicryl suture carefully. The dissection proceeds above the umbilicus to expose the rectus sheath and release any adhesions.

After musculofascial repair, the skin flap is advanced and amount of excess skin removal is marked. The key point is, not to displace the umbilicus beyond 2–3 cm as it may be too low in the abdomen. In a tall person umbilicus can be shifted upto 4 cm below the existing umbilical position. The umbilicus is fixated to the rectus sheath with 2-0 PDS. It is preferable to use sutures in all four corners at 12, 3, 6 and 9 o'clock position to prevent flushing of the umbilicus. Ensure that umbilicus is in the midline and appears symmetrical.

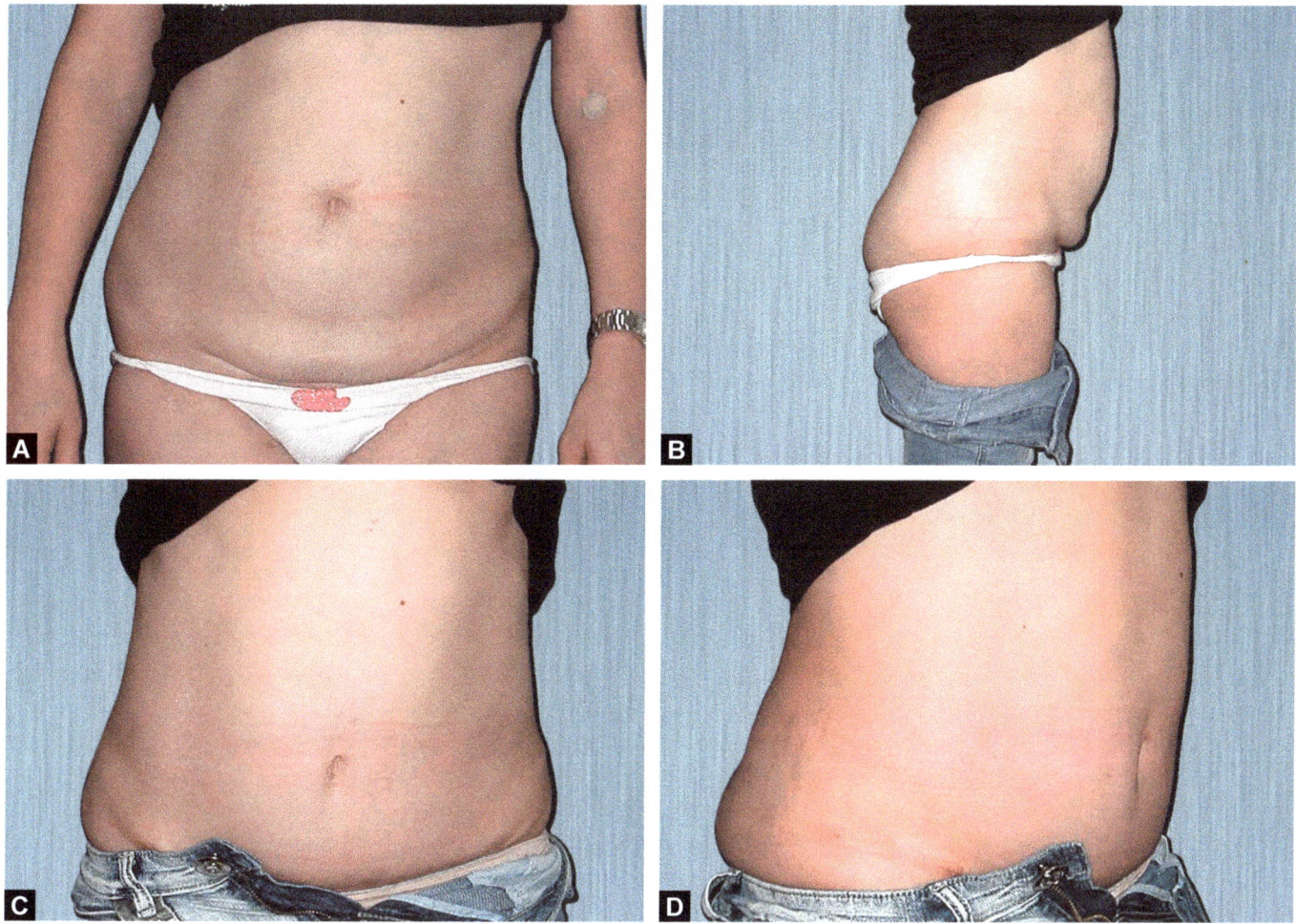

Figs. 14.4A to D: (A and B) Preoperative view of the patient with moderate supra and Infraumbilical skin excess. (C and D) Postoperative views after short scar abdominoplasty and "floating umbilicus' procedure.

This is followed by excision of the excess skin flap. The wound is closed in layers with vicryl and PDS sutures. Two corrugated drains coming out at the pubic area ensures a good drainage postoperatively (Figs. 14.4 A to D).

EXTENDED ABDOMINOPLASTY

Extended abdominoplasty addresses lateral skin excess and can also be used to lift the lateral thigh. In this procedure, the incision extends beyond the anterior superior iliac spine.

Indications

1. Panniculus extending laterally.
2. Large dog ears during the end of surgery.
3. Overweight and moderately obese patients.
4. Excess weight loss patients.

5. Simultaneous lateral thigh lift in excessive weight loss patients.
6. Existing rolls in the flank area.

Advantages

1. Preventing lateral dog ears.
2. Preventing bunching of the skin in the central abdomen.
3. Skin laxity correction in lateral trunk and lateral thigh.

Disadvantages

1. Extended scar.
2. Scar visible outside bikini line or low waist jeans.
3. Increased risk of complications.
4. Prolonged surgery and recovery.

▌CIRCUMFERENTIAL ABDOMINOPLASTY

It is also referred as body lift. In this procedure, the incision goes all around the trunk. This procedure allows maximal soft tissue resection with concurrent benefits to abdomen, waistline, back, and buttocks.

This procedure is a further advancement of "belt lipectomy" that was applied to address only the excess skin. With the addition of liposuction and contouring, the circumferential abdominoplasty gives a dramatic improvement in the torso. There are further modifications in this procedure applied to massive weight-loss situations that is out of the scope of this book.

Circumferential abdominoplasty can be performed as a one-stage or two-stage procedure based on patients' comfort, and surgeons' comfort.

Indications

1. Massive weight-loss patients with buttock and thigh ptosis is the primary indication of this procedure.

Limitations

1. Extensive operating time.
2. Increased risk of complications due to prolonged operating time and change of position intraoperatively.
3. It is difficult to control the position and symmetry of the scars due to change in positions.
4. High risk of hypertrophy of scar in lateral and posterior parts, particularly, in pigmented skin. This is due to frontal and lateral flexion movements of the patient.
5. Prolonged recovery time.

▌REVERSE ABDOMINOPLASTY

Since most of the patients have excess skin below the umbilicus, a conventional abdominoplasty is very effective. Some patients, however, are not ideal for lower abdominoplasty. Reverse abdominoplasty is suitable for patients who have predominantly excess skin in upper abdomen and there is minimal or no lower abdominal skin excess. This can be performed without umbilical shift.

The scar is placed in the inframammary fold. It may or may not extend in the xiphoid area of the sternum. The indications are limited, and the patient should be selected carefully. An ideal patient is the one who requires a combined breast lift procedure as well.

Disadvantages

1. Does not address lower abdominal skin excess.
2. Risk of hypertrophy of the scar, particularly in xiphoid area in darker skin patients.
3. Displacement of inframammary fold if it is not fixated well.
4. A patient with a low subcostal scar of previous surgery that cannot be excised is not a good candidate.

Technique

Careful patient selection and planning is the key to this procedure.

Marking is done in standing position. Both the inframammary folds are marked. If there is migration or ptosis of inframammary folds, the patient is asked to lift both the breasts up and mark new inframammary folds. The marking can be extended to the midline anteriorly or laterally in the axilla depending upon the indications.

Infiltration of solution and liposuction is performed as required.

Incision is made at the inframammary area. This is a very vascular zone and requires thorough hemostasis. The incision is inclined caudally at 45° angle to ensure the tough inframammary tissue is intact for fixation of the inframammary fold. The dissection continues with cautery keeping a layer of fat over the rectus sheath. The dissection continues to the umbilicus. It is not necessary to dissect below the umbilicus. Enough perforators are retained to vascularize the flap. Hemostasis is carefully achieved. If necessary rectus sheath can be plicated. I personally do not prefer to plicate the rectus sheath for two reasons. First the patient indicated for this procedure do not have a need for plication and secondly placating only the upper abdomen leaves behind bulging lower abdomen.

After dissection of the flap the excess skin is marked by pulling the flaps superolaterally. Maximum tension and amount of skin resection is preferred laterally than centrally. Minimal amount of skin if necessary is removed from the central part to prevent excessive tension and hypertrophy of the scars.

Fixation starts deep with number 0 vicryl. The flap is fixated all along the inframammary fold in a curvilinear pattern to give a natural look to the breasts. Second layer closure is performed with 2-0 vicryl and finally 3-0 PDO for subcuticular closure. The corrugated drains are inserted at the lateral ends of the incision.

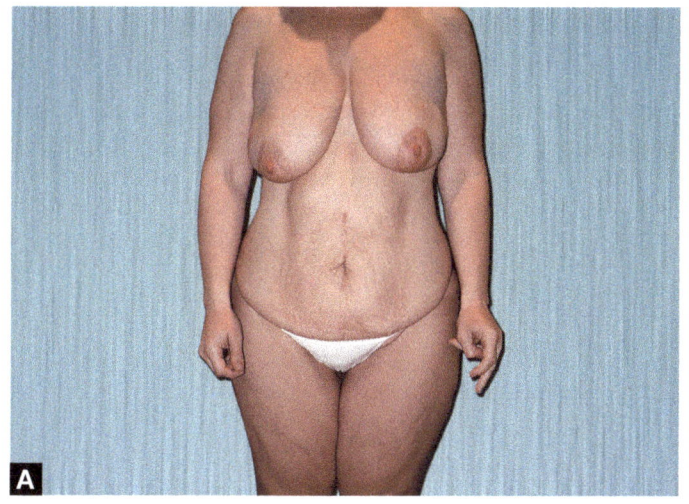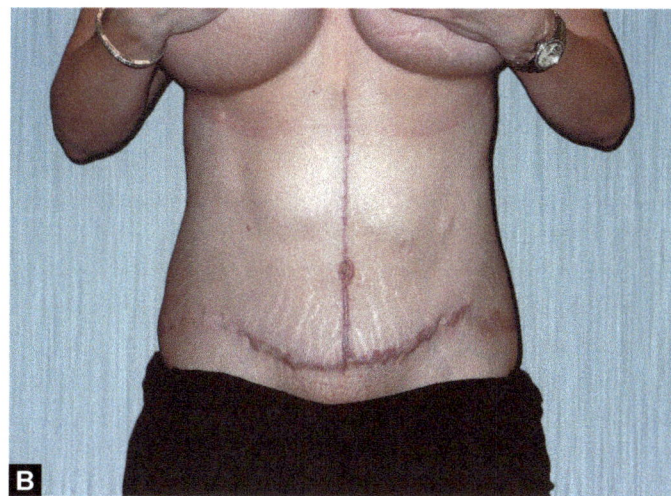

Fig. 14.5A and B: (A) Massive weight loss patient with vertical and horizontal skin excess in the abdomen. (B) Postoperative after fleur-de-lis abdominoplasty.

FLEUR-DE-LIS ABDOMINOPLASTY

Fleur-de-lis is a French word that means "lily flower" and the design of the incision is based on the symbol that is used in many coats of arms and flags.[9] The fleur-de-lis incision has been innovatively used in lip, breast, thoracic wall and lower back defect reconstruction, and increasingly today in abdominoplasty.[10,11]

So, fleur-de-lis abdominoplasty uses both horizontal and vertical incisions to remove skin excess in both the directions (horizontal and vertical) (Figs. 14.5A and B).

The commonest indication is in massive weight-loss patient; however, it may be required in patients with large ventral hernia to address the excess skin left behind after hernia repair.

Limitations

1. Extensive scarring.
2. Prolonged procedure time.
3. Risk of umbilical deformities.

HORSESHOE ABDOMINOPLASTY

It is a short scar modification described by Richard Moufarrège.[12] A horseshoe incision is marked around the pubis with a downward notch centrally, which gives a heart-shaped appearance. As second incision is made, it passes through the umbilicus. The whole flap is elevated; necessary muscle tightening is performed; excess skin is removed; and the incision is closed around the pubic

area by stealing principle of plastic surgery. This causes bunching of the skin and puckering that improves over 3–6 months.

If there is a horizontal skin excess, it adds a vertical component to the scar. I have never used this technique personally, but it was worth mentioning in this book.

SELECTION OF PATIENT AND PLANNING OF ABDOMINOPLASTY

A patient coming to our office for abdominal contouring needs to be assessed thoroughly. A systematic approach and planning ensures high satisfaction for both the patient and the surgeon likewise.

What are the Options We have?

1. *Lifestyle changes*: A patient who is undergoing weight changes is recommended to alter his/her lifestyle by focusing on healthy and balanced nutrition and regular physical exercise. This is also combined with any form of treatment that you recommend to your patient.
2. *Nonsurgical weight loss and body contouring*: As discussed earlier in the chapter of noninvasive modalities, we have enough scientific basis to recommend these options to the patient. However, explain the patient the pros and cons of nonsurgical management and extent of result that can be achieved.
3. *Liposuction and liposculpturing procedures*: Patients who have high expectations are not suitable for noninvasive methods. On the other hand, patients who are

reluctant to have abdominoplasty scars are not a good candidate for abdominoplasty and may well be indicated for liposculpting alone.

4. *Lipoabdominoplasty*: Patients who have triad of excessive skin of poor quality, muscle diversification, or laxity and hanging panniculus are best candidates for lipoabdominoplasty.

5. *Bariatric surgery*: Patients who generally have weight problem and has potential comorbid condition may be suitable for bariatric procedures.

There are three important stages to decide the type of procedure in a particular patient:

1. Consultation and counselling.
2. General evaluation and work-up.
3. Worksheet planning.

Consultation and Counselling

This is the time we listen to the patients and assess them.

1. History.
2. Primary concerns as narrated by the patient.
3. Psychosocial assessment of the patient by the surgeon during the process of consultation is important to identify red flags.
4. Lifestyle assessment is important to understand the weight pattern of the patient. Patient with healthy lifestyle tends to have more long-term results.
5. Expectations are carefully analyzed. Often patient are over expecting and our job is to bring their expectation down. However, we should focus on over delivering the result. This is the key to patient satisfaction.
6. Mutual decision will allow the patient to participate in decision making and leads to a more satisfied patient.
7. Detail explanation of the procedure and postoperative course will reduce their apprehension. Explaining the alternative methods of treatment with their expected outcome will allow the patient to make an informed decision. Note the following key points to be discussed in detail by the surgeon and the support staff to ensure patient is well aware and not taken by surprise postoperatively.
   a. Procedure
   b. Alternatives
   c. Risks
   d. Long-term outcome
   e. Financial responsibility
   f. Patient rights and responsibilities.

General Evaluation and Work-up

Consultation also involves getting a detailed medical history to rule out comorbid conditions and fitness for any type of procedure:

1. Weight loss history
2. Diet and exercise habits
3. Medical problems
   a. Neurological
   b. Cardiac
   c. Renal
   d. Hepatic
   e. Pulmonary
   f. Vascular
      Deep vein thrombosis (DVT)/Thromboembolic phenomenon
4. Previous surgery
5. Socioeconomic history
6. Physical examination
7. Laboratory work and specific studies often the treatment option changes on identifying medical comorbidity or psychological abnormality.

Worksheet Planning

The most important part is worksheet evaluation of the patient to systematically examine all elements and anticipate tissue response to any procedure that you may recommend to the patient. It is important to have a system that can be consistently used by you and the staff to evaluate the patient physically. The key elements of examination are described in Table 14.1.

Documenting Skin Excess (*see* Figs. 14.1A to I)

Photography is an important part of worksheet planning where we document all the details. Cardinal positions are required to document all aspects of the abdomen: frontal, right and left oblique, right and left profile, posterior, sitting position, grabbing the excess skin and divers view.

Many times it is difficult to assess excess skin in the abdomen particularly in standing position. Likewise, often in photographs, the patient may not appreciate the amount of excess skin she/he is having in the abdominal region. Sometimes additional positions such as sitting down and grabbing the skin are also necessary to document the skin excess.

In the forthcoming section, we will see some case studies and method of patient evaluation.

Table 14.1: Worksheet planning.

Frame of abdomen	Small	Medium	Large
Skin tone	Elastic/Normal	Moderate laxity	Flaccid
Contours	Irregularities	Flexion crease	Cellulite
Skin condition	Stria	Scars	Pigmentation
Umbilicus	Shape	Position	Depth
Fat distribution	Visceral	Subcutaneous	
	Upper abdomen	Lower abdomen	Waistline
Panniculus	Small	Medium	Large
Excess skin	Supraumbilical	Infraumbilical	
	Vertical	Horizontal	Global
Muscle	Lax	Diversification	Hernia
Posterior assessment	Skin	Muscle	Fat
Measurements	Circumferential (multiple levels)		
	Xiphoid to umbilicus		
	Umbilicus to pubic bone		
	Rectus diastasis		

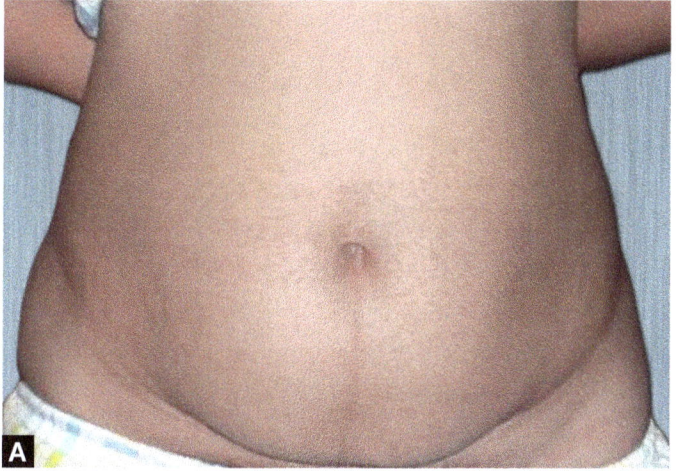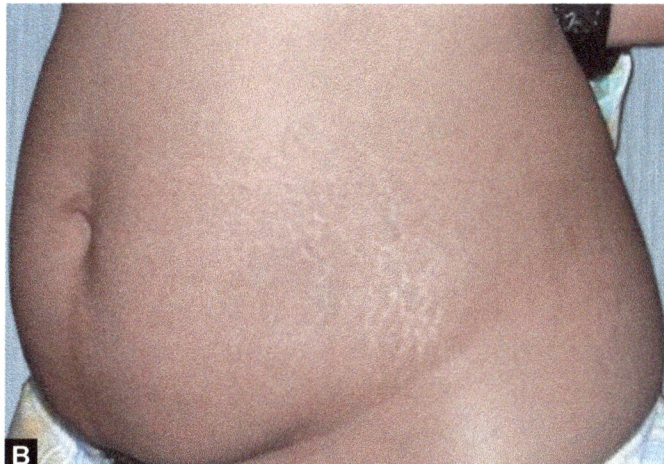

Figs. 14.6A and B: Case 1: A 32-year-old woman with two cesarean and moderate fat excess, moderate skin laxity, stretch marks, widening of waist line, and bulging of rectus muscle.

CASE 1 (FIGS. 14.6A AND B)

Consultation and Counselling

1. *History*: This is a 32-year-old woman with a history of two cesarean surgery. BMI is 25.6.
2. *Primary concerns*: Her concerns are large abdomen, increase in waistline, bulging muscle, and lax skin.
3. *Psychosocial assessment*: Confident lady.
4. *Lifestyle assessment*: Relatively healthy.
5. *Expectations*: High expectations but not looking for perfection. She is looking for flatter tummy, small waistline; does not want big scars; and wants quick recovery.
6. *Mutual decision*: After examination and discussion.

General Evaluation and Work-up

1. *Weight loss history*: Only after pregnancy otherwise stable weight.
2. *Diet and exercise habits*: Regular exercise, average dietary habit.
3. *Medical problems*: Nil.
4. *Previous surgery*: Two cesareans.

Worksheet Planning (Table 14.2)

We discuss the details of what is going on in the tummy area, what are the options for her, and pros and cons of each (Table 14.3).

Table 14.2: Summary of worksheet planning.

Frame of abdomen	Medium with good shape		
Skin tone	Moderate laxity		
Contours	Mild Irregularities lower abdomen		
Skin condition	Moderate stria	C-section scar is good	
Umbilicus	Deep and normal position		
Fat distribution	Small amount of visceral fat	Moderate subcutaneous fat	
	Upper abdomen	Lower abdomen	Waistline
Panniculus	Small lower abdomen		
Excess skin	Mild infraumbilical		
Muscle	Mildly lax		
Posterior assessment	Fat bulges		

Table 14.3: The patient is explained all the options with advantages and disadvantages.

Procedure options	Advantages	Disadvantages
Diet and exercise	Mandatory	
Nonsurgical:	Minimal risk, discomfort	Unpredictable result
Cavitation (HIFU)		May not meet expectations
CryoLipo		
Combination devices		
Vac/Rf/low-level laser		
Liposuction	Short anesthesia	Unpredictable skin tightening
	Early recovery	Muscle not addressed
	Less risk	May still need postsurgical skin tightening
	Minimal scars	and abdominoplasty
Lipoabdominoplasty	Removes extra skin	Major surgery
	Muscle repair	Pain/Risks
	Tummy appears flatter	Scars with potential additional scar of umbilical opening
		Leftover fat recurrence
Sequential procedure	Thorough lipo	Double surgery, etc
	Later only abdominoplasty	
	Better contour	
	Possibly shorter scars	

Mutual Decision

Based on the history and examination a mutual decision is made.

1. Three-dimensional liposuction followed by diet management, toning exercise and if necessary noninvasive technology-based skin tightening.
2. *If dissatisfactory outcome*: Short scar abdominoplasty.
3. *Procedure performed*: Infiltration anesthesia and intravenous (IV) sedation.
4. *Conventional liposuction*: Three-dimensionally.
5. Total aspirate 2,700 mL.

Results

1. Significant improvement in contour and skin tightening.
2. Mild unevenness acceptable to patient (Figs. 14.7A and B).
3. Long-term maintained result.

CASE 2 (FIGS. 14.8A AND B)

Consultation and Counselling

1. *History*: This is a 48-year-old woman with a history of two pregnancies. BMI is 32.

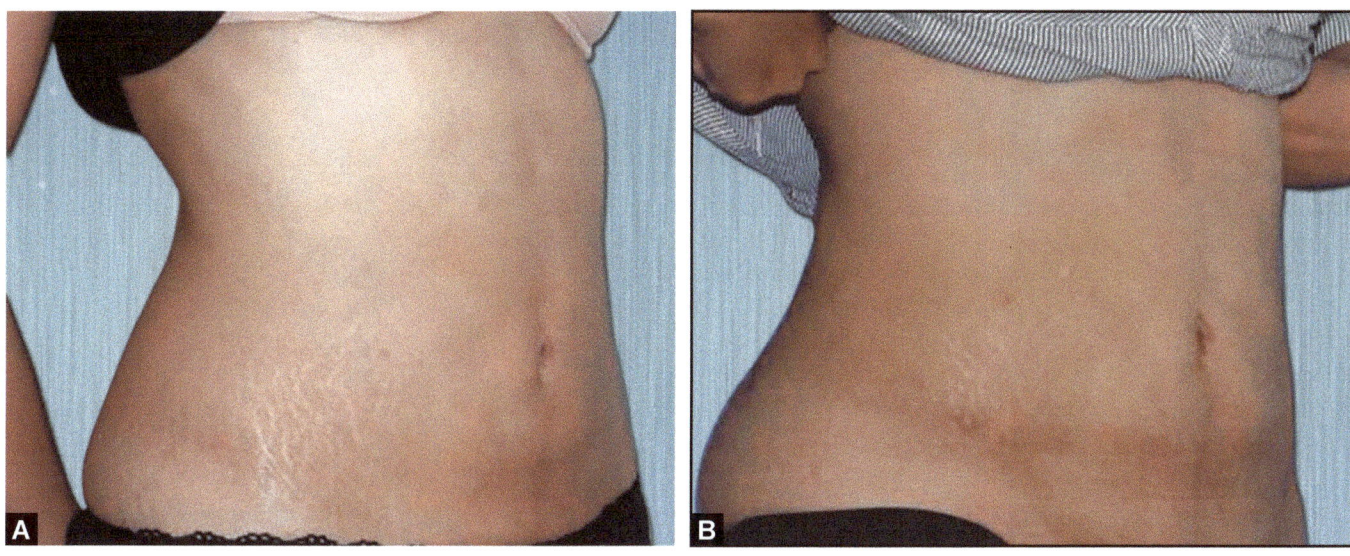

Figs. 14.7A and B: Three years and eight years postoperative after liposculpturing of abdomen and waistline. Same patient as in Figures 14.6A and B.

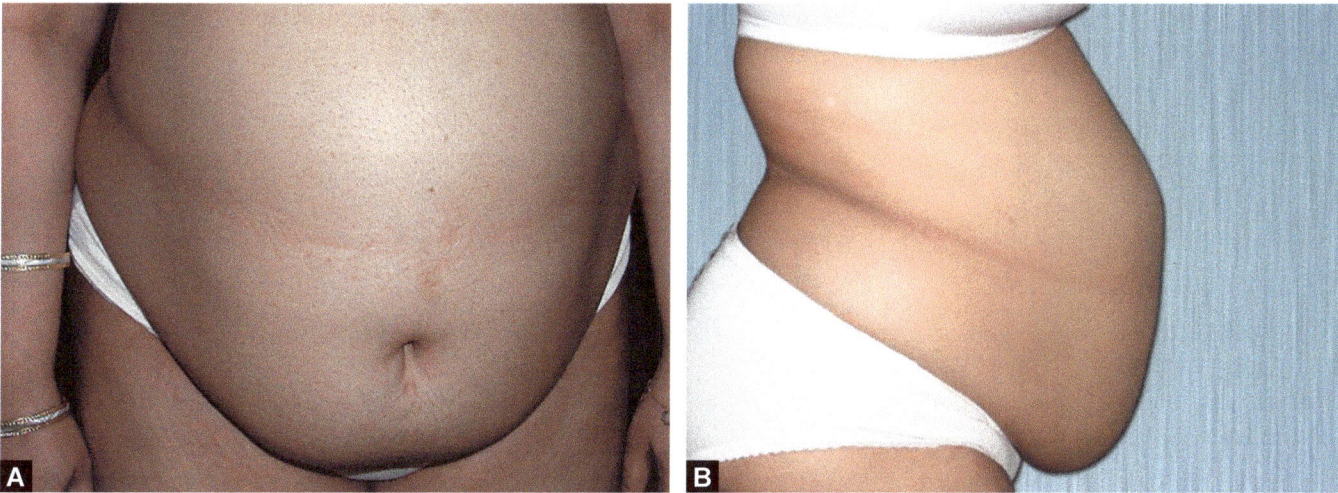

Figs. 14.8A and B: Case 2: An obese patient with large and bulging abdomen.

2. *Primary concerns*: Large and bulging abdomen, wide waist.
3. *Psychosocial assessment*: Depressed.
4. *Lifestyle assessment*: Not healthy, on and off diet management, cannot exercise.
5. *Expectations*: Wants smaller tummy and waist.
6. *Mutual decision*: After examination and discussion.

General Evaluation and Work-up

1. *Weight loss history*: Off and on.
2. *Diet and exercise habits*: Poor.
3. *Medical problems*: Diabetes, hypothyroidism.

Worksheet Planning

Detail analysis is performed (Table 14.4).

Options are discussed with pros and cons of each method of treatment (Table 14.5).

Mutual Decision

1. Three-dimensional liposuction.
2. Followed by diet management and exercise.
3. *If dissatisfactory outcome*: Consider bariatric surgery or abdominoplasty.
4. *Procedure performed*: General anesthesia.

Table 14.4: Summary of worksheet planning.

Frame of abdomen	Large and round		
Skin tone	Moderate laxity		
Contours	Normal		
Skin condition	Good, minimal striae		
Umbilicus	Deep and displaced inferiorly		
Fat distribution	Large amount of visceral fat		
	Large amount of subcutaneous fat all areas		
	Upper abdomen	Lower abdomen	Waistline
Panniculus	Large lower abdomen		
Excess skin	Significant supra- and infraumbilical		
Muscle	Very lax and bulging		
Posterior assessment	Fat bulges		

Table 14.5: Options.

Options	Advantages	Disadvantages
Nutrition and weight management	Loss of intra-abdominal fat	Patient already trying under medical supervision without much success
Exercise	Increase metabolism compliance	Needs lot of hard work, knee problems
Nonsurgical options	Cannot give the outcome	
Liposuction	Reduce a large volume skin contraction	Cannot address bulging muscle and intra-abdominal fat volume
Lipoabdominoplasty	Not indicated	Residual bulge Not great outcome
Sequential	Is an option	

5. *Conventional liposuction*: Three-dimensionally total aspirate 6,500 mL.
6. *Result*: Significant size reduction and gradual weight loss of 10 kg in 1 year (Figs. 14.9A and B).

▌ CASE 3 (FIGS. 14.10A AND B)

Consultation and Counselling

1. *History*: This is a 37-year-old woman with a history of two pregnancies. BMI is 28.
2. *Primary concerns*: Large abdomen, hanging skin.
3. *Psychosocial assessment*: Confident.
4. *Lifestyle assessment*: Healthy.
5. *Expectations*: Wants flat tummy, small waist, wants to wear "Sari" (Indian traditional Dress with exposed midrif).
6. *Mutual decision*: After examination and discussion.

General Evaluation and Work-up

1. *Weight loss history*: Off and on.
2. *Diet and exercise habits*: Good.
3. *Medical problems*: Nil.

Worksheet (Table 14.6)

Detail analysis is performed as a standard protocol. Options are discussed.

Mutual Decision

1. Lipoabdominoplasty.
2. Followed by diet management and exercise.
3. *Challenges explained*: Not enough supraumbilical skin to drape the abdomen.
4. Chances of additional scar of umbilicus or migration of scar superiorly.
5. *Procedure performed*: General anesthesia.
6. Conventional 3D liposuction (Judicious).
7. Subcostal release of upper abdominal flap.
8. No mobilization of pubic skin.
9. Fixation of flap to Scarpa's fascia.
10. Inward umbilical fixation.

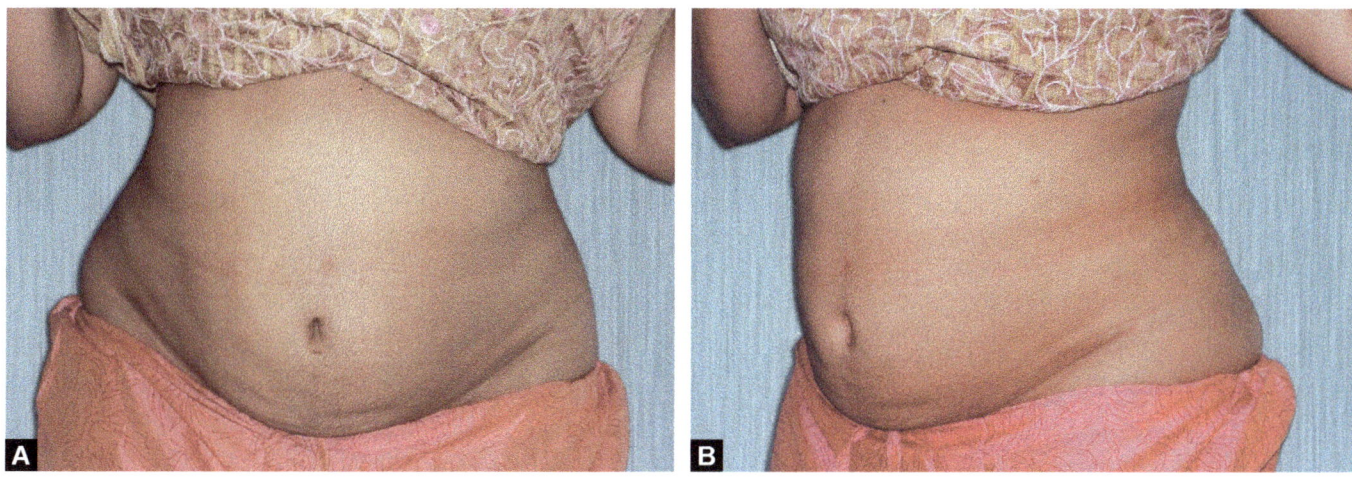

Figs. 14.9A and B: One year postoperative after three-dimensional liposuction. Same patient as in Figures 14.8A and B.

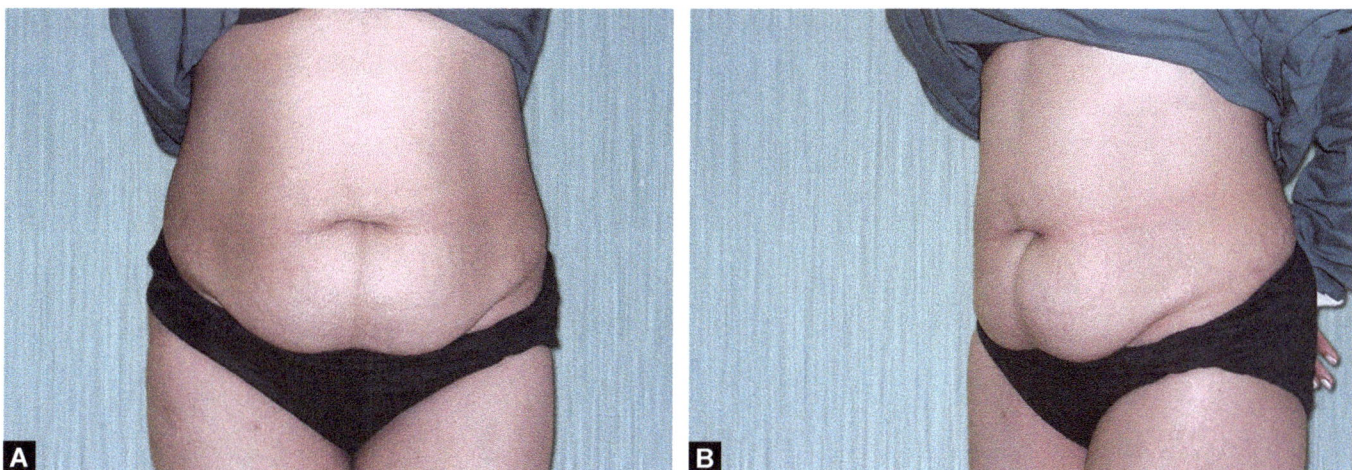

Figs. 14.10A and B: Case 3: A 37-year-old patient with two pregnancies, mild fat excess, moderate skin excess, infraumbilical skin flab, and muscle diversification.

Table 14.6: Summary of worksheet planning.			
Frame of abdomen	Moderate frame, poor waistline		
Skin tone	Moderate to poor skin tone with laxity		
Contours	Unevenness supraumbilical area and lower abdomen		
Skin condition	Extensive striae		
Umbilicus	Deep and mild inferior displacement		
Fat distribution	Mild visceral fat		
	Moderate subcutaneous fat all areas		
	Upper abdomen	Lower abdomen	Waistline
Panniculus	Moderate lower abdomen		
Excess skin	Mild to moderate supraumbilical skin excess and moderate to large infraumbilical		
Muscle	Moderate rectus diversification and laxity		
Posterior assessment	Moderate skin excess and fat bulges		

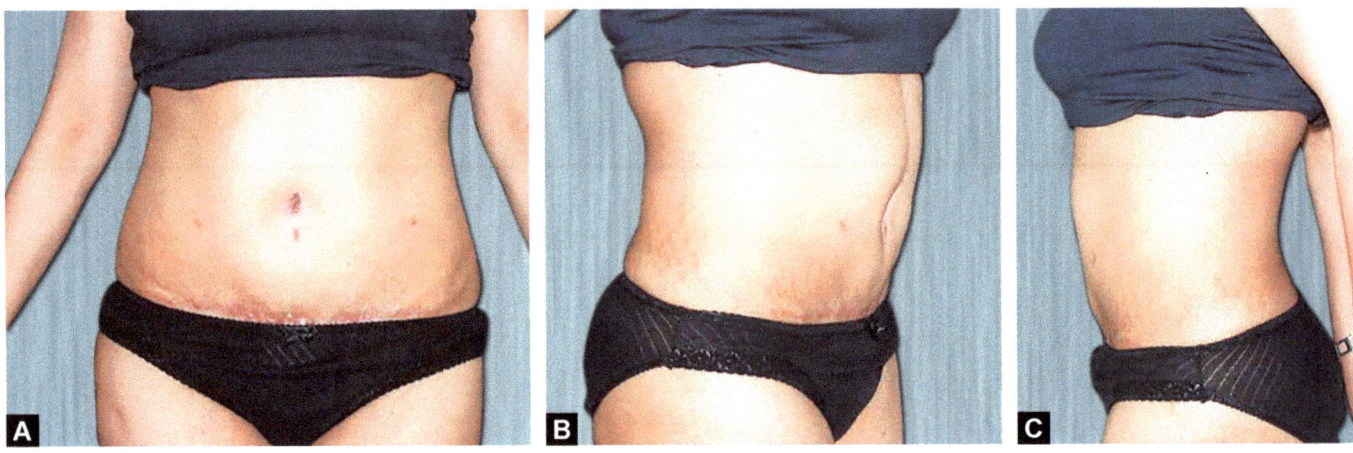

Figs. 14.11A to C: Eight months postoperative after lipoabdominoplasty.

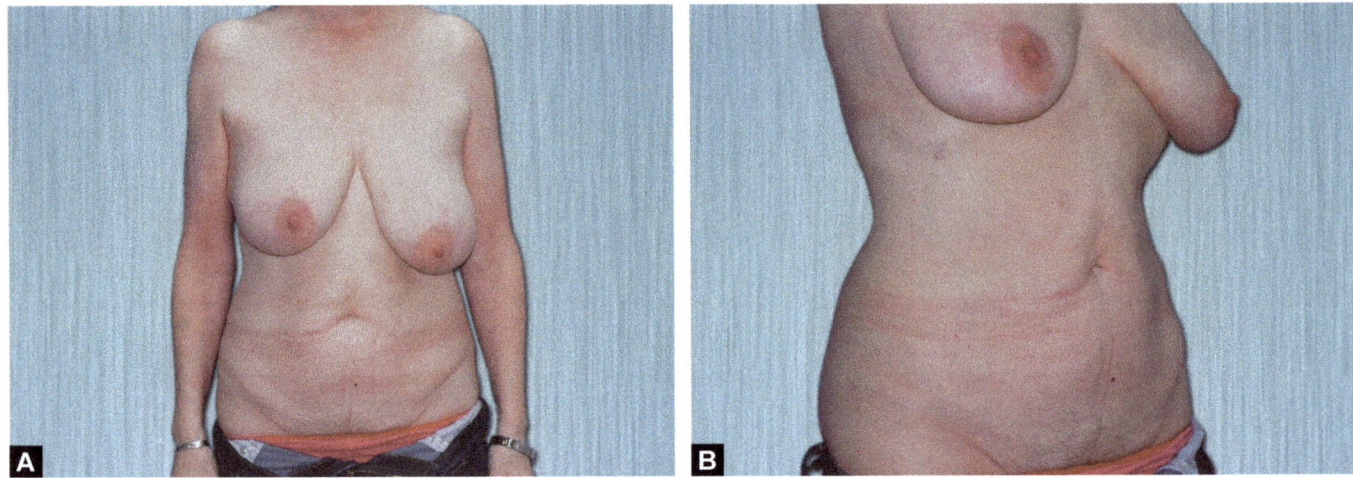

Figs. 14.12A and B: Case 4: A patient with excess weight loss and predominantly supraumbilical skin laxity with minimal laxity below the umbilicus.

Postoperative result: Improved waistline, low placed scar, " Innie" umbilicus (Figs. 14.11A to C).

CASE 4 (FIGS. 14.12A AND B)

Consultation and Counselling

1. *History*: This is a 56-year-old woman with a history of significant weight loss. BMI is 23.
2. *Primary concerns*: Lax skin in abdomen and breast sagging with asymmetry.
3. *Psychosocial assessment*: Confident.
4. *Lifestyle assessment*: Healthy.
5. *Expectations*: Wants skin tightening for tummy and breast lift, scar not a concern.
6. *Mutual decision*: After examination and discussion.

General Evaluation and Work-up

1. *Weight loss history*: Lost 35 kg weight.
2. *Diet and exercise habits*: Good.
3. *Surgery*: Sleeve gastrectomy 2 years ago.
4. *Medical problems*: Nil.

Worksheet (Table 14.7)

Detail physical analysis.

Mutual Decision

Reverse abdominoplasty with breast lift.

Table 14.7: Summary of worksheet planning.	
Frame of abdomen	Moderate frame, poor waistline
Skin tone	Moderate skin laxity, good skin tone
Contours	Supraumbilical skin fold
Skin condition	No striae
Umbilicus	Deep and no displacement
Fat distribution	Mild subcutaneous fat
Panniculus	No
Excess skin	Moderate supraumbilical skin excess and minimal infraumbilical skin excess
Muscle	Normal
Posterior assessment	Normal
Breast	Bilateral breast ptosis, grade 2, left breast is lower and larger

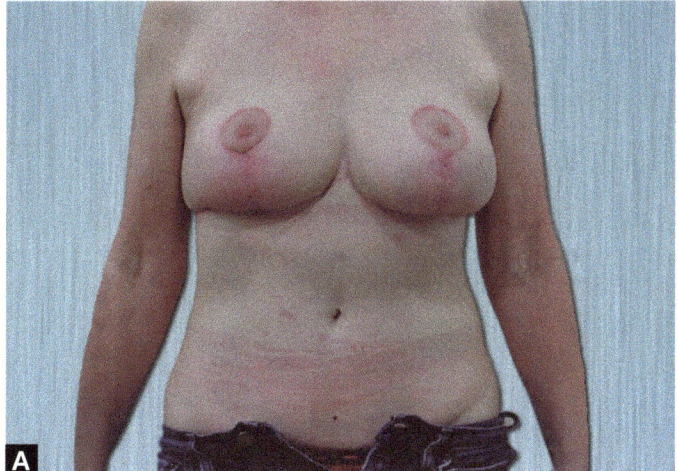
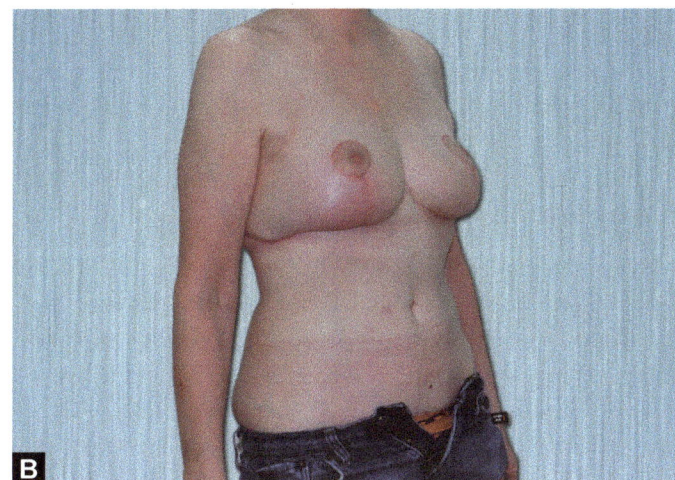

Figs. 14.13A and B: Three months postoperative after bilateral mastopexy and reverse abdominoplasty.

Limitations explained: Not enough supraumbilical skin to drape the abdomen, so standard abdominoplasty not appropriate. Reverse will not address lower abdominal skin.

Result: The surgery solved the problem of supraumbilical skin excess and breast sagging with a limited approach (Figs. 14.13A and B).

CONVENTIONAL ABDOMINOPLASTY (LIPOABDOMINOPLASTY)

Introduction

Conventional or complete abdominoplasty is the most commonly performed method of abdominoplasty. It addresses the following problems:

1. Excess skin removal.
2. Excess fat removal.
3. Correction of rectus diastasis.
4. Umbilical relocation.

Liposuction with or without ultrasound is now a routine part of abdominoplasty in our practice. It has improved the outcome of the surgery by contouring the abdomen, waistline, and back simultaneously along with skin tightening and muscle repair. This is possible due to our better understanding of the vascular anatomy of the abdominal region as described in Chapter 2.

Liposuction has other benefits that were missing in earlier days, and those are easy mobilization of the flap in a discontinuous way with preservation of perforators, rapid, and bloodless dissection of the flap and adequate thinning of the flap to drape the abdomen.

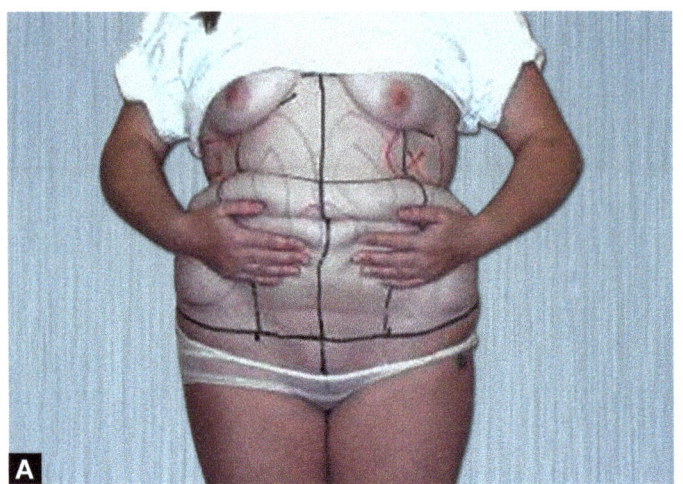 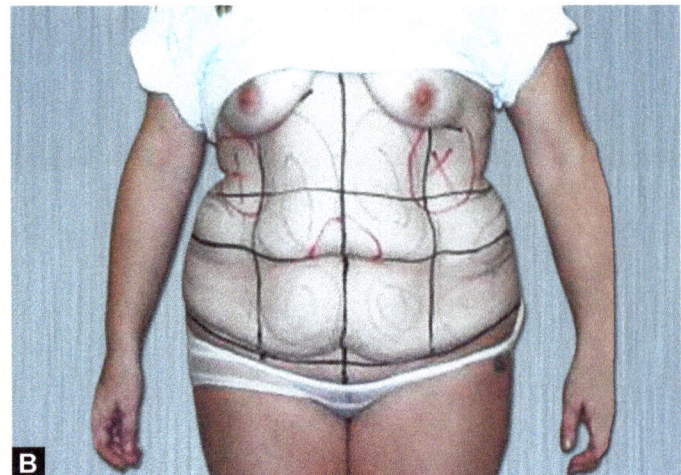

Figs. 14.14A and B: Markings for a typical lipoabdominoplasty surgery.

In patients with massive weight loss where we do not perform much liposuction, the surgery tends to be bloodier and time consuming.

Preoperative Consideration

It is discussed in great details in earlier chapters and should be a routine protocol for all kind of surgery. Diabetes and hypertension are not a contraindication as long as these medical conditions are under control with adequate medications. They do carry higher risk than an individual without any comorbid conditions. Smoking is of great concern; it increases the risk of bleeding, skin ischemia, fat necrosis, and pulmonary complications. In our preoperative written protocol, we keep reminding the patient to stop smoking at least 4–6 weeks prior to surgery. But it is not uncommon to find a noncompliant patient who continues to smoke. A written document ensures that they understand the risk associated with it and take full responsibility of the same.

Preoperative Protocol

1. Patient medical history.
2. Preoperative instructions.
3. Preoperative worksheet and planning.
4. American Society of Anesthesiologists' risk assessment.
5. Thromboembolic prevention protocol.
6. Postoperative instructions.
7. Consent forms.

    A routine checklist covering all the above ensures that all aspects are considered before the surgery. This will standardize the practice; ensure patient safety and superior outcome.

Worksheet Planning

I prefer to make an operative plan much ahead of the surgery along with all other preoperative protocol. This is recorded in charts and photographs. On the night before surgery, it is available in my computer/iPad with revision of the plan in my mind.

Preoperative Marking

Marking begins with a midline from xiphoid to pubic bone. Then I mark the costal margins and muscular outline. The patient is asked to lift his/her abdomen with both hands symmetrically (Figs. 14.14A and B).

Incision site is marked as low as possible in a straight line. This varies if the distance between umbilicus and pubic bone is long and I anticipate difficulty in draping the abdomen without additional scar of umbilical closure. This may also differ in patients requiring monsplasty or patient preferring a different bikini line scar.

The upper incision is marked in a curved fashion from one of the lower incision to the other, either passing above, at or below the umbilicus depending upon excess skin. High lateral tension incision marking is preferred if the patient insists on smaller scar or if there is excess skin in the waistline area. In my opinion, the high lateral tension causes significant bunching in the central abdomen that may take long-time to settle down.

Other marking includes areas of liposuction, adhesive bands, or rolls that may require special attention. If there

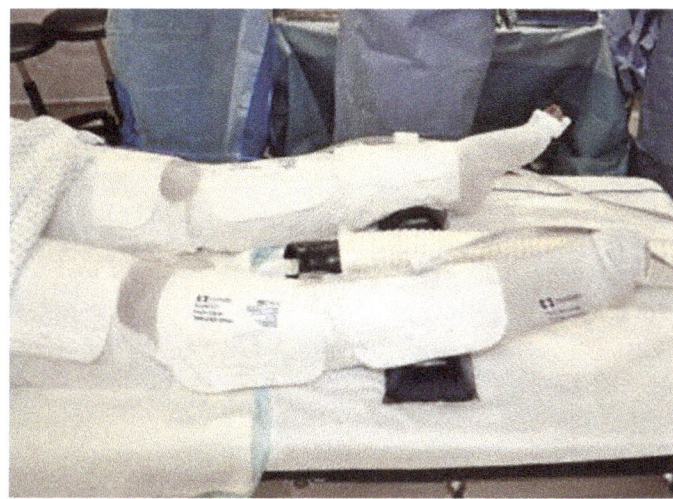

Fig. 14.15: Sequential pneumatic compression device in place prior to the induction of anesthesia.

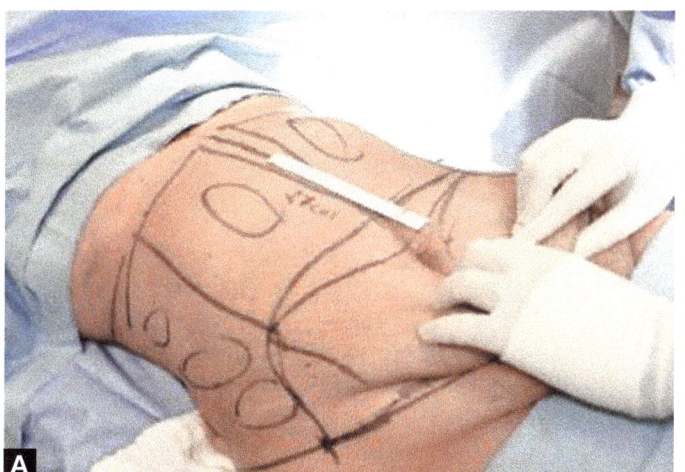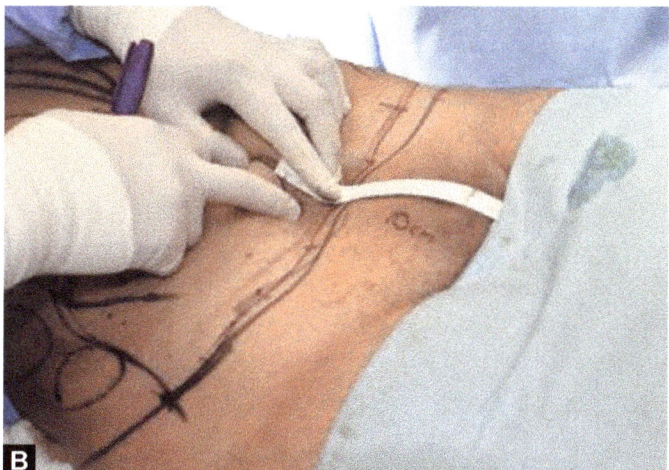

Figs. 14.16A and B: Intraoperative marking as the situation changes when patient is in supine position.

is diversification, the medial edges of the muscle are marked in lying down position.

The markings are confirmed and measured on the table to achieve symmetry.

Intraoperative Steps

The patient lies in supine position on the operating table. He/She is given compression stockings in the ward. In addition to that, we apply sequential pneumatic compression device and patient warming device (Fig. 14.15). General anesthesia, IV antibiotics, and steroids are administered.

Intraoperative Marking (Figs. 14.16A and B)

All the markings are confirmed in supine. Measurement of skin in stretched position is done from xiphisternum to the umbilicus. Measurement of distance between xiphisternum process and pubic bone will give us an estimate of skin excision and availability of skin flap to cover the abdomen. This is an important decision to decide how low you can make the incision with removal of umbilical opening.

INFILTRATION AND LIPOSUCTION

Superwet infiltration is performed in all the areas of the abdomen, waistline, flanks, and pubic areas. Any other areas to be liposuctioned are also infiltrated. After a waiting period of 20 minutes, liposuction is performed. Separate small incisions are made within the excision area and some incisions in the flank, pubic, and submammary areas. These incisions are left open postoperatively; it allows free drainage and helps in minimizing bruising and swelling.

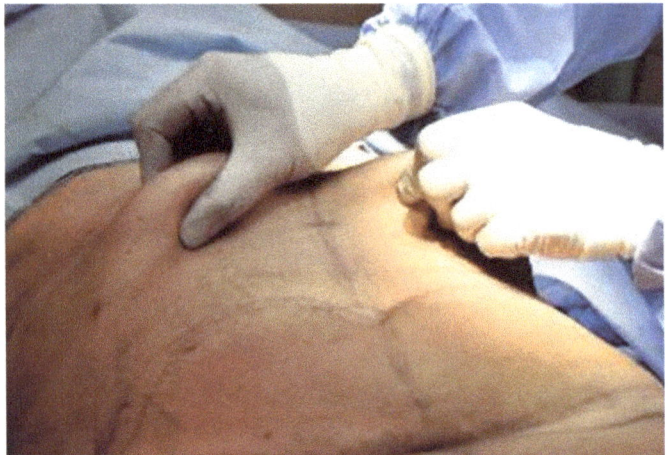

Fig. 14.17: Flap thinning after liposuction.

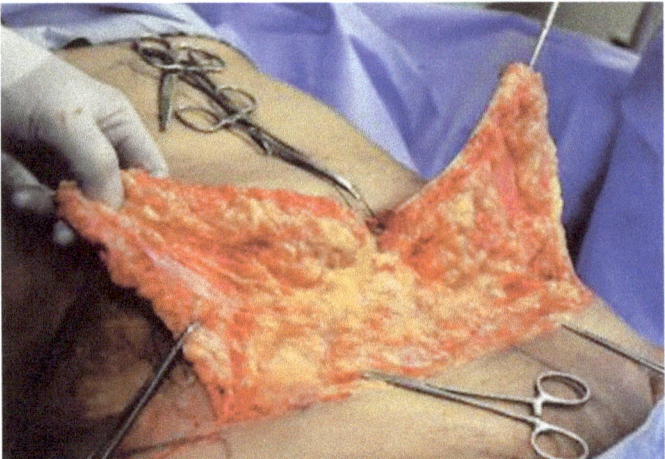

Fig. 14.18: Flap elevated with a thin layer of adipose tissue on the rectus sheath to prevent seroma.

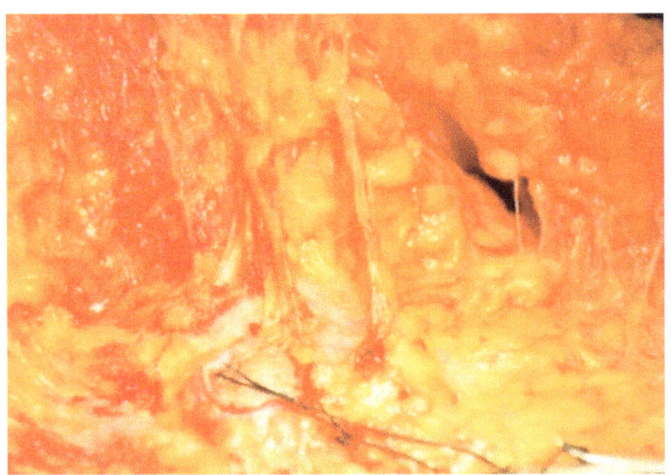

Fig. 14.19: Periumbilical perforators at least 2 to 3 left intact on each side.

Liposuction is performed as in the three-dimensional sculpting procedure described earlier. In most areas superficial, medium, and deep liposuction are performed. In some areas I do judicious liposuction and prevent excessive thinning of the flap such as just above the umbilicus to prevent suprapubic depression and lateral costal areas to preserve the vascular network. The musculocutaneous perforators arise through interdigitations of serratus anterior and external oblique muscle along the lateral aspect of abdomen and it is an important source of cutaneous supply.

Overall the skin flap can be thinned down to 2 cm (Fig. 14.17).

Incision starts at the lower part of the abdomen initially with a scalpel then with electrocautery. It is easy to identify the superficial epigastric vascular pedicle. I prefer to ligate or transfix it, as it can open up later once the adrenaline effect is over or if the patient's blood pressure shoots up postoperatively. The incision continues down to Scarpa's fascia. The flap is then elevated leaving a small amount of fat over the rectus sheath. This is a different approach unlike past where the aponeurosis was cleanly dissected. This leads to potential seroma formation (Fig. 14.18).

There are perforators around the umbilicus. Some of these perforators can be preserved; they supply blood to the distal part of the flap and this is the key to a good liposuction that can be performed without the concern of flap devascularization (Fig. 14.19). The perforators that are sacrificed for flap mobility are securely transfixed with 2–0 vicryl suture.

After dissecting the flap till the umbilicus, two skin hooks are applied at 12 and 6 o'clock positions and is circumscribed with 11 number scalpel (Figs. 14.20A and B).

Silk sutures are applied at 12 o'clock and 6 o'clock positions of the umbilicus for orientation purpose. The umbilicus is dissected out with a pair of scissor leaving a small amount of fat in the stalk. The flap is then dissected in a tunnel fashion centrally keeping tissues attached at both the sides. Enough dissection is performed for rectus plication. A combination of sharp and blunt dissection is done to mobilize the flap. Laterally, it is easy to mobilize the flap with Lockwood dissector that easily releases the costal attachment of the flap (Figs. 14.21A and B).

Rectus muscle border is marked with a marker. It is plicated with a double loop number 0 ethilon starting from the costal region. Ensure that the first suture is high

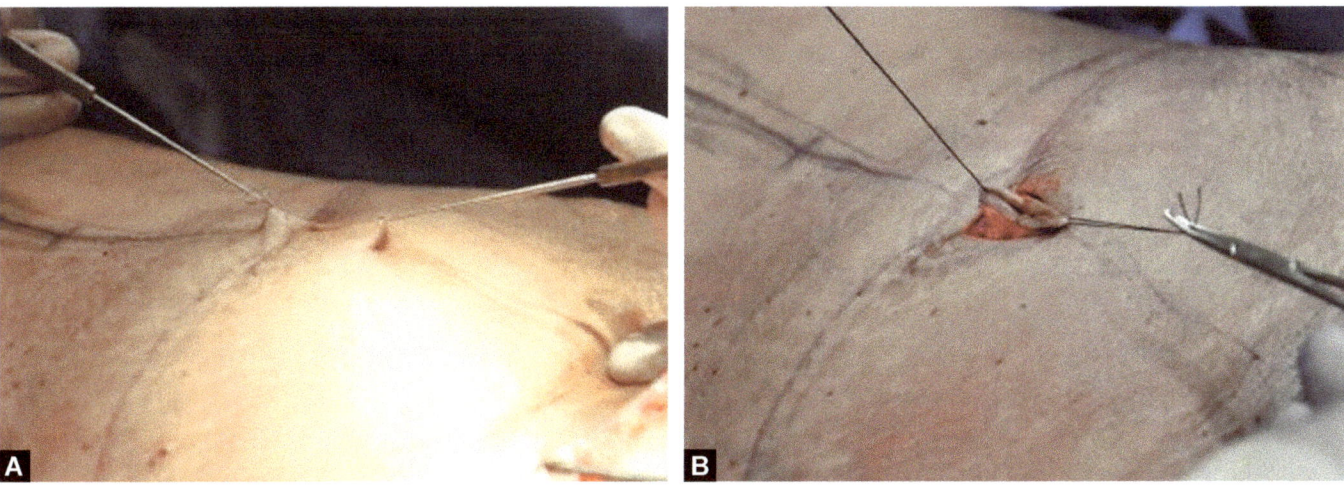

Figs. 14.20A and B: Circumscribing the umbilicus in a vertical elliptical shape and applying silk sutures for correct orientation.

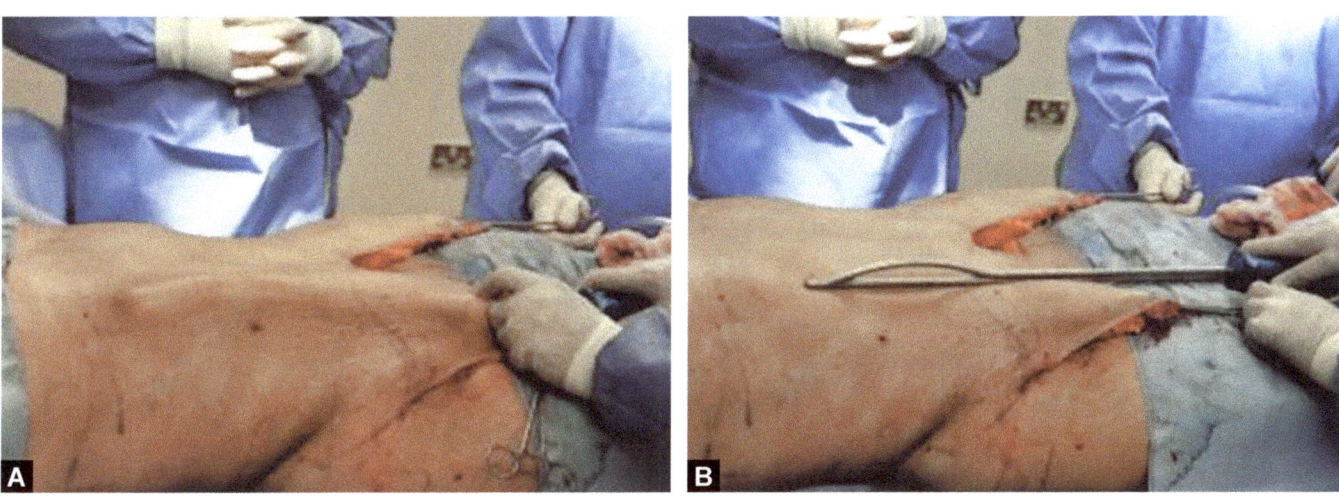

Figs. 14.21A and B: Use of Lockwood's dissector to release the abdominal flap.

enough to prevent abnormal bulge above the first suture placement. More importantly get a good bite of the rectus sheath or else this part of the suture cuts through the fat and becomes loose forming a groove postoperatively. I do not go through the muscle as it can cause intramuscular hematoma and pain postoperatively. Take a good bite of the rectus sheath. As you reach the umbilicus you can circumvent the umbilicus and continue with the same suture until the pubic bone (Figs. 14.22A to C).

If there is large intra-abdominal volume or significant myofacial laxity (massive weight loss, patient). I prefer two-layer closure of the rectus sheath. The second layer can be interrupted using 2–0 Ethibond sutures. Ensure to bury all the knots deep inside the rectus sheath. In thin patients, the suture knots can be palpable and bothersome for long time.

The amount of skin flap excision is estimated by using flap markers (Figs. 14.23A to C). I personally do not prefer to flex the OR table significantly, particularly in dark skin patients to prevent scar migration superiorly. It is very important to excise the flap in appropriate amount to prevent over excision.

Careful blunt dissection to break the fibrous bands can help advance the flap further. I mobilize the lower flap only if I am unable to close the wound with usual maneuvers. The wound is temporarily closed in the center to mark the location of the umbilicus. Pitanguys tissue demarcator is used to determine the location of umbilical opening (Figs. 14.24A and B). A vertical ellipse of skin is excised and flap is defatted around the opening. Three key sutures are placed at 3, 6 and 9 o'clock position from subcutaneous tissue of flap and umbilical skin and is fixated to the rectus sheath to achieve a dip in the umbilicus (Figs. 14.25A to C). The temporary sutures are removed and flap is elevated.

At this stage, I ask the anesthesiologist to increase the blood pressure to 100–120 mm Hg to look for any bleeders. This is the key to prevent hematoma. The perforators either

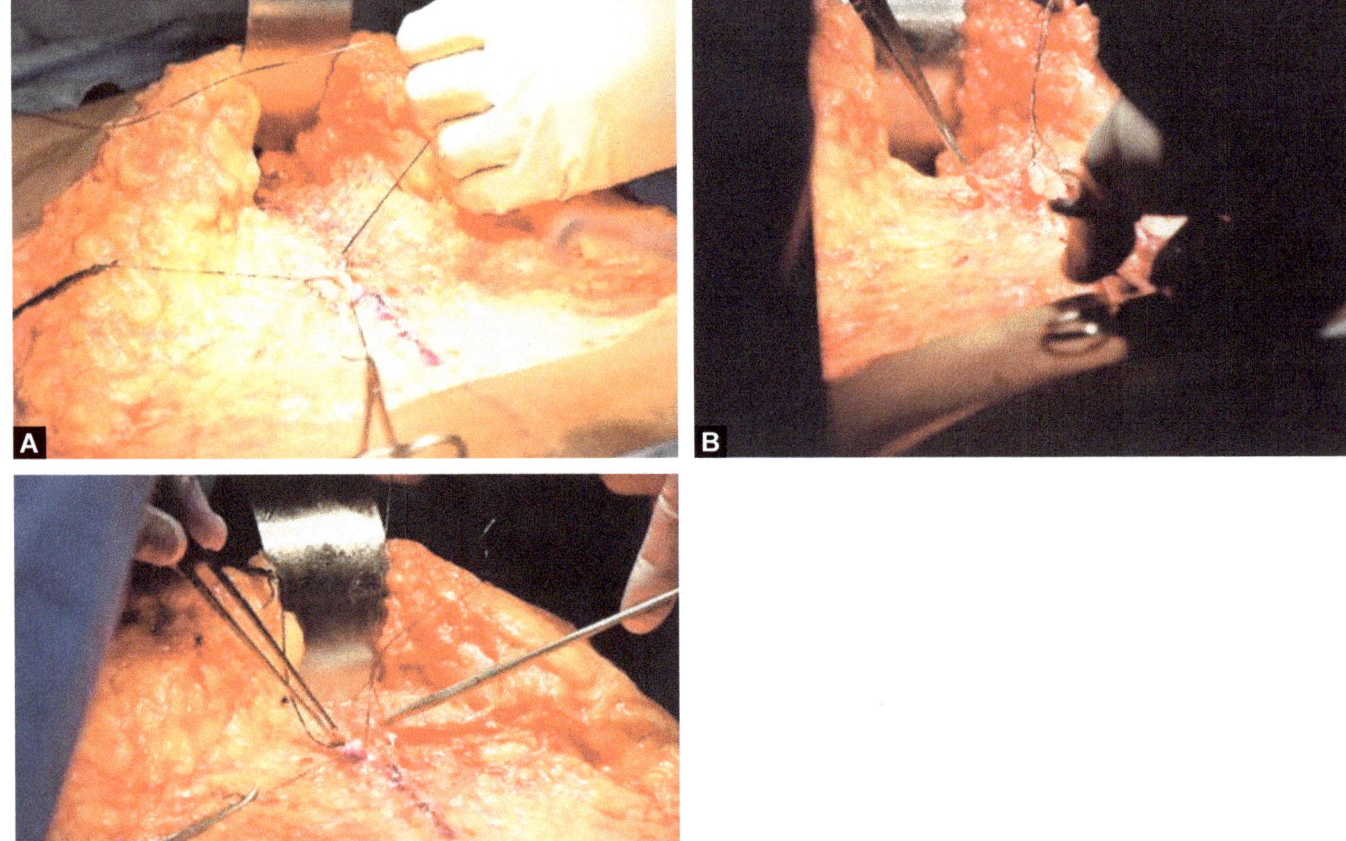

Figs. 14.22A to C: Rectus sheath plication using number 0 double loop ethilon. It is circumvented around the umbilicus to complete the suture in the pubic area.

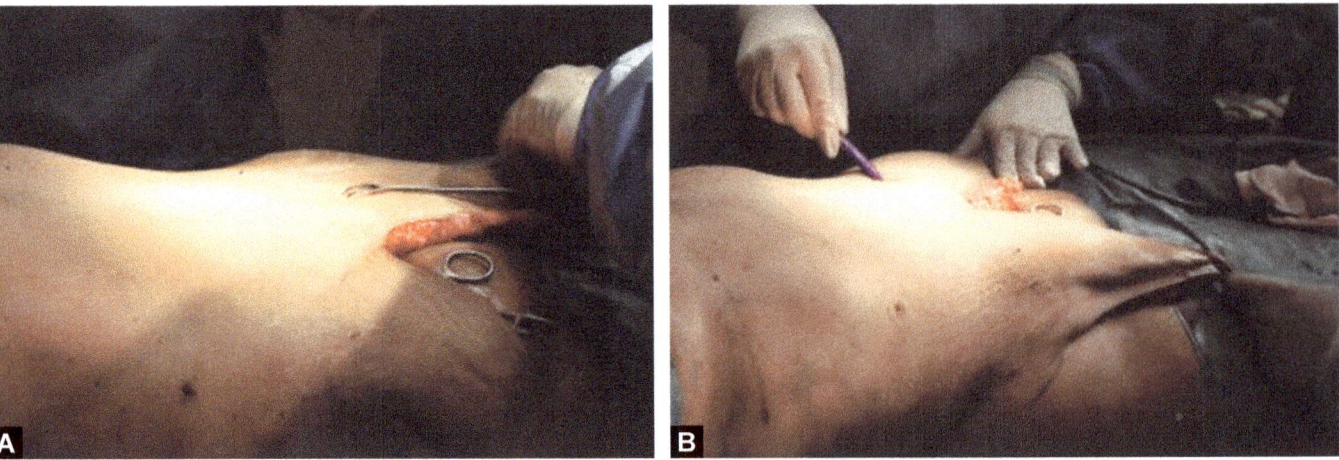

Figs. 14.23A and B

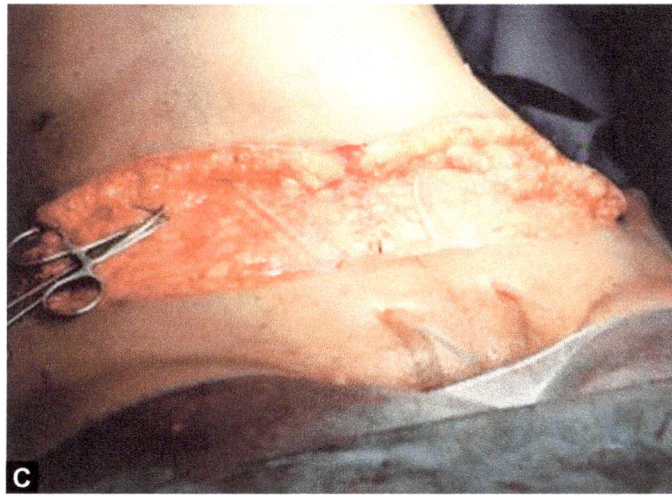

Figs. 14.23A to C: (A) Flap marker is used to mark the excess skin keeping patient in neutral position. (B) Marking of the skin excision. (C) Excision of the excess skin without flexing the OR table.

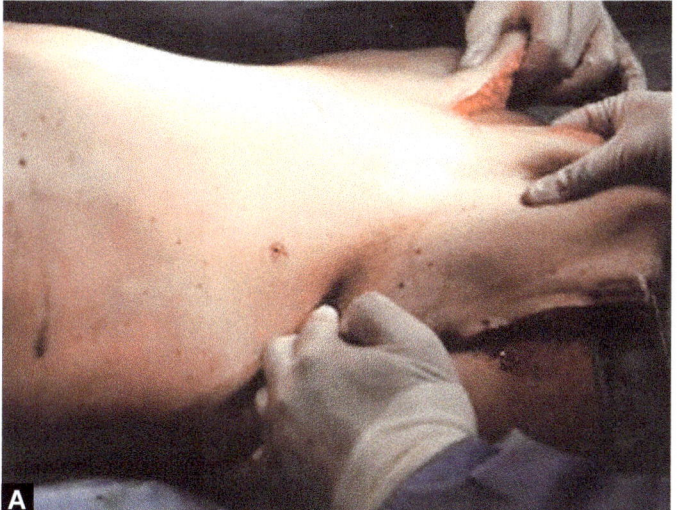
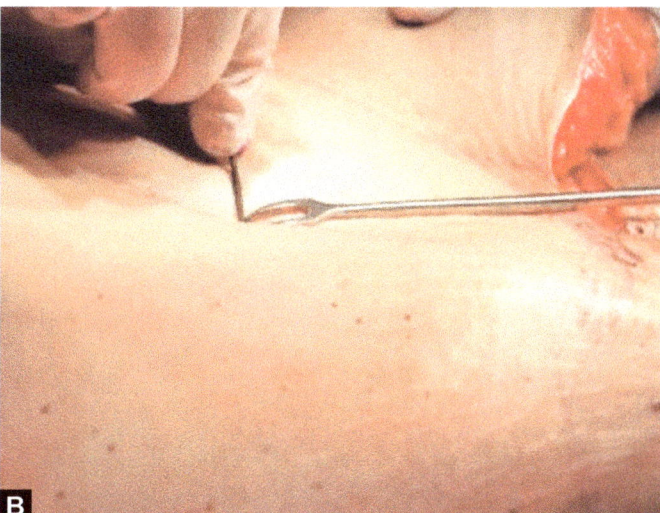

Figs. 14.24 A and B: Marking the position of umbilical opening. (A) Umbilicus is approximately at the level of highest point of iliac creast. (B) The position is confirmed by using Pitanguys marker.

are retracted or constricted due to adrenaline and they open up after the effect of adrenaline weans off or if the blood pressure shoots up postoperatively.

The subscarpal fat is easily identified as pale fat; this is conservatively excised mostly in the lateral part of the abdominal flap. The central part is conservatively excised to prevent depression and flap devascularization.

The integrity of the rectus plication is ensured; marcaine is injected in the rectus sheath (5–10 mL of 0.25% without adrenaline). Personally, I prefer a silicone corrugated drain that is placed through small stab incisions in the pubic region. I have done many cases without any drain, but I realized the swelling and bruising are more if the fluid/blood is retained under the flap. More than the

risk of hematoma, the fluid and blood are drained out in first 24–48 hours, and the abdomen looks less tense postoperatively.

I do not prefer Jackson Pratt drain because it often gets blocked and gives a false security to the surgeon and nurses.

Quilt sutures using 2-0 rapid vicryl are placed in an advancing manner in the midline above the umbilicus and medially and laterally in the lower abdomen. The suture bites in the flap are not very deep to prevent visible dimpling. The midline is first closed and suturing starts with Scarpa's fascia approximation using number 0 vicryl (Figs.14.26A and B). The flap is advanced medially to prevent dog ears. Fixation to the Scarpa's fascia ensures good

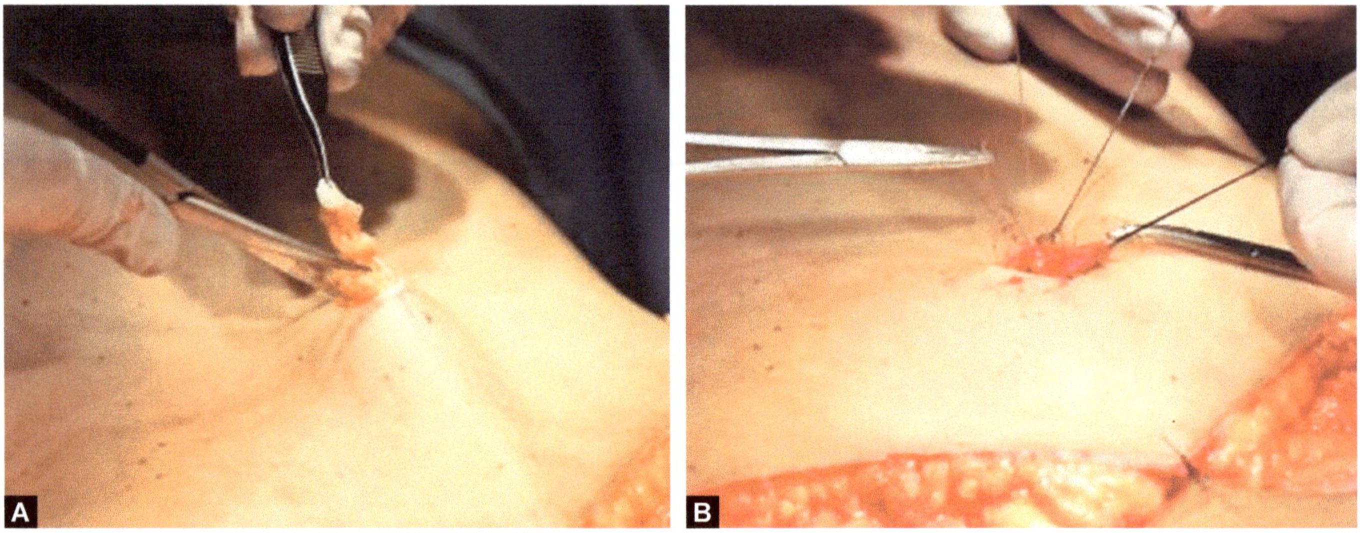

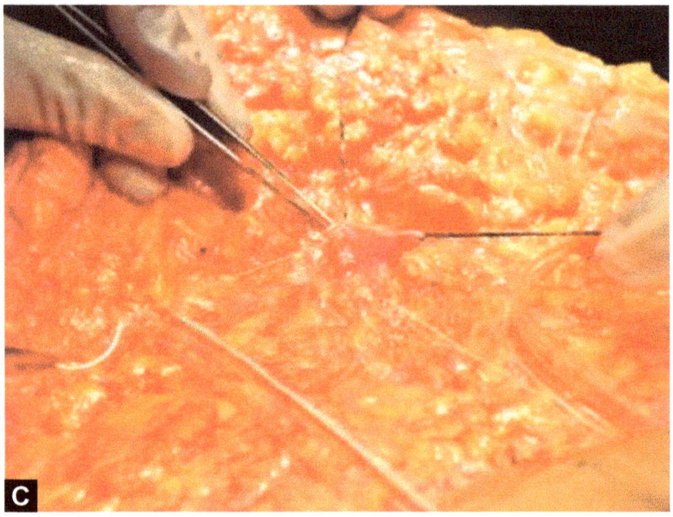

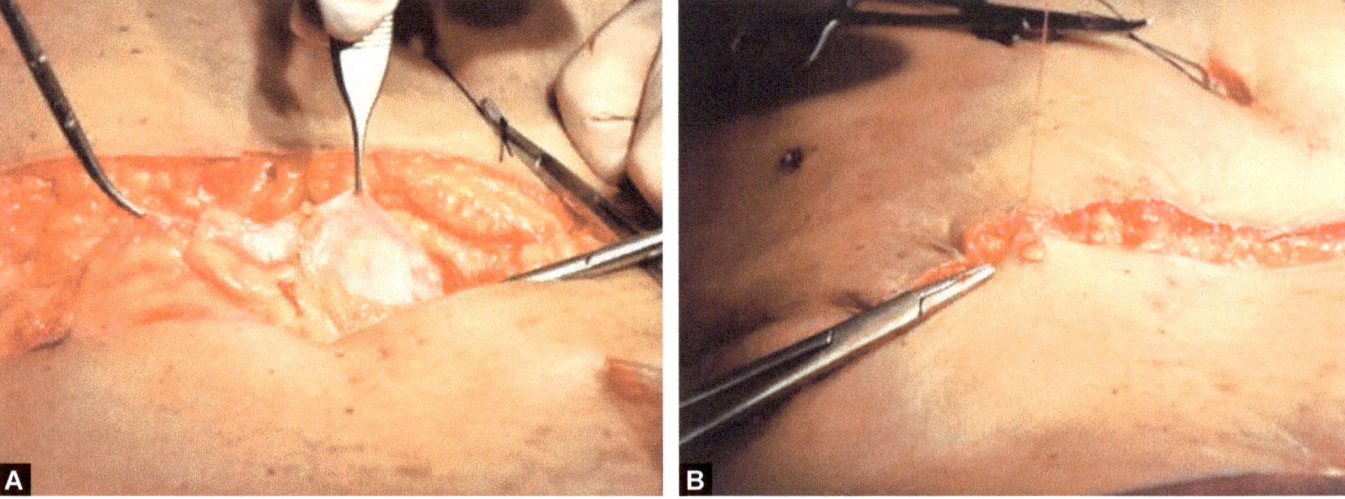

Figs. 14.25A to C: (A) A excision of elliptical skin and de fattening of the flap for umbilical fixation. (B) Key sutures are placed at 3, 6 and 9 o'clock position. (C) If the flap is too thick the umbilicus can be fixed to rectus sheath with 3 key sutures by elevating the flap.

Figs. 14.26A and B: (A) Scarpa's fascia (B) Second layer of flap suturing.

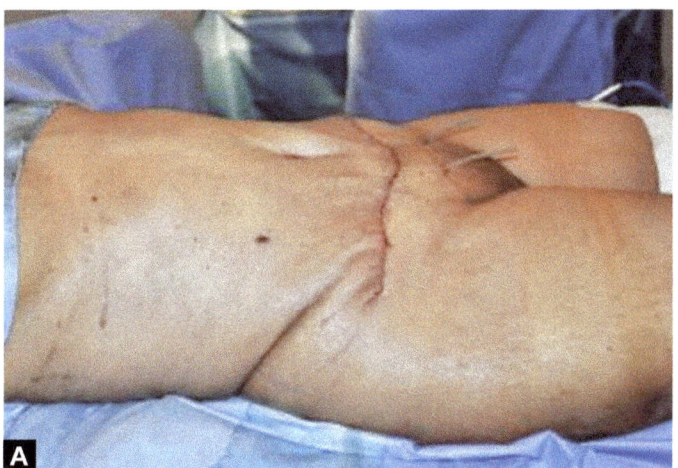 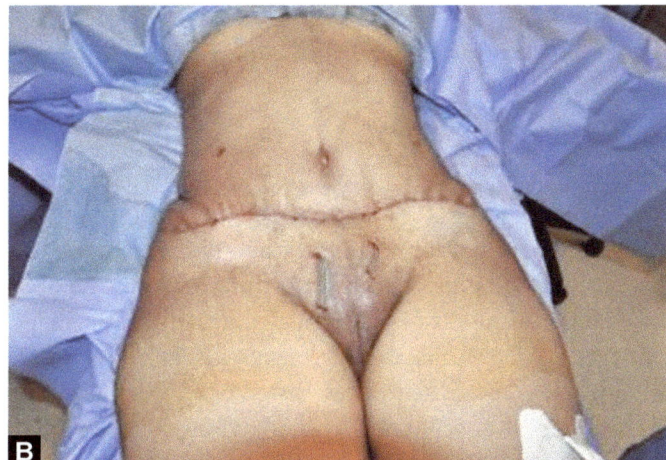

Figs. 14.27A and B: Final closure of the skin, the subcuticular PDO sutures in neutral position of patient.

stability to the flap and prevents its retraction proximally. If the skin quality is poor with extensive stretch marks, I do not prefer to advance the flap medially as the bunching and skin wrinkling can persist for long-time. I prefer to extend the incision laterally and keep the abdomen contour uniform.

This is followed by the second line of closure with 2-0 vicryl ensuring the sutures are placed deep to prevent "suture spitting" postoperatively. Finally a continuous intradermal 4-0 polydioxanone (PDS) suture is used to close the skin (Figs. 14.27A and B).

The umbilicus sutures depend upon the thickness of the flap and tension in the umbilical region. In dark skin patients and if there is excessive tension on the umbilicus I do not anchor the umbilicus to the rectus sheath. Excessive tension in the umbilical area leads to wound breakdown, umbilical discoloration, and hypertrophic scar.

The detail of umbilical closure is covered in subsequent sections.

POSTOPERATIVE CARE

Maintaining temperature is important to prevent shivering and hypothermia. I do not recommend cleaning the patient with wet sponges excessively; we just remove the blood stains and dry the skin and apply padded dressing with adhesive plaster. The patient is nursed in 30° sit up position with pillows under the knee to prevent tension in the suture line. Nurses are instructed to encourage patient to do deep breathing exercise, move knees and ankles, and turn to sides time to time. They are ambulated after 4–6 hours. Urinary catheter is used only to drain the urine

immediately after the surgery and is not retained in unless the situation demands.

The initial process of ambulation requires assistance by nurse to prevent postural hypotension and syncope. The patient's first sit up with legs hanging out of the bed and take deep breaths. If they feels dizzy, they return back to supine position. If the patient feels fine then he/she is asked to stand up. This is the time we see corrugators drain blood and fluid. It should be padded enough so that the patient does not see blood drainage. These steps are repeated until the patient feels comfortable. Patients stay overnight in the hospital for fluid and pain management.

Most patients are discharged next day with drains removed and a pressure garment. They are given postoperative instruction in written form with emergency contact details.

UMBILICAL RECONSTRUCTION IN ABDOMINOPLASTY

Many authors have proposed various types of incisions and fixation around the umbilicus. Umbilical appearance is one of the most challenging parts of abdominoplasty because any deformities and scar formation results in unaesthetic appearance.

Umbilical Changes in Abdomen

The umbilicus goes through changes when the patient gains weight and subsequently loses it. Depending upon the accumulation of fat (intra- and versus extra-abdominal) the umbilicus may appear shallow and flushed or deep and long. The presence of hernia and old scars may further distort the shape of the umbilicus.

Umbilicus Location

Umbilical location varies from person to person; some may have it highly placed whereas in others it may be low in the abdomen. Abdominoplasty method may depend on the location of the umbilicus. If the umbilicus is stretched and long or located low in the abdomen, it can be easily managed by classical abdominoplasty and a translocation method. If there is a significant distance between umbilicus and pubic bone, particularly without much excess skin in the lower abdomen, there may be an additional scar required to close the umbilical opening.

Marking of New Umbilicus Position

Marking of new umbilical position on the flap is based on following landmarks:
1. *Exact position of the umbilicus attachment to the rectus*: This is marked on the flap using Pitanguy's marker.
2. At the level of iliac crest.
3. At least 6–8 cm above the lower edge of abdominal flap.

Characteristics of an Aesthetic Umbilicus

1. *Small size*: Small umbilicus is considered more aesthetically pleasing. Therefore, the ideal skin ellipse should not be wider than 1.5 cm and longer than 2.5 cm.[13]
2. *Superior hooding*: It is considered as an essential factor for creating a natural umbilicus. Some authors suggest thinning the flaps. Niranjan in 2004 suggested a different technique where instead of suturing the dermis of the skin of flap and umbilicus to the rectus sheath, he sutures the superficial fascia of abdominal skin to the dermis of the flap. This composite tissue is then sutured to the umbilical skin.[14] I prefer to suture this composite tissue to the rectus sheath to prevent stretching of the umbilicus in future.
3. *Periumbilical concavity*: This is created by excising the fatty tissue under the flap and fixing the skin to the rectus fascia. This gives an aesthetic depression in the umbilical region.
4. *Aesthetic umbilical scar*: Hypertrophic scar in dark skin people can impair the final appearance of the umbilicus. It is important to prevent tension in the skin edges while suturing. All the tension should be transmitted

to the rectus sheath, and skin is closed with subcuticular running suture.

INCISION TECHNIQUES

There are different incision patterns:
1. Vertical elliptical.
2. Inverted Y-incision.
3. Double inverted Y-incision.

Inverted Y-incision has advantages of breaking the scar continuity and creating a seamless umbilicus inferiorly.

Fixation Technique

Suture fixation starts before the abdominal flap is closed. Umbilical stalk is shortened if it is long by using plication suture. Sutures are taken at 3, 6, and 9 o'clock position by passing through the edge of the umbilical opening of the flap, the umbilical dermis, and the rectus sheath. These sutures are left long and brought out of the flap opening for tightening later after the initial abdominal flap closure.

Once the central part of the flap is closed, the sutures are tied ensuring there is adequate inversion of the edges. This is followed by some deep vicryl sutures to reduce the tension on the skin. Finally a running PDS suture is used for skin approximation.

COMPLICATIONS OF ABDOMINOPLASTY

To minimize the complications of abdominoplasty we need to understand the causes of the complications; based on that we can take preemptive measures to prevent complications.

Mohan published a classification system in 2008.[15] Complications in abdominoplasty have many implications such as delayed recovery, unnecessary expenses, poor scar, compromised result, and psychological trauma to the patient. I believe a patient who has undergone complication loses faith in the doctor and their practice and is not a good word of mouth source of referral.

In our center, we follow a rigid protocol pre, intra, and postoperatively to prevent any complications.

Classification of Complications

1. General
   a. Hypothermia
   b. Sepsis

c. DVT and thromboembolic phenomenon
d. Fat embolism.
2. Local complications.
3. Major complications requiring emergency surgery
   a. Skin necrosis
   b. Infection, necrotizing fasciitis
   c. Bleeding and hematoma
   d. Visceral damage
   e. Pulmonary complications.
4. Major complications requiring revision surgery/Procedure
   a. Seroma
   b. Fat necrosis
   c. Cellulitis
   d. Abscess
   e. Extensive contour deformities and lumpiness
   f. Skin excess
   g. Wrinkling.
5. Minor complications
   a. port infection
   b. Scars
   c. Induration
   d. Pigmentation problems
   e. Hyposthesia
   f. Chronic pain
   g. Suture granulomas and spitting.

Hypothermia

It is defined as a minimum temperature of 35°C or lower. Previous randomized trials have demonstrated that hypothermia is associated with a variety of complications, such as seroma, bleeding, surgical wound infection, and cardiac events.[16,17] In the body contouring procedure, the chances of hypothermia are increased due to the exposure of the body parts, use of antiseptic solution, tumescent infiltration, and duration of surgery. The author adopts following measures to prevent reduction in body temperature:
1. Body warmer.
2. Higher ambient temperature of operating room.
3. Warm antiseptic application.
4. Fluid warmer for infiltration fluid and IV fluid.
5. Postoperative drying the patient with dry warm pads.

Deep Vein Thrombosis

Abdominoplasty carries a significant risk of deep venous thrombosis and pulmonary embolus. Thromboembolic risk increases when abdominoplasty is combined with other procedures and significantly more when combined with intra-abdominal procedures such as hysterectomy.

The protocol and preventive measures is discussed in earlier chapters. Patient education is essential for prompt evaluation and treatment. The patients are warned to report any signs of dyspnea, dizziness, tachycardia, pain, and swelling in the legs.

Hematoma

The following are the common causes of hematoma in abdominoplasty:
1. *Bleeding vessels*: Perforators around umbilicus, superficial inferior epigastric vessels, superficial circumflex vessels, and veins in the lateral part of the abdominal incision are the commonest source of bleeding intra or postoperatively. Because of hypotensive anesthesia and vasoconstricting effect of epinephrine these vessels may skip our attention. Massive weight loss patient often tends to have large veins increasing the risk of hematoma. The author prefers to underrun the bleeders with 2-0 vicryl and ensure adequate hemostasis after increasing the blood pressure prior to closure of the wounds.
2. *Rectus sheath hematoma*: This can occur if the perforators are transected close to the rectus sheath and retract inside or due to needle injury to the perforators of deep epigastric vessels while plicating the rectus sheath. The author prefers to transect and ligate a few millimeters above the sheath and pass the needle carefully through the rectus sheath during plication.

There are two kinds of hematoma. These are as follows:
1. Expanding hematoma with drop in blood pressure and tachycardia needs an emergency operation to evacuate and stop the active bleeders.
2. Stable hematoma without alteration of hemodynamics can be observed and eventually drained under local anesthesia without wound exploration.

Seroma

Seroma is the accumulation of fluid under the abdominal flap that requires repeated aspiration. There are many contributing factors to seroma.
1. Undrained hematoma.
2. Electrocautery injury to the tissues.
3. Excessive ultrasonic energy during liposuction.
4. Traumatic liposuction with the use of curetting cannulas or large cannulas.
5. Tissue dissection baring the aponeurosis delays tissue adhesion and is potential space for seroma.
6. Excessive tumescence without any drainage postoperatively.

Treatment of seroma involves aspiration under sterile technique, adequate compression, and regular follow-up.

Fat Necrosis

Fat necrosis can be a problem in obese individuals with excessive fat and thick abdominal flap. The most vulnerable part of the adipose tissue is the fat around the umbilicus and under the Scarpa's fascia. If you see the anatomy carefully, the subscarpal fat receives its blood supply from deep epigastric perforators. If the flap is elevated close to the aponeurosis, the fat on the undersurface of the Scarpa's fascia is deprived of its perforator supplies from deep vascular system. And carries a high risk of necrosis. Fat necrosis presents postoperatively as; induration, cellulitis, discharging wound, and infection and eventually leads to depressed scars or residual fibrous lump. To prevent this problem excise the subscarpal fat from the undersurface of the flap prior to flap closure.

The treatment involves opening the wound and debriding the fat sequentially. A secondary correction may be required to improve the contour.

Scar Problems

Excessive scar formation or hypertrophy, stretched scars, asymmetrical scars, depressed scars, umbilical scars, displaced scars are some of the common problem of the abdominoplasty.

To minimize scar is a huge challenge particularly in pigmented skin people.

Let us analyze the causes of scars in abdominoplasty patients:

1. *Skin type*: Darker skin has more tendencies for hypertrophy; however, even fair skin can have unsightly scars. The plan of the surgery is modified according to the skin type. If hypertrophy is anticipated, the author prefers to minimize the amount of skin excision and focus on securing deep sutures to prevent tension on skin edges.
2. *Improper placement of incision*: Incision should be as low as possible in the pubic region and laterally in the inguinal region. It may wary depending upon the dress patients want to wear such as bikini style, low waist jeans, and sari (Indian traditional wear). Various incision lines have been described in the literature and each one has special indications.[6]
3. *Excessive skin tension*: Overexcision of the skin is the primary cause of excessive skin tension. Other causes

are improper distribution of tension while closing deeper layers of the skin and poor suturing technique. A proper estimate of the amount of skin excision will prevent over resection. An adequate release of the flap from its costal attachment and pre-existing folds are also important steps to advance the flap and minimize skin tension.

4. Complications such as hematoma, infection, ischemia, and suture spitting are other causes of poor scar formation. Hence, minimizing the complications is the key to reduce unaesthetic scars.
5. *Poor closure technique*: Although it is rare as plastic surgeons are trained in meticulous closure but we do see time to time poor wound closures.

Umbilical Complications

1. *Displaced umbilicus*: The umbilicus may be off center to right or left or it may be too low in the abdomen. Umbilical landmark, orientation, and proper placement and fixation are the key to avoid the complications.
2. *Umbilical scar*: Tension in the umbilical suturing can lead to hypertrophy or hyperpigmentation of the scar.
3. *Umbilical stenosis*: If the umbilical opening is small and circular, the scar can contract and cause umbilical stenosis.
4. *Stretching of umbilicus*: A large umbilicus can further stretch after the swelling subsides and may appear unaesthetic.
5. Ischemic changes can occur in umbilicus leading to problems from discoloration to necrosis. This is due to excessive skeletonizing of the stalk, strangulating rectus placating sutures or excessive tension on the skin.

▮ REFERENCES

1. Demars, Marx. In: Voloir P (Ed). Opérations Plastiques Sus-Aponévrotiques sur la Paroi Abdominale Antérieure. Paris: Thése;1960.
2. Kelly H A. Report of gynecological cases (excessive growth of fat). Johns Hopkins Med J. 1899;10:197.
3. Passot R. Chirurgie Esthetique Pure. Paris:Doin;1931. pp. 260-7.
4. Thorek M. Plastic surgery of the breast and abdominal wall. Springfield, I11:Charles C Thomas;1924.
5. Vernon S. Umbilical transplantation upward and abdominal contouring in lipectomy. Am J Surg. 1957;94:490.
6. Hunstad JP, Repta R. History. In: Atlas of Abdominoplasty. Amsterdam: Elsevier Inc, 2009, pp. 1-5.
7. Somalo M. Cruciform ventral dermal lipectomy swallow-shaped incision. Prensa Med Argent 1946;33:75.

8. Gonzalez-Ulloa M. [Circular lipectomy with transposition of the umbilicus and aponeurolytic plastic technic] (in Spanish). Cir Cir. 1959;27:394-409.

9. Pastoureau M, Garvie F. Heraldry: Its Origins and Meaning. Trans. London, UK: Thames and Hudson;1997. p. 98.

10. Millard DR Jr. A lip fleur-de-lis flap. Plast Reconstr Surg. 1964;34:34-6.

11. Dellon AL. Fleur-de-lis abdominoplasty. Aesthetic Plast Surg. 1985;9:27-32.

12. Moufarrège R. The Moufarrège horseshoe abdominoplasty Aesthet Surg J. 1997;17(2):91-6.

13. Craig SB, Faller MS, Puckett, CL. In search of the ideal female umbilicus. Plast. Reconstr. Surg. 2000;105:389.

14. Niranjan NS, Staiano JJ. An anatomical method for resiting the umbilicus. Plast Reconstr Surg. 2004;113(7):2194-8.

15. Rangaswamy M. Minimising complications in abdominoplasty: an approach based on the root cause analysis and focused preventive steps. Indian J Plast Surg. 2013;46(2): 365-76.

16. Kurz A, Sessler DI, Lenhardt R. Perioperative normothermia to reduce the incidence of surgical-wound infection and shorten hospitalization. Study of Wound Infection and Temperature Group. N Engl J Med. 1996;334:1209-15.

17. Schmied H, Kurz A, Sessler DI, et al. Mild hypothermia increases blood loss and transfusion requirements during total hip arthroplasty. Lancet. 1996;347:289-92.

Index